Bone Resorption

Felix Bronner, Mary C Farach-Carson and
Janet Rubin (Eds)

Bone Resorption

Volume 2 in the Series
Topics in Bone Biology

Series Editors:
Felix Bronner and Mary C. Farach-Carson

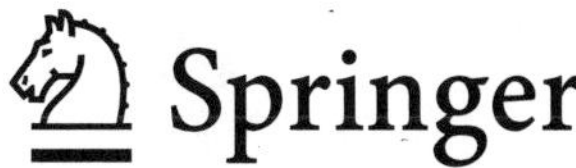

Felix Bronner, PhD
Department of BioStructure and Function,
Department of Pharmacology,
University of Connecticut Health Center,
Farmington, CT,
USA

Mary C Farach-Carson, PhD
Department of Biology,
University of Delaware,
Newark, DE, USA

Janet Rubin, MD
Division of Endocrinology and Metabolism,
Emory University School of Medicine,
Veterans Affairs Medical Center,
Decatur, GA,
USA

British Library Cataloguing in Publication Data
A catalogue record for this book is available from the British Library

Library of Congress Control Number: 2005924008

ISBN 1-85233-812-1
Springer Science+Business Media
springeronline.com

Typeset by SNP Best-set Typesetter Ltd., Hong Kong
Printed and bound in the United States of America
28/3830-543210 Printed on acid-free paper SPIN 10943977

Preface

Bone Resorption, the second volume of the series *Topics in Bone Biology,* is centered on the osteoclast, the bone-resorbing cell. The volume thus complements the first volume of the series, *Bone Formation,* which discussed origin, function, and pathology of the bone-forming cell, the osteoblast. Both volumes are addressed to scientists and clinicians who are active in or wish to enter the field of skeletal function; this group encompasses a wide variety of specialties, including orthopaedics, rheumatology, endocrinology, nephrology, oncology, dentistry, nursing, and chiropractic medicine.

Rubin and Greenfield, in the first chapter, discuss the origin and differentiation of the osteoclast. Recognized as a multinuclear cell about 150 years ago, its origin was not uncovered until a century later when, as a result of an experiment in which quail and chicken cells were co-cultured, it became clear that osteoclasts arose from hematopoietic stem cells. The authors then discuss the osteoclastogenic factor, now known as RANKL; the inhibitory binding protein, osteoprotegerin (OPG); and the complex signaling pathway that leads to differentiation and late differentiation of this complicated cell. A section of the chapter is devoted to a concise discussion of regulators and repressors of osteoclast differentiation, including sex steroids, calcitonin, nitric oxide, and mechanical factors. The chapter concludes that the osteoclast modulates bone development, bone growth, and bone disease.

Bone cells resorb bone by spreading their membrane over the bone surface and then secreting enzymes that cause bone salt to be solubilized and the organic matrix to be disassembled. Oursler, in Chapter 2, discusses the osteolytic enzymes of the osteoclast. One pivotal enzyme is the tartrate-resistant acid phosphatase, yet its precise role remains unresolved. Recent data indicate that this enzyme can dephosphorylate osteopontin and may therefore play a role in suppressing bone resorption. Oursler proceeds to discuss the cathepsins and points out the important role of cathepsin K in basic bone resorption. Although most matrix metalloproteases (MMPs) are produced by osteoblasts, osteoclasts produce MMP 1 and 9, which may therefore be implicated in osteoclast-mediated bone degradation. As yet it is difficult to generalize about the roles played by MMPs and cathepsins. Future studies may reveal that different molecules of these two enzyme classes bring about osteolysis when resorption is due to remodeling, as compared to the molecules that are implicated in disuse or other bone-destroying processes.

How osteoclast activity is regulated is discussed by Baron and Horne in the third chapter. Five steps are required for the bone-resorbing cell to do its job: migration to the portion of bone that is to be resorbed, adhesion of the podosome membrane, secretion of the various lytic and other enzymes, acidification of the fluid under the podosome, and internalization, i.e., retrograde transport or transcytosis of some products under the podosome.

The essentiality of these five steps becomes obvious when constituent steps or molecules are genetically altered. The authors discuss the many signaling molecules and cascades that regulate these five steps. They conclude that signaling from the integrins and from the receptors for RANK, M-CSF, and calcitonin constitute the key regulatory pathways and that most signaling cascades involve sequential phosphorylation and dephosphorylation events. As these steps are identified, they may then become targets for therapeutic approaches that attempt to re-equilibrate the relationship between bone formation and resorption.

For bone tissue to be able to change its shape and structure, pre-existing bone mineral and matrix must first be removed. Bain and Gross, in the fourth chapter, provide an overview of the structural aspects of bone remodeling, with specific focus on how the osteoclast modulates bone mass and architecture. In cortical bone, the activation of the osteoclast machinery leads to a linear cellular assembly that can tunnel through the cortex. This osteoclast-generated tunnel then is filled by osteoblastic bone formation, leading to the formation of what is called a bone structural unit (BSU). The authors indicate that on the basis of available data a cortical BSU has a life span of 200 days and suggest that the bone-remodeling rate has been genetically programmed to maintain the skeletal competence of the skeleton. In cancellous bone, the BSU is hemi-osteonal in nature; and, rather than boring a tunnel, the osteoclasts effect a trench-like structure on the surface of cancellous bone. In contrast with the relatively long time period it takes for bone loss to weaken the structure of bone as a result of aging or of the hormonal changes due to the menopause, loss of bone mass due to disuse is rather rapid, the result of profound osteoclastic resorption on endo-and intracortical surfaces. As a result of disuse, bone porosity is twice as great as normal. Hyperactive osteoclasts and excessive bone resorption can lead to irreversible bone loss and structurally weakened bone.

The role of inflammatory cytokines in bone disease is discussed in Chapter 5 by Nanes and Pacifici, who emphasize that inflammatory cytokines play a major role in bringing about bone disease. For example, estrogen deficiency, typical of the menopause, leads to the elevated production of the tumor necrosis factor (TNF) and of interleukin-1 (IL-1). These in turn stimulate osteoclastogenesis and inhibit osteoblast differentiation and function. The signaling pathways of TNF and IL-1, though different, converge, activating a transcription factor and stimulating a mitogen-activated protein kinase. The chapter reviews in detail the data on the effect of estrogen deficiency on cytokine production; on the central role for TNF, its source, on estrogen regulation of T cell clonal expression; and on interferon gamma and the skeletal effects of this interferon. TNF signaling and its relation to IL-1 signaling, and to RANKL, is detailed, and the authors discuss how osteoclast survival is enhanced by the effects of these cytokines. A section on the effects of cytokines on osteoblast differentiation, function, and survival concludes the chapter.

A detailed analysis and description of how mutations affect the various aspects of osteoclastogenesis and osteoclast function as delineated in transgenic mouse models is provided in Chapter 6 by Horowitz, Kacena, and Lorenzo. In the early part of the chapter the authors describe transcriptional regulation, based in part on events occurring in the course of the more widely explored B-cell differentiation. The authors cover over-expression of some transcription factors, the role of proto-oncogenes, e.g., c-fos, and the effects of nuclear-factor-activated T cells—c1, a critical signaling molecule in osteoclastogenic responses. Although the initial response of the bone-resorbing cell to signals is mediated by surface membrane receptors, the initial signals are followed by intracellular events that are then described. An example is the colony-stimulating factor-1 (CSF-1 or MCSF) that may play a role in minimizing osteoclast apoptosis. The role of OPG and its relationship to RANK and RANKL and their function in osteoclastogenesis is described in detail. This is followed by discussion of the roles of tumor necrosis factor (TNF), the interleukins, prostaglandins, and prostaglandin receptors. The last part of the chapter deals with specific mutations and their effects on the development and function of the mutant mice and on specific bone-resorbing processes. The role and function of cathepsin K is illustrated by discussion of what happens to cathepsin K knockout mice. A final section deals with the role of integrins in bone resorption.

Rubin and Nanes, in Chapter 7, discuss diseases of unchecked osteoclast activity that lead to a marked increase in bone fragility, as well as conditions and diseases of too little osteoclast activity, in which bone mineral content has increased beyond the normal and bone structure has become disordered. Diseases of relatively excessive osteoclastic activity include postmenopausal osteoporosis, hyperparathyroidism, and Paget's disease. The latter is an example of a genetic disorder. Other inherited diseases with an overactive osteoclastic phenotype that are discussed are familial expansile osteolysis, Nasu–Hakola disease, and Rett syndrome. Inherited diseases with an under-active osteoclastic phenotype include three types of malignant osteopetrosis, two types of osteopetrosis that are autosomal dominant, as well as the rare diseases pycnodysostosis, osteopetrosis with renal tubular acidosis, and Cammurati–Engelmann disease. The chapter discusses the known genetic basis in detail and functional and clinical aspects of these diseases, whether relatively common, e.g., hyperparathyroidism, or quite rare, as are the osteopetroses. The chapter contains illustrations of many of these conditions.

Osteoporosis is the most common bone disease that affects people over 50 years of age. Because the bone resorption rate exceeds that of bone formation, pharmaceutical research has been directed at agents that target recruitment and function of the osteoclast. Fitzpatrick, in Chapter 8, reviews the principal compounds that have been tested and have become drugs used to treat bone loss. A major category of these drugs includes the bisphosphonates, reviewed in the chapter as a class and invidually, including alendronate, risedronate, ibandronate, etidronate, tiludronate, and zolendroic acid. Clinical trials involving these drugs are described and their results analyzed and evaluated. Because bisphosphonates are relatively new drugs, their long-term efficacy, not yet well known, is discussed and evaluated. Estrogens and estrogen-like compounds are an entirely different class of agents that are used or proposed as anti-resorptive agents. Results from the Women's Health Initiative have demonstrated unequivocally that estrogen reduces fracture risk and the details of that study and related studies of selected estrogen receptor modulators (SERMs) are discussed, as are the results of treatment with calcitonin and of combination antiresoptive therapies. The chapter concludes with a brief outlook of future therapies.

The last chapter, by Clines, Chirgwin, and Guise, describes and analyzes the role of the osteoclast in causing skeletal complications of malignancy. The principal syndromes discussed are bone metastases, the most common, the hypercalcemia of malignancy, and oncogenic osteomalacia. The authors discuss humoral mediators of malignancy, i.e., parathyroid hormone-related protein, 1,25-dihyroxyvitamin D_3, parathyroid hormone, as well as some cytokines, the tumor necrosis factor, and the granulocyte-colony stimulating factor. The authors then outline treatment of hypercalcemia due to malignancy and proceed to a discussion of solid tumor metastases in which they classify them, describing the clinical consequences, the steps leading to the metastases, and the development of the skeletal lesions. They illustrate the vicious cycle between tumor cells and the skeleton and then turn to osteoblastic and mixed metastases. The chapter concludes with a discussion of experimental and clinical therapies and an evaluation of how therapy affects the skeleton of cancer patients who have lost bone.

All chapters contain extensive bibliographies, thereby permitting the interested reader to explore a given topic further. Illustrations and summarizing tables are in included in many chapters. We thank the contributing authors for their willingness to undertake the task of making available to the scientific community their knowledge and experience in this fast-developing field and for providing a rational summary of what is known or yet to be known, thereby contributing to the long-term quality of life for patients with skeletal disease. We also thank the publisher for being patient and for helping us to make this a pleasing and readable book

May, 2005.

Felix Bronner   Mary C Farach-Carson   Janet Rubin
Farmington, CT   Newark, DE   Decatur, GA

Contents

Contributors

Steven D. Bain, PhD
SkeleTech, Inc
Bothell, WA
USA

Roland Baron, DDS, PhD
Department of Orthopedics and Rehabilitation
Department of Cell Biology
Yale University School of Medicine
New Haven, CT
USA

Felix Bronner, PhD
Department of BioStructure and Function
Department of Pharmacology
The University of Connecticut Health Center
Farmington, CT
USA

John M. Chirgwin, PhD
Department of Internal Medicine
Division of Endocrinology
University of Virginia
Charlottesville, VA
USA

Gregory A. Clines, MD, PhD
Department of Internal Medicine
Division of Endocrinology
University of Virginia
Charlottesville, VA
USA

Mary C. Farach-Carson, PhD
Department of Biology
University of Delaware
Newark, DE
USA

Lorraine A. Fitzpatrick, MD
Global Development
General Medicine Therapeutic Area
Amgen, Inc.
Thousand Oaks, CA
USA

Edward M. Greenfield, PhD
Department of Orthopedics
Case Western Reserve University
Cleveland, OH
USA

Ted S. Gross, PhD
Department of Orthopedics and Sports Medicine
University of Washington
Seattle, WA
USA

Theresa A. Guise, MD
Department of Internal Medicine
Division of Endocrinology
University of Virginia
Charlottesville, VA
USA

William C. Horne, PhD
Department of Orthopedics and Rehabilitation
Yale University School of Medicine
New Haven, CT
USA

Mark C. Horowitz, PhD
Department of Orthopedics and Rehabilitation
Yale University School of Medicine
New Haven, CT
USA

Melissa A. Kacena, PhD
Department of Orthopedics and Rehabilitation
Yale University School of Medicine
New Haven, CT
USA

Joseph A. Lorenzo, MD
Department of Medicine
Division of Endocrinology
University of Connecticut Health Center
Farmington, CT
USA

Mark S. Nanes, MD, PhD
Department of Medicine
Division of Endocrinology and Metabolism
Veterans Affairs Medical Center
Emory University School of Medicine
Decatur, GA
USA

Merry Jo Oursler, PhD
Endocrine Research Unit
Mayo Clinic College of Medicine
Rochester, MN
USA

Roberto Pacifici, MD
Department of Medicine
Division of Endocrinology and Metabolism
Emory University School of Medicine
Atlanta, GA
USA

Janet Rubin, MD
Division of Endocrinology and Metabolism
Emory University School of Medicine
Veterans Affairs Medical Center
Decatur, GA
USA

1.

Osteoclast: Origin and Differentiation

Janet Rubin and Edward M. Greenfield

Introduction

The skeleton is an engineering feat: it is strong but light enough to permit locomotion, rigid to allow muscles to be fixed but capable of bending without breaking, and its structure is programmed for variable loading (Figure 1.1). In addition to its structural role, the skeleton serves as a reservoir and sink for calcium, an ion that plays an important role in cell metabolism and function. This means that bone must be malleable, that its calcium stores must be accessible, and that its structure can be sampled, adapted, or fine-tuned, in a process termed remodeling. The primary step in remodeling is the resorption of bone. The multinucleated osteoclast, a highly specialized cell, is responsible for resorbing the mineral phase of the skeleton.

The osteoclast, therefore, is a basic element in skeletal physiology. Abnormalities in osteoclast development or function that severely limit its ability to resorb bone are incompatible with normal locomotion, and, if severe enough, with life. Defects in osteoclastogenesis can result in lethal neonatal disease because the bones lack a marrow space for hematopoiesis. Milder defects in osteoclastogenesis lead to crippling skeletal lesions in childhood. In adulthood, excess osteoclast action – due either to the presence of too many osteoclasts or hyperactivity of those present – is the predominant cause of most skeletal pathology. Within the past ten years, research into the origin of the osteoclast and the signals that direct its formation at a specific

hydroxyapatite surface has led to a fuller understanding of this important cell.

In this introductory chapter we set out the basic aspects of osteoclast origin and differentiation. Beginning with a description of the multinuclear cell found in bone and a brief introduction to its typing through functional characteristics, we discuss developing research from a historical viewpoint. However, attention will be focused on the current understanding of osteoclastogenesis, shown in Figure 1.2.

The Osteoclast: Lineage of the Multinucleated Macrophage

The osteoclast was recognized in 1873 as the principal multinuclear cell that digested bone [87], but its origin was not uncovered until more than a century later. Kahn and Simmons were able to separate the lineage of osteoclasts from the other key cell in remodeling, the osteoblast, with a clever experiment in 1975. They took advantage of the morphological differences between cell nuclei of quail and chicken by growing quail bone rudiments on well-vascularized portions of chorioallantoic membranes of chicken embryos. The osteoblasts appearing a week later were of quail origin, but the nuclei of the osteoclasts had a predominantly chicken morphology [75]. This was the first convincing evidence that osteoclasts were hematogenous in origin. Several years later, building on work showing that cure of osteopetrosis in mice was possible by transplantation of

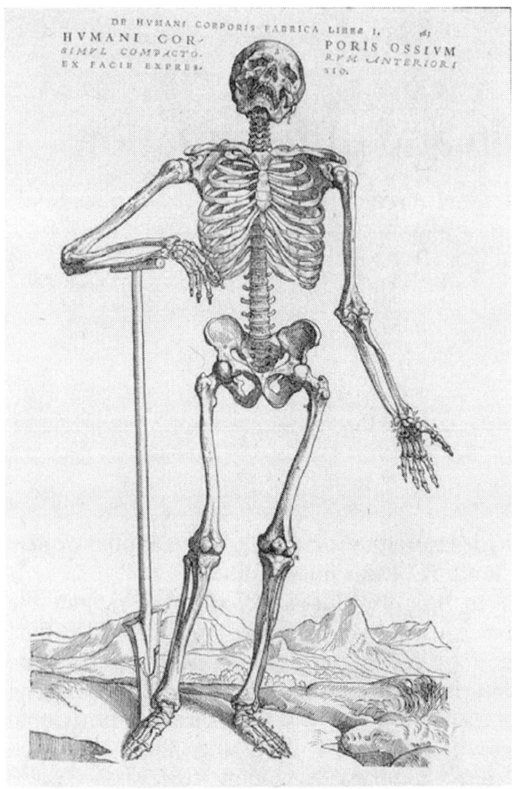

Figure 1.1 The skeleton as interpreted by Vesalius.

normal bone marrow [187], the first successful bone-marrow transplantation was performed in a female human infant with malignant osteopetrosis. In the normally remodeling bone, the osteoclasts appearing in situ lacked Barr bodies, as would be expected in male nuclei: indeed, the bone marrow had been harvested from the patient's brother [24].

With evidence that the osteoclast arose from fusion of hematogenous cells, the next step in determining the lineage was to develop an *in vitro* process to obtain polykaryons capable of resorbing calcified bone matrix. Neither monocytes nor macrophages fit this definition, although they are able to resorb some mineral. Burger et al. [17], culturing hematopoietic tissue, showed that at two weeks the culture consisted largely of immature and mature mononuclear phagocytes, but contained no osteoclast-like cells. When, however, stripped bone rudiments were added to the hematopoietic cell culture, osteoclasts appeared in close contact with the calcified matrix [17]. This demonstrated that recreation of the bone environment provided sufficiency for transformation of hematologic precursors into osteoclasts. The need for elements of the bone environment to allow osteoclastogenesis has become key to understanding the intricate relationship between bone osteoblasts/stromal cells and osteoclasts.

The understanding that osteoclasts arose from hematopoietic stem cells (HSC) created a need for adequate typing to ensure that multinucleated "osteoclasts" were not other cells arising from the HSC. Indeed, many characteristics of osteoclasts are shared by macrophages, including the ability to fuse with like cells and the ability to phagocytose. However, macrophages associated with bone surfaces do not have the ruffled border that is characteristic of the osteoclast, nor do they respond to calcitonin with a change in shape. Moreover, and most convincingly, macrophages are unable to rescue an osteopetrotic deficit [184]. Cell morphology, staining for functional characteristics such as tartrate resistant acid phosphatase, and the ability to respond to calcitonin, were all found to be useful for differentiating osteoclasts from macrophages. Many laboratories contributed to a more exacting definition of cell type by examining cell surface characteristics. For instance, osteoclasts lack the Fc and C3 surface receptors that typify macrophages. As pre-osteoclasts differentiate, they loose their early macrophage characteristics, decreasing expression of macrophage-specific surface antigens F4/80, Mac-1. Their ability to phagocytose is also diminished [20, 185]. In comparison with macrophage polykaryons, osteoclasts express a variable but restricted range of macrophage-associated antigens (e.g., CD13, CD15A, CD44, ICAM-1), whereas macrophage polykaryons strongly express CD18, CD14, CD31 [10]. This allows for a discrete separation of osteoclasts from macrophage multinuclear cells.

Cell typing that largely pertains to the available and developed antibodies has led to further demarcation between osteoclasts and cells of macrophage lineage [59, 60]. Currently markers used during flow cytometry delineate the extended progression from stem cell to the osteoclast phenotype. Indeed these steps constitute a road map of the differentiation program. (These are shown along the top of Figure 1.2.)

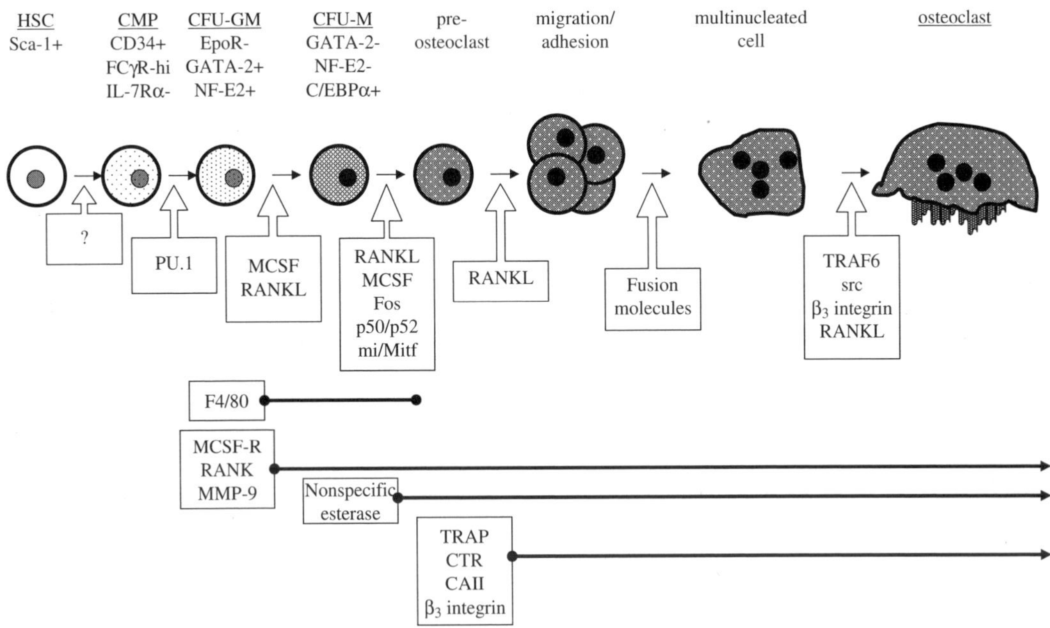

Figure 1.2 Osteoclast Differentiation. The diagram shows the progression from the hematopoietic stem cell (HSC) through the common myeloid progenitor (CMP) to the colony-forming unit for granulocytes and macrophages (CFU-GM) to the CFU for macrophages and into the osteoclast lineage. Markers that can be used to identify early stem cells are shown above the cells. Factors that stimulate progressing are shown in the arrowed boxes. The boxes on the bottom of the diagram show appearance of markers associated with osteoclast lineage.

In vitro co-culture systems that adequately simulate the bone microenvironment have been a major tool for study of progression along the osteoclast lineage. Using variations on the Dexter marrow culture [28, 29], bone biologists found that it was possible to generate osteoclasts in the presence of osteoclastogenic agents in primate [141], feline [65], and murine cultures [95, 162, 168]. Such culture systems allowed the identification of factors that enhanced osteoclast development such as 1,25-dihydroxyvitamin D [141], prostaglandins [5], and cyclic AMP [148], as well as parathyroid hormone [6]. Within the context of murine marrow cultures, other cytokines such as IL-6 and TNF have also been shown to regulate osteoclast differentiation [3, 182]. Dexter's culture [29] had opened the way to understanding the role of colony-stimulating factors (CSFs) in blood cell proliferation and differentiation. It therefore seemed logical to expect that colony-stimulating factors would also play a role in osteoclast development. Macrophage CSF (MCSF) was found to be essential for osteoclastogenesis [86] and granulocyte-macrophage-CSF (GM-CSF) was shown to enhance osteoclast formation [95]. The effect of these CSFs gave support to the idea that macrophages and osteoclasts share a common origin. Experiments also made it possible to identify three stages in osteoclast differentiation: early differentiation, where hematopoietic stem cells proliferate within the macrophage lineage [53]; progression into the early osteoclast precursor stage with expression of calcitonin receptors and TRAP [51]; and a later stage where fusion occurs [13]. The extensive osteoclastogenic marrow culture literature adds to the conclusion that the osteoclast precursor begins as a nonadherent hematopoietic stem cell and progresses through the colony-forming unit for granulocytes and macrophages (CFU-GM) to become a CFU-macrophage (CFU-M) before entering the osteoclast lineage.

As stated above, accessory cells representing bone stromal elements are necessary for osteoclast formation. In addition, cell–cell contact is required between the myelocytic precursor and the bone stroma [163, 203]. The critical factor contributed by bone stromal cells for terminal osteoclast differentiation was identified in 1998 as RANKL, a member of the tumor necrosis factor family [97, 206]. The discovery of this factor has permitted osteoclast biology to shift into high gear, as will be described below.

Early Differentiation

The first process we will examine is the progression from the pluripotent hematopoietic stem cell to the colony-forming unit for macrophages.

Myeloid Differentiation

The pluripotent hematopoietic stem cell (HSC) in the marrow cavity awaits signals that direct its development into the myeloid lineage. This requires expression of molecules that allow response to osteoclastogenic factors. The HSC bears stem cell antigen-1 (Sca-1+), which indicates a self-renewing capacity [135, 159]. The first way station in HSC differentiation is a choice between entry into the myeloid or the lymphoid progenitor pool. Expression of the interleukin-7 receptor α-chain (IL-7Rα) differentiates the common lymphoid progenitor (CLP) that reconstitutes T-cells, B-cells, and natural killer cells from cells of the myeloid lineage [88].

The immediate precursor of the myeloid progenitor population is identified by the absence of the IL-7Rα. In a search for the earliest myeloid cell, Akashi and colleagues recently used cell sorting to discard IL-7Rα-positive cells that have entered lymphoid lineage. They next selected an IL-7Rα-negative fraction expressing the myelomonocytic Fcγ receptor [4]. In the presence of GM-CSF and a mixture of cytokines (steel factor, Flt-3 ligand, IL-11, IL-3, erythropoietin, and thrombopoietin) 80% of this fraction commits to myeloid lineage [4]. If this lineage is further separated into a fraction with high FcγR expression that also expresses the cell surface molecule sialomucin CD34, this fraction becomes almost exclusively myeloid. FcγR^{hi}CD34$^+$ cells divide into three lineages that contain macrophages and/or granulocytes, i.e., CFU-M, CFU-G, and CFU-GM. In contrast the FcγR^{lo}CD34$^+$ behave like HSCs, and the FcγR^{lo}CD34$^-$ give rise to colonies that contain only megakaryocytes and/or erythrocytes. Thus, Akashi was able to differentiate the common

myeloid precursor, "CMP," from the common lymphoid precursor as an IL-7Rα-, GATA-2+, NF-E2+, GATA-1+, GATA-3- cell [4]. It is this cell that responds to signals that generate proliferation of the CFU-GM, as distinguished from the lineage providing cells for megakaryocyte or erythrocyte lineage, or the earlier fork where the HSC enters the lymphoid pathway.

Interestingly, the absence of the Pax5 gene, a key to the B-lymphoid lineage, leads to enrichment of the myeloid lineage in transgenic Pax5$^{-/-}$ animals [132]. The Pax5$^{-/-}$ pro-B cells respond to M-CSF with expression of macrophage markers Mac-1 and F4/80, and, in the presence of RANKL, into osteoclasts. Although scientists were unable to force the pro-B cells into erythroid or megakaryocytic lineage, pro-B cells clearly maintain a degree of plasticity even after they are committed to a lymphoid lineage [132].

The factors responsible for herding HSC into the common myeloid progenitor lineage and then into the CFU-GM are multiple and very likely redundant. By means of targeted deletions of early lineage markers from embryonic stem cells, GATA-2 and SCL/tal-1 were shown to be important for early development [202]. The SCL/tal-1 transcription factor was first described as an abnormal translocation in T-cell leukemia and is necessary for generation of all hematopoietic cells. GATA-2, while not necessary for later expansion of osteoclast progenitors, has some role in separating CFU-M from those cells that are most responsive to RANKL. The colony-stimulating factors for macrophage and/or the granulocyte lineage cause cultured osteoclast numbers to swell in numbers by increasing the number of precursors [34, 53, 95, 160, 167, 175].

Becoming a Macrophage Progenitor

As the colony differentiates, a number of markers identify the emergence of the macrophage lineage. Macrophage colonies are readily identifiable because they express a non-specific esterase, along with the receptor for the macrophage colony-stimulating factor. The movement from the common myeloid precursor (CMP) through the CFU-GM and into the macrophage lineage is in fact, largely due to the macrophage colony-stimulating factor (MCSF). The importance of MCSF to osteoclast lineage became apparent as the result of the discovery that the osteopetrotic (op/op) mouse, whose marble bone disease and lack of dental eruption are lethal consequences of total osteoclast deficiency, has a mutation in the gene that codes for MCSF [193, 208]. Similarly, in the toothless rat, which displays the osteopetrotic phenotype, a frameshift mutation in the MCSF gene causes a loss of function that brings about a profound deficiency of osteoclasts and macrophages [186]. In culture, MCSF is more potent than GM-CSF or interleukin-3 in stimulating osteoclast formation in primate bone marrow [137]. GM-CSF cannot rescue the op/op MCSF deficient mouse, but does support the development of osteoclast-like cells if vitamin D is present in the culture [93]. In contrast, VEGF can substitute for MCSF when administered to op/op mice and appears to be the molecule responsible for the age-related resolution of osteopetrosis seen in mice nursed through their early otherwise lethal inability to wean [131].

MCSF has importance as a growth and differentiating factor. It is also required for survival of cells of the macrophage lineage [175]. In a culture containing high levels of MCSF, monocytes will increase in number at the expense of osteoclastogenesis, probably because MCSF strongly promotes the development of mononuclear monocytes [34, 136]. Yet, in the case of estrogen deficiency, increased levels of MCSF in bone marrow may enhance osteoclastogenesis [81]. These discrepancies may be due to differences in the expression patterns of MCSF, resulting from at least two splice variants. One of these is a secreted soluble factor. The other, representing a much smaller amount of the total MCSF, ~5%, is expressed on the surface of bone stromal cells [35, 204]. Because the insoluble form of MCSF is anchored and displayed by cells within bone, this isoform may represent a local signal that regulates osteoclast development. Indeed in the op/op MCSF-deficient mouse, the membrane-bound form of MCSF can correct the osteoclast defect [205]. Perhaps the best way to summarize the literature is to state that MCSF expands the precursor pool capable of responding to osteoclastogenic signals from the bone marrow and, at the same time, enhances macrophage differentiation and survival.

The CFU-GM expresses the MCSF receptor, which is a membrane tyrosine kinase encoded by the gene *c-fms* [153]. Multiple second messengers that are activated through this membrane tyrosine kinase receptor trigger proliferation of the CFU-M [155]. The downstream proliferative response to the MCSF ligand includes induction of G2 progression through activation of cyclin genes. It is difficult to separate the differentiative from the proliferative responses in MCSF-R-bearing cells [74, 154]. Myeloid cells become macrophage, in part, because the myeloid and B-cell-specific transcription factor PU.1 also increases. The finding that PU.1-deficient mice have a decreased number of macrophages and no osteoclasts gives support to the role played by PU.1 in macrophage recruitment [179].

The transcription factor *fos*, and perhaps other members of the AP-1 transcription factor family, play an important role in osteoclast differentiation. It has been long known that the v-fos oncogene induced by murine sarcoma virus causes osteosarcoma and that overexpression of the cellular homolog, c-fos, led to the development of bone tumors [149]. Because these fos lesions were in osteoprogenitor cells, not in the osteoclast lineage or in HSCs, it was surprising that mice lacking c-fos developed osteopetrosis, essentially an overgrowth of bone [48]. In fact, c-fos is not required for normal osteoprogenitor development but is required for osteoclast differentiation: c-fos-negative HSC progress normally into CFU-M and from there to become terminally differentiated macrophages, but osteoclasts are totally absent in this mouse. Whether the requirement for *fos* is in the stromal accessory cell (e.g., for normal expression of RANKL), or only in the osteoclast progenitor (e.g., required for response to osteoclastogenic signals) has not yet been worked out. However, overexpression of c-fos in osteoclast precursors can increase osteoclast differentiation [122] and RANKL does induce transcription of genes through c-fos activation. This suggests a link between RANKL signaling and c-fos activation [115]. RANKL has, in fact, been shown to induce interferon-B in osteoclast precursor cells. This interferes with RANKL-induced expression of c-fos and decreases osteoclastogenesis [172].

Other members of the AP-1 family are also involved: Fra-1 can rescue the c-fos defect in osteoclast precursors [38]; this may suggest some redundancy between AP-1 members in intracellular signaling leading to osteoclastogenesis. Overexpression of Fra-1 by itself, also, leads to increased osteoblast differentiation and thus to a progressive increase in bone mass [73].

Expression of AP-1 proteins therefore plays critical roles in osteoclast and osteoblast progenitors and is necessary for normal coupling between the remodeling cells.

CFU-M into Pre-Osteoclast: The RANKL:RANK Signal

RANKL Comes Calling

The progression of the macrophage colony-forming unit into the osteoclast lineage has been traditionally characterized by development of a panel of osteoclastic phenotypic features. These include expression of the calcitonin receptor, of enzymes such as tartrate-resistant acid phosphatase and carbonic anhydrase II, and the ability to resorb bone [12, 52, 102, 103]. Other established markers are the vitronectin receptor and the vacuolar-type proton pump [94]. Although the progression from the monocytic precursor to the osteoclast progenitor was thus clearly established, the critical factor responsible for this metamorphosis was unknown.

Experiments had shown that when the CFU-M (or its earlier precursors) collected from bone marrow or spleen was added to a culture of osteoprogenitor cells, to which any one of a handful of osteoclastogenic hormones or cytokines was added, osteoclastogenesis could proceed [112]; the osteoclastogenic factors acted synergistically [139] and furthermore appeared to target the stromal accessory cells, since the accessory cells could be pretreated with agents such as 1,25-dihydroxyvitamin D and fixed prior to culture with the hematogenous precursors [35, 190]. Moreover the accessory cells actually had to be in direct contact with the osteoclast progenitor cells. Separation by a membrane prevented the process [164]. This meant that the stimulated stromal cells, even when fixed, provided a contact signal to the CFU-M. What was this signal?

Laboratories working in Japan and California discovered the answer simultaneously. TNF-related activation-induced cytokine, or TRANCE, originally described as a factor that activated signals in T-lymphocytes [197], was found to be the osteoclastogenic factor that is now known as Receptor Activator of NFκB Ligand or RANKL [97, 206] (Figure 1.3). Discovery of RANKL involved similar strategies by both groups, using a previously identified inhibitory binding factor to screen for the osteoclastogenic factor. Yasuda's team used an osteoclast inhibitory factor from bone-cell-conditioned media that eventually was shown to be the TNF-R-like decoy receptor osteoprotegerin, to tag expression libraries encoding the ligand partner for the inhibitory protein [206]. They called their gene product "osteoclast differentiation factor" and showed that it induced osteoclast formation from spleen cells in the absence of stromal elements. Osteoclast differentiation factor expression was upregulated in stromal cells by osteoactive factors such as parathyroid hormone and 1,25-dihydroxyvitamin D. Lacey's group in California had discovered the same soluble inhibitory binding protein, named it osteoprotegerin (OPG), and showed that it prevented osteoclastogenesis *in vivo* [157]. Searching for the binding partner of OPG, they cloned "osteoprotegerin-ligand" (OPGL) from a murine expression library [97]. OPGL bound to hematopoietic progenitor cells

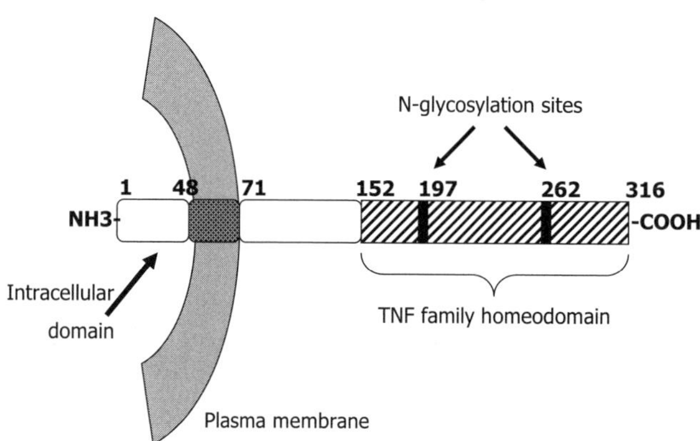

Figure 1.3 RANKL. The drawing shows the protein structure of RANKL.

and rapidly induced osteoclast genes. The final selection of the term RANKL, or receptor activator of NFκB ligand [7] as the name of the OPG binding partner in place of ODF, OPGL or the earliest manifestation, TRANCE, helped to clear the alphabet confusion.

RANKL thus was identified as a membrane-associated protein of the TNF ligand family that is expressed by stromal cells after stimulation by bone resorbing cytokines/hormones. Anderson et al. also cloned by direct expression a gene that they called RANKL (the earliest and final designation) as the ligand partner to a receptor termed RANK, that they had previously characterized [7]. The RANKL cDNA clone has an open reading frame that encodes a 316 amino acid type II transmembrane protein (Figure 1.4). A 48 amino acid intracellular amino-terminus precedes the 24-residue hydrophobic domain that passes through the plasma membrane. The carboxy-terminal residues have significant homology to members of the TNF ligand family. Wong et al. remark on similarity of the mouse TRANCE with TRAIL, FasL, and TNF, especially in those regions that form the beta strands seen in the TNF crystal structure [197]. Furthermore, there are putative N-linked glycosylation sites, all of which are highly conserved between mouse and human. Lam and colleagues successfully crystallized the ectodomain of murine RANKL [98]: RANKL associates into a homotrimer, similarly to other TNF molecules with four unique surface loops that are necessary for full activation of RANK.

Once the identity of RANKL as the factor necessary for osteoclastogenesis was confirmed, osteoclast biology became much more transparent. First, the role of the accessory cell, and indeed the cell–cell contact necessary between the support cells and the osteoclast precursors, was found to be a function of the presence of RANKL expressed on the accessory cell membrane. Indeed, RANKL *is* the bone environment. When RANKL was expressed in non-bone cells osteoclastogenesis was induced [101]. Furthermore it was possible to fix these non-bone cells with paraformaldehyde prior to adding the HSC responders [206], as is also true for bone cells [35]. Interestingly, the need for a stromal cell could also be overcome by the addition of the extracellular domain of RANKL [97, 206]. MCSF, which also is made by the stromal cells, is necessary for proliferation of the progenitor pool, as well as for survival of cells of macrophage lineage; in the absence of stromal cells, a source of MCSF must also be provided [181]. Soon it was realized that "soluble RANKL," either secreted directly by some cells [89], or cleaved from its membrane position by a metalloproteinase [110, 129], also had a role in osteoclastogenesis. Bone stromal cells have not been shown to generate secreted RANKL under

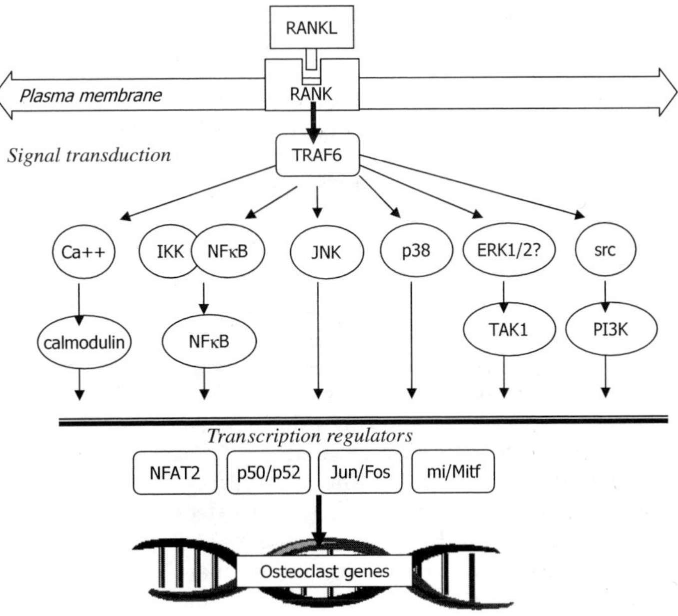

Figure 1.4 RANK signal transduction. RANK signaling is complex and involves multiple cascades. This diagram does not rule out interaction between the signals, some of which may be redundant.

known osteoclastogenic stimuli: conditioned media from stromal cells are ineffective in generating osteoclastogenesis. Spot cultures of stromal cells, in fact, generated osteoclasts only in the local area of RANKL-expressing cells. This further underscores that cell–cell interactions are involved in bone cell RANKL:RANK signaling [69].

The murine gene for RANKL exists as a single copy of five exons spanning about 40 kilobases [85]. The intracellular and transmembrane domains are encoded in the first exon, with the important ligand domain beginning in the first exon and continuing through the fifth. The organizational structure is similar to that of the other members of the TNF family, with mouse RANKL having most homology to CD40L, which also has five exons. Both molecules play a role in dendritic cell function [85]. Ablation of the RANKL gene led to some surprising phenotypic effects in the transgenic mouse [90]. The RANKL-null mouse had severe osteopetrosis due to a complete absence of osteoclasts, but it also had unexpected defects in both T and B lymphocytes and no lymph nodes. The relevance of RANKL's regulation of lymph-node organogenesis for osteoclastogenesis has not yet been worked out, but may be important in situations where osteopetrosis is accompanied by impaired lymphocyte development.

Control of RANKL Expression by Accessory Cells

Before RANKL, the response of the osteoclast-generating unit, i.e., HSC plus accessory cells, was studied as a response of one or both of these elements to agents known to increase bone resorption in the whole animal. Thus, hormones such as 1,25-$(OH)_2D_3$ and PTH were known to stimulate osteoclastogenesis, as were inflammatory cytokines, such as tumor necrosis factor and many of the interleukins [163, 165]. Of the factors that increase osteoclastogenesis in culture, most, if not all, increase RANKL expression by the accessory cell. Parathyroid hormone increases RANKL expression in a dose-dependent fashion within at least 24 hours [105], as does 1,25-$(OH)_2D_3$ [61, 147]. The major exception to this paradigm is stimulation of osteoclast differentiation by TNF. Although TNF stimulates RANKL expression, its primary target during stimulation of osteoclast differen-

tiation appears to be the osteoclast precursors themselves, rather than the accessory stromal cells [99, 139].

RANKL mRNA expression by stromal cells has become a reliable marker of the osteoclastogenic potential of the microenvironment or culture system. IGF-I, which stimulates long bone apposition during growth, upregulates RANKL [144]. Equally important is the fact that when a load is applied to cultured cells, RANKL expression decreases [146], whereas when weightlessness is simulated in culture, RANKL increases [76]. Disease states are also associated with changes in RANKL expression. In Paget's disease, where localized and intense bone remodeling occurs, RANKL expression is increased in marrow samples from affected, but not from unaffected, bones [120]. The expression of RANKL in the estrogen deficiency state, where increased resorption leads to decreased bone mass, was not convincingly increased in the marrow [156]. Rather, as discussed below, the response of the osteoclast precursor to RANKL signaling via RANK is diminished.

Both early bone stromal cells and osteoblasts express RANKL, and several authors have suggested that the differentiation state of the bone cell may affect the level of response to the stimulatory agent. While this certainly would hold in terms of response to PTH, where PTH-R are not expressed until after the cell is well on its terminal differentiation path [117], this is less clear for unstimulated expression of RANKL. RUNX2, an essential transcription factor for osteoblast differentiation, must be present before RANKL is expressed [42]. This suggests that the earliest stromal cells may not have the machinery to induce RANKL transcription. However, less mature osteoprogenitor cells may have an increased basal expression of RANKL [44, 178].

It should be noted that it has been difficult to measure RANKL <u>protein</u> in stromal cells. While soluble RANKL can be measured by a commercial ELISA, both ELISA and Western analysis of membrane-associated RANKL have been exceedingly difficult. An OPG-based pull-down assay echoing original strategies for identifying RANKL has been useful in some cases [130] but its tendency to bind other members of the TNF family limits its usefulness. Because there exist three isoforms of RANKL, one with a shorter intracellular domain, and one with no transmembrane domain at all that may represent the secreted factor [66], the assay is complicated further.

Despite problems with measurement of the RANKL protein, the endogenous mRNA for RANKL in stromal cells responds to stimulation by increasing robustly. This in turn is associated with an increase in the culture's potential to generate osteoclasts from precursor cells [147]. Attention to the RANKL promoter should therefore have led to an understanding of the mechanism by which bone stromal cells regulate RANKL expression. This has not been the case. Nearly 1,000 base pairs of murine and human RANKL promoters were cloned shortly after RANKL was identified [82]. However, RANKL expression should be tissue restricted, and the available promoter sequences are not sufficient to limit expression or to provide the expected response to agents known to increase RANKL mRNA expression [133]. Novel methods, perhaps involving study of the local chromatin structure, may be needed to understand tissue expression and its regulation.

In vivo, non-bone cells can also express RANKL, as shown by localization in white cells and the effects of RANKL in lymph nodes and dendritic cells [7, 191, 197]. T-lymphocytes secrete a soluble form of RANKL into inflamed rheumatic joints, causing osteoclastic bone destruction [89]. There is evidence that T cells with RANKL expression may be key elements in the bone loss caused by estrogen deficiency [19, 180].

RANK: RANKL Signal Transduction in the Monocytic Cell

Stimulation of the Receptor Activator of NFκB, or RANK, with activation of NFκB, leads to the development of the full osteoclast phenotype, including fusion. RANK signaling also increases the net resorptive activity, and, like MCSF, promotes the survival of osteoclast cells. RANK was first identified in dendritic cells, whose immune surveillance mechanism processes and presents antigens to T cells [7]. The osteoclast precursor sequentially expresses the receptor for MCSF and then RANK [8]. RANK is highly expressed in isolated bone marrow-derived osteoclast progenitor cells, as well as in mature osteoclasts [62]. Cognate ligand binding has been shown to activate multiple downstream signaling cascades, including NFκB, c-jun N-

terminal kinase (JNK), ERK1/2 kinase, p38 kinase, and c-src (see Figure 1.4).

The extracellular domain of RANK binds both the membrane and soluble forms of RANKL as well as other members of the TNF family. The intracellular portion of the molecule has domains that interact with the TRAF family (TNFR-associated factor) proteins. TRAF proteins serve as adaptor proteins that recruit and activate downstream transducers [62, 198]. The amino termini of TRAFs are characterized by a RING finger domain that is required for interaction with other proteins, and for the subsequent release of NFκB from its cytoplasmic anchor. The signal cascade activated through TRAF binding is complex, but certainly involves TRAFs 2, 5, and 6 through multiple associations on the RANK intracellular domain [26]. TRAF2 knockout mice do not have obvious problems with osteoclast recruitment [128, 207], while TRAF6 knockout mice have osteopetrosis [106]. TRAF6 thus is recognized as the key adaptor to activated RANK.

Experiments using RANK constructs mutated for selective binding of various TRAF proteins have shown that while some TRAF proteins are redundant, TRAF6 was absolutely required for the formation of cytoskeletal structures and to permit the osteoclast to resorb bone [9]. Kobayashi's study of TRAF6 structure suggests that the RING finger domain of the protein, while necessary for IL-1 and LPS signal activation of NFκB, may not be required for early osteoclast maturation [84]. Thus, while in the absence of the RING finger several osteoclast marker genes such as cathepsin K, calcitonin receptor and TRAP, are expressed, the actin-sealing machinery necessary to complete the seal of the resorption pit is not functional. The RING mutant TRAF still activates NFκB, but perhaps does not allow association with a significant adapter protein required for late differentiation. TRAF6 also activates transforming growth factor β-activated kinase 1 (TAK1). Interestingly TAK1 mediates JNK and p38 MAP-kinases. This may explain the ability of transforming growth factor β to enhance osteoclastogenesis in the presence of RANKL [152]. To complicate issues, MAPK activates TAK1! Thus Kobayashi's finding that TRAF6 was necessary for the terminal maturation steps, as well as Wong's earlier work that showed TRAF activated c-src, a kinase necessary for the actin ring structure of the osteoclast [196], suggest that

TRAF6 is a specific transducer of later effects of RANKL.

The TRAFs have also been implicated in modulating the effects of many of the bone active cytokines. For instance, interferon-gamma strongly suppresses osteoclastogenesis by silencing RANK signal transduction. This process invokes interferon-gamma activation of a ubiquitin-proteasome system, whereby TRAF6 signals are abrogated when TRAF6 is degraded [173].

The rest of the seemingly redundant TRAFs play roles in the earlier stages of osteoclast formation [9, 26]. Because multiple signaling cascades are involved, (e.g., NFκB, JNK, p38), one approach to disentangling the important signals is to perform gene expression profiling after RANKL stimulation of RANK. Four of more than 100 early RANKL-inducible genes have been found to be linked to induction of osteoclast maturation [67]. One important gene candidate arising from that study was NFAT2 (nuclear factor of activated T cells-2); suppression of NFAT2 with antisense interfered with osteoclast formation. NFAT2-deficient embryonic stem cells do not respond to RANKL with formation of osteoclasts. Moreover, overexpression of NFAT differentiates precursors in the absence of RANKL [171]. NFAT molecules act as co-factors with AP-1 or fos/jun proteins to bind to regulatory cis DNA elements [171]. NFATs may one day be shown to be part of the pathophysiology responsible for the osteopetrotic phenotype seen in the *fos*less mouse [48]. What are the postulated targets and partners of NFAT2? Clearly osteoclast marker genes such as TRAP, calcitonin receptor and carbonic anhydrase II have multiple sites recognized by NFAT as well as its partner AP-1 [171].

P38 MAPK is another important downstream signal of RANK, as it is involved in expression of carbonic anhydrase II and TRAP through activation of mi/Mitf [113]. As will be discussed below, estrogen may exert its effects by damping the action of the p38 MAPK.

Osteoprotegerin: A Second Binding Partner for RANKL

Osteoprotegerin (OPG) is the third element of the RANK: RANKL: OPG triumvirate. Simonet originally identified OPG as a novel member of the TNFR superfamily through sequence homology [157]. Its importance was recognized even before its target ligand was identified, when OPG was used to identify RANKL as its binding partner in experiments using expression libraries. The binding of RANKL by this soluble decoy receptor served to prevent RANKL binding to its target on the osteoclast precursor – thus the name, osteoprotegerin (OPG), signifies that it preserves bone. Indeed, OPG is often regulated *in vivo* and *in vitro* in inverse proportion to the levels of RANKL [57].

OPG contains 401 amino acids, with a signal peptide encoding its status as a secreted molecule expressed in many tissues including liver, lung, heart, and kidney and, importantly in bone and cartilage. It contains no hydrophobic amino acids that would make for a transmembrane-spanning domain, so after secretion it is not cell-associated. The N-terminal protein has high homology with other members of the TNFR superfamily, allowing binding of RANKL [97] and of at least one other TNF family member, TRAIL [30].

Transgenic mice that overexpress OPG in the liver under the control of the human apolipoprotein E gene promoter display increases in bone density, even osteopetrosis, if the hepatic OPG output is very high [157]. Recombinant OPG can be used to simulate the phenotype of OPG-overexpressing transgenic mice. It protects rats against ovariectomy-associated bone loss. Osteoclastogenesis can be entirely inhibited if OPG is added to culture or is expressed by stromal cells and osteoblasts [183]. Conversely, OPG-deficient mice develop an early-onset osteoporosis [16]. In fact, many studies have shown that OPG regulates osteoclastogenesis both *in vivo* and *in vitro*; it does so by preventing the effects of RANKL [96, 183, 210]. Interestingly, endothelial cells also express OPG. This local OPG expression appears not only to modulate inflammatory bone states [25] but can also prevent the calcification of arteries as encountered in atherosclerosis [121]. OPG-deficient mice exhibit calcification of the large arteries [16].

The regulation of osteoprotegerin secretion from bone cells is thus of great interest. The OPG promoter has twelve RUNX2 binding elements that underwrite OPG's strong expression in osteoblasts, which express RUNX2 after differentiation. Not surprisingly then, overexpression of RUNX2 increases OPG promoter activity [177]. Transforming growth factor-β, which can both stimulate and inhibit osteoclastogenesis, increases OPG expression [170]. Estradiol stimulates OPG expression *in vitro* [150] and may increase OPG levels *in vivo* [166]. Leptin, a hormone of lipid metabolism that modulates bone remodeling by an as yet poorly understood mechanism, also increases OPG [18]. As expected, factors that increase osteoclastogenesis and bone resorption decrease OPG secretion by bone cells. Glucocorticoids, which cause osteoporosis by stimulating bone resorption and inhibiting bone formation, inhibit OPG while also stimulating RANKL expression [56]. Parathyroid hormone also decreases OPG and increases RANKL *in vitro* [104]. It does so also *in vivo*, provided the hormone is administered continuously [111]. Insulin-like growth factor-I (IGF-I) also appears to downregulate OPG *in vitro* and *in vivo*. This may account for the remodeling and increase in bone markers seen in trials where IGF-I was given in an attempt to increase bone density [144].

There is a growing appreciation of the role of OPG in rare metabolic bone diseases. In the autosomal recessive Juvenile Paget's disease, also known as hyperostosis corticalis deformans juvenilis, a progressive osteopenic skeletal deformity arises out of intense bone remodeling. Two unrelated patients with this disease were shown to have a defect in the OPG gene, resulting in undetectable serum OPG levels [192]. Autosomal dominant familial expansile osteolysis is another rare bone disorder associated with focal areas of osteolysis that arise from a deletion of the OPG coding sequence [64].

Exceptions: Osteoclastogenesis Without RANKL:RANK

Although RANKL and MCSF are sufficient to induce osteoclast differentiation in cell culture, it would be surprising, given the complexity of most other paracrine regulatory systems, if the control of osteoclast differentiation *in vivo* involved only these two factors. The best-characterized exception to the RANKL/MCSF paradigm is stimulation of osteoclast differentiation by TNFα. Although TNFα stimulates RANKL expression by stromal cells, it can induce osteoclast differentiation in the absence of both accessory cells and exogenous RANKL [11, 83]. OPG, moreover, does not block osteo-

clast differentiation induced by TNFα [139]. Studies using either stromal cells [99] or osteoclast precursors [139] from mice lacking TNF receptors have shown that it is the osteoclast precursors rather than the accessory stromal cells that are the primary target of TNFα stimulation. However, TNFα cannot fully replace RANKL during osteoclast differentiation. Rather, the action of TNFα requires that a permissive amount of RANKL either be present in the culture or be added with the TNFα [139]. Recent studies have shown that molecules other than TNFα are synergistic with, or can replace, RANKL or MCSF in stimulating osteoclast differentiation. These molecules include TGFβ [41, 152], BMP-2 [68], activin A [40], VEGF [131], flt3 ligand [100], MIP-1α [49], and prostaglandin E2 [188]. Even this more complex view of the regulation of osteoclast differentiation is likely to be an oversimplification. For example, the effect of TGFβ appears to depend on the mixture of cell types and cytokines that are present in the microenvironment in which osteoclast differentiation occurs [114]. *In vivo* osteoclast differentiation therefore must involve multiple cytokines acting in a complex regulatory network. Nonetheless, it is the balance between RANKL and OPG that must be considered the primary regulator of osteoclastogenesis.

Late Differentiation

Once the CFU-M has been exposed to RANKL and has committed to osteoclast lineage, additional differentiation steps must occur, the most striking of which is fusion of multiple committed cells into the osteoclast polykaryon. The number of osteoclast nuclei that occupy the same fused cell appears to influence the ability of the polykaryons to resorb bone. For instance, in Paget's disease, those pagetic osteoclasts responsible for site-specific increases in bone turnover have more nuclei than normal osteoclasts [91]. The increase in activity associated with a cell that contains several nuclei may be due to the increase in cytoplasm and membrane area, allowing for the formation of resorption pits in the bone area covered by the osteoclast [31]. It may also be due to the fact that the nuclei continue to be transcriptionally active [14]. Indeed, the calcitonin-mediated decrease in osteoclast resorptive activity appears due to a decrease in transcription by the osteoclast nuclei [14].

Fusion of Mononuclear Osteoclast Precursors

Cell fusion is not a widespread phenomenon. As a rule skeletal myoblasts, syncytial trophoblasts, megakaryocytes, and cells of macrophage lineage are the only cells that fuse. It is likely that the fusion processes in these cells and in the fusion of spermatocyte with oocyte or of enveloped viruses with host cells involve similar mechanisms. Cell fusion involves many factors, including proteins that dissolve discrete areas of membrane. An example of the latter is disintegrase meltrin-alpha [199], a molecule that is also expressed by osteoclast precursors [2]. Other molecular factors are the receptor-ligand partners such as the HIV gp160 envelope glycoprotein and the CD4 molecule that are expressed in virus-induced cell fusion and in the osteoclast [124]. Syncytin, an aptly named protein expressed by trophoblasts, stimulates cell:cell fusion and is also expressed by retrovirus [209].

Ketoconazole, long known to inhibit cell fusion, also diminishes the fusion of osteoclasts in culture [33]. Ketoconazole inhibits HMG-CoA reductase, thus decreasing cholesterol biosynthesis and the production of N-linked oligosaccharides necessary for the fusion of myoblasts in culture [71]. Mannose is an oligosaccharide that is expressed on the outer membrane of osteoclast precursors; mannose residues are necessary for the osteoclast fusion process [92], probably the mannose receptor enhances cell–cell binding [125]. Interleukin-13 increases fusion of macrophages through upregulation of the mannose receptor [27]. This may be an important mechanism by which inflammatory cytokines upregulate pathologic bone loss. In fact, decreasing the oligosaccharide binding partners of the mannose receptor decreases bone loss. Interestingly, cholesterol depletion by means of an HMG-CoA reductase inhibitor like that used to treat hypercholesterolemia also decreases the fusion of TRAP-positive mononuclear cells [151]. The ability of bisphosphonates to inhibit cholesterol synthesis may in fact contribute to their inhibition of osteoclast differentiation, doing so by preventing the expression of membrane signals necessary to induce fusion [37].

The disintegrin eichistatin, derived from snake venom, inhibits alpha(v)beta3 integrin ($\alpha v\beta 3$) by blocking RGD (arginine-glycine-asparagine) sites to which the integrin binds. Eichistatin binds to osteoclast membranes and completely inhibits the formation of multinucleated osteoclasts, even though it cannot do so when introduced in an earlier step of osteoclast differentiation [127]. Eichistatin action is partly due to inhibition of migration, a process that allows precursor cells to co-locate, and partly to detrimental effects on the fusion process itself.

The extracellular matrix, upon which the precursor cells are located, is also important in supporting fusion. This is illustrated by the role of ascorbic acid which, when present in the culture, causes the fusion of precursors to increase [138]. E-cadherin, which binds to cell adhesion molecules and is expressed in marrow mononuclear cells, is also involved in the fusion process [116].

The macrophage fusion receptor, also called SHPS-1, is another transmembrane glycoprotein that appears to have a role in macrophage fusion leading to multinucleation [50]. The absence of SHIP, a protein that blocks PI-3 kinase signaling in transgenic animals, leads to enlarged osteoclasts that may contain upwards of 100 nuclei; clearly when precursors undergo excessive fusion, excessive bone resorption results [174]. The purinergic receptor expressed on cells of macrophage lineage is another target of anti-fusogenic factors [32].

The control of osteoclast fusion thus involves multiple membrane proteins that regulate cell migration, cell–cell attachment, and intracellular signaling processes. RANKL [72] and 1,25-$(OH)_2D_3$ [1] are the major determinants of cell fusion and the differentiation pathway.

MITF Involvement in Late Differentiation

Interestingly, the mi/mi microphthalmic mouse held a clue to late differentiation events well before any of these events were understood. Examination of osteoclasts in these osteopetrotic mice revealed that mi/mi osteoclasts were mononuclear and lacked ruffled borders [176], even though they expressed other osteoclast enzymes [45, 54]. Other aspects of the mi/mi phenotype, such as reduced eye size and pigmentation, involve expression of a gene that encodes a basic helix-loop-helix-leucine zipper transcription factor [55], now known as micropththalmia transcription factor, or MITF.

MITF plays a role in osteoclastogenesis, by increasing the expression of TRAP through a conserved sequence (GGTCATGTGAG) that is located in the TRAP proximal promoter [108]. It also interacts with the PU.1 transcription factor [109]. MCSF, another early differentiation factor, induces phosphorylation of MITF, thereby triggering recruitment of the transcriptional co-activator, p300 [189]. Cathepsin K is downstream from these partners, as MITF upregulates expression of this important osteoclast enzyme [126].

Other Factors in Late Differentiation

Other factors that act on late differentiation continue to be discovered through screening osteoclast libraries. One such factor cloned from an immortalized murine osteoclast precursor is ADAM8, a disintegrin-like meltrin (see above). ADAM8 increases osteoclast formation during the later stage by an as yet unknown mechanisms [22].

Matrix recognition, needed to accomplish fusion or to identify bone, is a function of cell surface integrins or adhesion molecules. As noted above, the alpha(v)β3 integrin (αvβ3) has been implicated in bone resorption. Mice, in whom the β3 integrin subunit was deleted, develop osteosclerosis notwithstanding an increased number of multinucleated osteoclasts [118]. These β3 subunit null osteoclasts do not adequately resorb bone due to a cytoskeletal defect leading to dysfunctions in their ability to spread and form the actin ring/ruffled borders that are necessary for sealing and bone excavation. For osteoclasts to function, therefore, the entire resorptive apparatus must be expressed. Any one of multiple osteoclast enzyme deficiencies, even if the deficiency does not affect osteoclast recruitment, can lead to osteopetrosis due to defective bone resorption. For instance, a defect in cathepsin K results in the curious disease of pycnodyostosis [43], typified by osteosclerosis and short stature, and thought

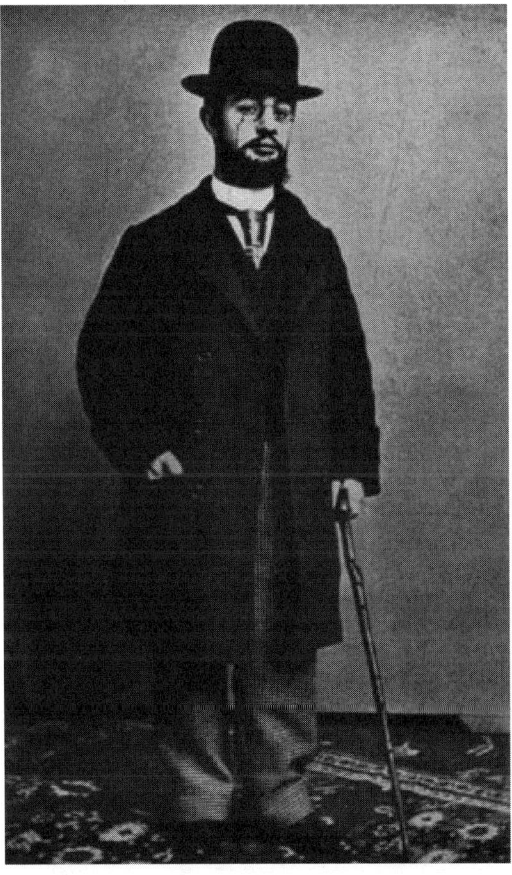

Figure 1.5 Toulouse-Lautrec: pycnodyostosis phenotype.

to be the phenotype exhibited by the great French painter, Toulouse-Lautrec (Figure 1.5). Another unexpected requirement is for the ubiquitous intracellular tyrosine kinase *c-src*, which is needed to form the ruffled borders that seal the resorption bay at the basal surface of the osteoclast [15, 158].

Stimulators and Repressors of Osteoclast Differentiation

Of the many regulators of osteoclast differentiation, some of the more important are discussed briefly below, in an effort to provide an overview of the large number of factors that affect osteoclastogenesis.

Hormones

Sex Steroids

Estrogen deficiency has long been known to cause a resorptive osteoporosis. While estrogen may modulate the action of T-lymphocytes and T-lymphocyte expression on RANKL [140, 191], it also dampens the RANKL-stimulated signal cascade. It does so by decreasing c-Jun expression and its phosphorylation by c-Jun N-terminal kinase [156]. Androgen deficiency also results in bone resorption and osteoporosis through the loss of androgen dampening of RANK activation of c-Jun [63].

Gonadal steroids also affect osteoclast recruitment by regulating the expression of osteoprotegerin. In ovariectomized rats, both RANKL and OPG are upregulated. This suggests that estrogen deficiency stimulates the entire RANKL system [66]. In men, serum OPG increases with age, while resorptive markers decrease [166]. In men made acutely hypogonadal, serum OPG increases. This suggests a response to an upregulated resorptive system [79]. Alternatively, estrogen appears to upregulate OPG expression by bone cells [58, 150]. These and other studies suggest that OPG is modified with respect to the bone remodeling rate [78].

Parathyroid Hormone and Vitamin D

Vitamin D is a potent stimulator of osteoclastogenesis and bone resorption. It acts by increasing MCSF [145] and RANKL [206] levels locally and decreasing OPG [61]. Parathyroid hormone, when administered continuously at high concentrations, has effects similar to those of vitamin D in terms of MCSF [190] and RANKL:OPG [61, 105], leading to increases in bone resorption. While both PTH and vitamin D alter cytokine levels, such as that of IL-6 [46, 47], it is their effect on the RANKL:OPG equilibrium that is the major factor by means of which they control osteoclast formation.

The expression of fibroblast growth factor 2, which potently induces osteoclast formation, is stimulated by PTH and may serve as a secondary mechanism to increase bone resorption. In bone marrow cultures made from the FGF-2 null mouse, PTH was less effective in stimulating osteoclast formation [134]. Interestingly, PTH stimulated RANKL to the same degree in the FGF-2-replete and FGF-2-null cultures. The RANKL:OPG equilibrium was shifted away from resorption due to a 30-fold increase in osteoprotegerin. This result indicates that FGF-2 enhances the inhibitory effect of PTH on OPG gene expression. FGF-2 is required in PTH-induced hypercalcemia, as evidenced by the resistance of the FGF-2 null animal to PTH-induced hypercalcemia [134]. Whether this effect is entirely due to FGF-2 mediated bone remodeling, or whether FGF-2 also promotes the PTH induced increase in renal calcium excretion, is not known.

Insulin-like Growth Factor-I

Insulin-like growth factor-I (IGF-I) is secreted during puberty, inducing long bone growth [200]. Because of its anabolic effects on bone, increasing bone density [201], it was thought that IGF-I should have salutary effects in osteoporosis. Surprisingly, in clinical trials, IGF-I caused an elevation of bone markers without significant increases in bone density [39]. This may be the result of IGF-I action on osteoclastogenesis. Addition of IGF-I to osteoclast-generating systems increased the numbers of osteoclasts, as well as the pit area per osteoclast [123]. In culture IGF-I increased RANKL expression and decreased OPG [144]. It is likely that the pleiotropic effects of IGF-I in bone allow for bone remodeling, rather than pure anabolism of bone.

Calcitonin

Calcitonin, a 32-amino-acid peptide secreted from the C-cells of the thyroid, has been used in hypercalcemia of malignancy to curtail osteoclastic bone resorption. Osteoclasts express receptors for calcitonin during early differentiation and maintain these throughout their life [103]. Thus calcitonin decreases the activity of mature osteoclasts, but also inhibits early differentiation events [168].

Prostaglandins

Prostaglandins may have biphasic effects on bone remodeling, dependent on the local microenvironment. Addition of PGE_2 to murine osteoclast generating systems *in vitro* stimulates osteoclast formation [5] and increases RANKL expression [206]. PGE_2 does, however, inhibit osteoclast formation in cultures of human cells [21]. Many of prostaglandin's variable effects may be due to differential or temporal expression of the many prostaglandin receptor types.

Secreted Factors other than Cytokines

Nitric Oxide and other Reactive Oxygen Species

Nitric oxide (NO) has effects in nearly every tissue in the body, including bone. One of the earliest reports linking NO to bone remodeling showed that inhibition of NOS, the enzyme that synthesizes NO from L-arginine, potentiates bone resorption in ovariectomized rats [77]. Since then, studies have shown that NO can slow bone loss in animals and humans [70, 194, 195]. NO alters osteoclast indices *in vitro*: osteoclastic resorption is potentiated during NOS inhibition [77]. This could result from effects on osteoclast activity, because NO induces a shape change in the osteoclasts associated with a reduction in bone resorption. Nitric oxide also decreases osteoclast recruitment and subsequent bone resorption [107]. The effect of NO on osteoclast recruitment is likely through alteration in the RANKL/OPG equilibrium as NO has been shown to both decrease RANKL and increase OPG expression in bone stromal cells [36].

Other reactive oxygen species induced by stress or as byproducts of nitric oxide are active in cells as well. Hydrogen peroxide has been shown to increase osteoclast differentiation, either directly or in combination with 1,25-dihydroxyvitamin D [161].

Factors Secreted by Osteoclasts: Annexin II and Legumain

Annexin II was identified as a candidate gene in the stimulation of osteoclast formation from a mammalian osteoclast cDNA expression library [169]. Purified recombinant AXII induced osteoclast formation in the absence of 1,25-dihydroxyvitamin D, probably acting on the proliferative stage of osteoclast precursors, and enhancing the growth of the CFU-GM [119]. Annexin II appears to stimulate the secretion of GM-CSF from T-cells and thus may have a role in inflammatory bone loss.

The osteoclast cDNA expression library [169] from which AXII was initially isolated also yielded an inhibitor of osteoclast formation found to be identical to human legumain, a cysteine endopeptidase [23]. Legumain can be detected in human marrow plasma from normal donors. When human marrow cultures are treated with an antibody to legumain, osteoclast formation is enhanced in the absence of 1,25-dihydroxyvitamin D.

Cytokines

A host of cytokines, including tumor necrosis factor and interleukins-1, -4, -6, -11, -18, have both positive and negative effects on osteoclastogenesis. These are dealt with in chapter 5.

Osteoclast-Associated Receptor Ligand

Other factors produced by osteoblasts and stromal cells have been identified through finding binding partners of discrete osteoclast receptors. One of the most interesting is the "osteoclast-associated receptor," or OSCAR, representing a novel member of the leukocyte receptor complex [80]. OSCAR expression varies from the usual immunoglobulin-like surface receptors typical of leukocytes by being expressed only in pre-osteoclasts and mature osteoclasts. The ligand for OSCAR (OSCAR-L) is expressed in osteoprogenitor cells. This is a developing area of research that may help to link the immune system genes more closely to bone remodeling.

Mechanical Factors

A major function of the skeletal structure is to provide support for locomotion. To adapt to functional loading, the skeleton has evolved a finely tuned response system that recognizes mechanical input. Unloading leads to bone resorption and loading to bone apposition and preservation. The cells of bone must thus be able to respond to unloading by initiating bone resorption. The results of bone resorption are seen in the skeletons of paraplegics and of astronauts, and quite readily in situations where unloading was generated experimentally [142, 143]. Thus, the recruitment of additional osteoclasts involved in unloading-associated resorption probably occurs via changes in the dominant RANKL:OPG equilibrium. Experimental studies with cells subject to loading suggest that loading stromal cells decreases their expression of RANKL through a pathway that involves activation of MAP-kinases [146, 147].

Conclusion

Resorption of the calcified surface of bone involves the orchestrated action of a large variety of enzymes and disposal mechanisms. Interference with, or overactivity of, any of these processes, leads to dysregulation of bone remodeling. Thus regulation of both the formation and action of the osteoclast modulates bone development, bone growth, and bone disease.

References

1. Abe E, Miyaura C, Tanaka H, Shiina Y, Kuribayashi T, Suda S, et al. (1983) 1 alpha,25-dihydroxyvitamin D3 promotes fusion of mouse alveolar macrophages both by a direct mechanism and by a spleen cell-mediated indirect mechanism. Proc Natl Acad Sci USA 80: 5583–7.
2. Abe E, Mocharla H, Yamate T, Taguchi Y, Manolagas SC (1999) Meltrin-alpha, a fusion protein involved in multinucleated giant cell and osteoclast formation. Calcif Tissue Int 64:508–15.
3. Abu-Amer Y, Erdmann J, Alexopoulou L, Kollias G, Ross FP, Teitelbaum SL (2000) Tumor necrosis factor receptors types 1 and 2 differentially regulate osteoclastogenesis. J Biol Chem 275:27307–10.
4. Akashi K, Traver D, Miyamoto T, Weissman IL (2000) A clonogenic common myeloid progenitor that gives rise to all myeloid lineages. Nature 404:193–7.
5. Akatsu T, Takahashi N, Debari K, Morita I, Murota S, Nagata N, et al. (1989) Prostaglandins promote osteoclastlike cell formation by a mechanism involving cyclic adenosine 3′,5′-monophosphate in mouse bone marrow cell cultures. J Bone Miner Res 4:29–35.
6. Akatsu T, Takahashi N, Udagawa N, Sato K, Nagata N, Moseley JM, et al. (1989) Parathyroid hormone (PTH)-related protein is a potent stimulator of osteoclast-like multinucleated cell formation to the same extent as PTH in mouse marrow cultures. Endocrinology 125: 20–7.
7. Anderson DM, Maraskovsky E, Billingsley WL, Dougall WC, Tometsko ME, Roux ER, et al. (1997) A homologue of the TNF receptor and its ligand enhance T-cell growth and dendritic-cell function. Nature 390:175–9.
8. Arai F, Miyamoto T, Ohneda O, Inada T, Sudo T, Brasel K, et al. (1999) Commitment and differentiation of osteoclast precursor cells by the sequential expression of c-Fms and receptor activator of nuclear factor kappaB (RANK) receptors. J Exp Med 190:1741–54.
9. Armstrong A, Tometsko M, Glaccum M, Sutherland C, Cosman D, Dougall W (2002) A RANK/TRAF6-dependent signal transduction pathway is essential for osteoclast cytoskeletal organization and resorptive function. J Biol Chem 277:44347–56.
10. Athanasou NA, Quinn J (1990) Immunophenotypic differences between osteoclasts and macrophage polykaryons: immunohistological distinction and implications for osteoclast ontogeny and function. J Clin Pathol 43:997–1003.
11. Azuma Y, Kaji K, Katogi R, Takeshita S, Kudo A (2000) Tumor necrosis factor-alpha induces differentiation of and bone resorption by osteoclasts. J Biol Chem 275:4858–64.
12. Biskobing DM, Fan D, Fan X, Rubin J (1997) Induction of carbonic anhydrase II expression in osteoclast progenitors requires physical contact with stromal cells. Endocrinology 138:4852–7.
13. Biskobing DM, Fan X, Rubin J (1995) Characterization of MCSF-induced proliferation and subsequent osteoclast formation in murine marrow culture. J Bone Miner Res 10:1025–32.
14. Boissy P, Saltel F, Bouniol C, Jurdic P, Machuca-Gayet I (2002) Transcriptional activity of nuclei in multinucleated osteoclasts and its modulation by calcitonin. Endocrinology 143:1913–21.
15. Boyce BF, Yoneda T, Lowe C, Soriano P, Mundy GR (1992) Requirement of pp60c-src expression for osteoclasts to form ruffled borders and resorb bone in mice. J Clin Invest 90:1622–7.
16. Bucay N, Sarosi I, Dunstan CR, Morony S, Tarpley J, Capparelli C, et al. (1998) osteoprotegerin-deficient mice develop early onset osteoporosis and arterial calcification. Genes Dev 12:1260–8.
17. Burger EH, Van der Meer JW, van de Gevel JS, Gribnau JC, Thesingh GW, van Furth R (1982) In vitro formation of osteoclasts from long-term cultures of bone marrow mononuclear phagocytes. J Exp Med 156: 1604–14.
18. Burguera B, Hofbauer LC, Thomas T, Gori F, Evans GL, Khosla S, et al. (2001) Leptin reduces ovariectomy-induced bone loss in rats. Endocrinology 142:3546–53.
19. Cenci S, Weitzmann MN, Roggia C, Namba N, Novack D, Woodring J, et al. (2000) Estrogen deficiency induces bone loss by enhancing T-cell production of TNF-alpha. J Clin Invest 106:1229–37.
20. Chambers TJ, Owens JM, Hattersley G, Jat PS, Noble MD (1993) Generation of osteoclast-inductive and osteoclastogenic cell lines from the H-2KbtsA58 transgenic mouse. Proc Natl Acad Sci USA 90:5578–82.
21. Chenu C, Kurihara N, Mundy GR, Roodman GD (1990) Prostaglandin E2 inhibits formation of osteoclastlike cells in long-term human marrow cultures but is not a mediator of the inhibitory effects of transforming growth factor beta. J Bone Miner Res 5:677–81.
22. Choi SJ, Han JH, Roodman GD (2001) ADAM8: a novel osteoclast stimulating factor. J Bone Miner Res 16: 814–22.
23. Choi SJ, Reddy SV, Devlin RD, Menaa C, Chung H, Boyce BF, et al. (1999) Identification of human asparaginyl endopeptidase (legumain) as an inhibitor of osteoclast formation and bone resorption. J Biol Chem 274:27747–53.
24. Coccia PF, Krivit W, Cervenka J, Clawson C, Kersey JH, Kim TH, et al. (1980) Successful bone-marrow trans-

plantation for infantile malignant osteopetrosis. N Engl J Med 302:701–8.

25. Collin-Osdoby P, Rothe L, Anderson F, Nelson M, Maloney W, Osdoby P (2001) RANKL and OPG expression by human microvascular endothelial cells, regulation by inflammatory cytokines, and role in human osteoclastogenesis. J Biol Chem 23:23.

26. Darnay B, Ni J, Moore P, Aggarwal B (1999) Activation of NF-kappaB by RANK requires tumor necrosis factor receptor-associated factor (TRAF) 6 and NF-kappaB-inducing kinase. Identification of a novel TRAF6 interaction motif. J Biol Chem 274:7724–31.

27. DeFife KM, Jenney CR, McNally AK, Colton E, Anderson JM (1997) Interleukin-13 induces human monocyte/macrophage fusion and macrophage mannose receptor expression. J Immunol 158:3385–90.

28. Dexter TM (1979) Haemopoiesis in long-term bone marrow cultures. A review. Acta Haematol 62:299–305.

29. Dexter TM, Allen TD, Lajtha LG, Schofield R, Lord BI (1973) Stimulation of differentiation and proliferation of haemopoietic cells in vitro. J Cell Physiol 82:461–73.

30. Emery JG, McDonnell P, Burke MB, Deen KC, Lyn S, Silverman C, et al. (1998) Osteoprotegerin is a receptor for the cytotoxic ligand TRAIL. J Biol Chem 273:14363–7.

31. Fallon MD, Teitelbaum SL, Kahn AJ (1983) Multinucleation enhances macrophage-mediated bone resorption. Lab Invest 49:159–64.

32. Falzoni S, Munerati M, Ferrari D, Spisani S, Moretti S, Di Virgilio F (1995) The purinergic P2Z receptor of human macrophage cells. Characterization and possible physiological role. J Clin Invest 95:1207–16.

33. Fan X, Biskobing DM, Bain S, Rubin J (1996) Ketoconazole and phorbol myristate acetate regulate osteoclast precursor fusion in primary murine marrow culture. J Bone Miner Res 11:1274–80.

34. Fan X, Biskobing DM, Fan D, Hofstetter W, Rubin J (1997) Macrophage colony stimulating factor downregulates MCSF-receptor expression and entry of progenitors into the osteoclast lineage. J Bone Miner Res 12:1387–95.

35. Fan X, Fan D, Gewant H, Royce C, Nanes M, Rubin J (2001) Increasing membrane-bound MCSF does not enhance OPGL-driven osteoclastogenesis from marrow cells. Am J Physiol Endocrinol Metab 280: E103–11.

36. Fan X, Zhu L, Roy E, Murphy TC, Hart CM, Rosen C, Nanes MS, Rubin J (2004) Nitric oxide decreases RANKL and increases OPG expression in bone stromal cells Endocrinology 145:751–759.

37. Fisher JE, Rogers MJ, Halasy JM, Luckman SP, Hughes DE, Masarachia PJ, et al. (1999) Alendronate mechanism of action: geranylgeraniol, an intermediate in the mevalonate pathway, prevents inhibition of osteoclast formation, bone resorption, and kinase activation in vitro. Proc Natl Acad Sci USA 96:133–8.

38. Fleischmann A, Hafezi F, Elliott C, Reme CE, Ruther U, Wagner EF (2000) Fra-1 replaces c-Fos-dependent functions in mice. Genes Dev 14:2695–700.

39. Friedlander AL, Butterfield GE, Moynihan S, Grillo J, Pollack M, Holloway L, et al. (2001) One year of insulin-like growth factor I treatment does not affect bone density, body composition, or psychological measures in postmenopausal women. J Clin Endocrinol Metab 86:1496–503.

40. Fuller K, Bayley KE, Chambers TJ (2000) Activin A is an essential cofactor for osteoclast induction. Biochem Biophys Res Commun 268:2–7.

41. Fuller K, Lean JM, Bayley KE, Wani MR, Chambers TJ (2000) A role for TGFbeta(1) in osteoclast differentiation and survival. J Cell Sci 113 (Pt 13):2445–53.

42. Gao YH, Shinki T, Yuasa T, Kataoka-Enomoto H, Komori T, Suda T, et al. (1998) Potential role of cbfa1, an essential transcriptional factor for osteoblast differentiation, in osteoclastogenesis: regulation of mRNA expression of osteoclast differentiation factor (ODF). Biochem Biophys Res Commun 252:697–702.

43. Gelb BD, Shi GP, Chapman HA, Desnick RJ (1996) Pycnodysostosis, a lysosomal disease caused by cathepsin K deficiency. Science 273:1236–8.

44. Gori F, Hofbauer LC, Dunstan CR, Spelsberg TC, Khosla S, Riggs BL (2000) The expression of osteoprotegerin and RANK ligand and the support of osteoclast formation by stromal-osteoblast lineage cells is developmentally regulated. Endocrinology 141:4768–76.

45. Graves L, 3rd, Jilka RL (1990) Comparison of bone and parathyroid hormone as stimulators of osteoclast development and activity in calvarial cell cultures from normal and osteopetrotic (mi/mi) mice. J Cell Physiol 145:102–9.

46. Greenfield EM, Horowitz MC, Lavish SA (1996) Stimulation by parathyroid hormone of interleukin-6 and leukemia inhibitory factor expression in osteoblasts is an immediate-early gene response induced by cAMP signal transduction. J Biol Chem 271:10984–9.

47. Greenfield EM, Shaw SM, Gornik SA, Banks MA (1995) Adenyl cyclase and interleukin 6 are downstream effectors of parathyroid hormone resulting in stimulation of bone resorption. J Clin Invest 96:1238–44.

48. Grigoriadis AE, Wang ZQ, Cecchini MG, Hofstetter W, Felix R, Fleisch HA, et al. (1994) c-Fos: a key regulator of osteoclast-macrophage lineage determination and bone remodeling. Science 266:443–8.

49. Han JH, Choi SJ, Kurihara N, Koide M, Oba Y, Roodman GD (2001) Macrophage inflammatory protein-1alpha is an osteoclastogenic factor in myeloma that is independent of receptor activator of nuclear factor kappaB ligand. Blood 97:3349–53.

50. Han X, Sterling H, Chen Y, Saginario C, Brown EJ, Frazier WA, et al. (2000) CD47, a ligand for the macrophage fusion receptor, participates in macrophage multinucleation. J Biol Chem 275:37984–92.

51. Hattersley G, Chambers TJ (1989) Calcitonin receptors as markers for osteoclastic differentiation: correlation between generation of bone-resorptive cells and cells that express calcitonin receptors in mouse bone marrow cultures. Endocrinology 125:1606–12.

52. Hattersley G, Kerby JA, Chambers TJ (1991) Identification of osteoclast precursors in multilineage hemopoietic colonies. Endocrinology 128:259–62.

53. Hattersley G, Owens J, Flanagan AM, Chambers TJ (1991) Macrophage colony stimulating factor (M-CSF) is essential for osteoclast formation in vitro. Biochem Biophys Res Commun 177:526–31.

54. Helfrich MH, Mieremet RH (1988) A morphologic study of osteoclasts isolated from osteopetrotic microphthalmic (mi/mi) mouse and human fetal long bones using an instrument permitting combination of light and scanning electron microscopy. Bone 9:113–19.

55. Hodgkinson CA, Moore KJ, Nakayama A, Steingrimsson E, Copeland NG, Jenkins NA, et al. (1993) Muta-

tions at the mouse microphthalmia locus are associated with defects in a gene encoding a novel basic-helix-loop-helix-zipper protein. Cell 74:395–404.

56. Hofbauer LC, Gori F, Riggs BL, Lacey DL, Dunstan CR, Spelsberg TC, et al. (1999) Stimulation of osteoprotegerin ligand and inhibition of osteoprotegerin production by glucocorticoids in human osteoblastic lineage cells: potential paracrine mechanisms of glucocorticoid-induced. Endocrinology 140:4382–9.

57. Hofbauer LC, Heufelder AE (2001) Role of receptor activator of nuclear factor-kappaB ligand and osteoprotegerin in bone cell biology. J Mol Med 79:243–53.

58. Hofbauer LC, Khosla S, Dunstan CR, Lacey DL, Spelsberg TC, Riggs BL (1999) Estrogen stimulates gene expression and protein production of osteoprotegerin in human osteoblastic cells. Endocrinology 140: 4367–70.

59. Horton MA, Pringle JA, Chambers TJ (1985) Identification of human osteoclasts with monoclonal antibodies. N Engl J Med 312:923–4.

60. Horton MA, Rimmer EF, Lewis D, Pringle JA, Fuller K, Chambers TJ (1984) Cell surface characterization of the human osteoclast: phenotypic relationship to other bone marrow-derived cell types. J Pathol 144:281–94.

61. Horwood N, Elliott J, Martin T, Gillespie M (1998) Osteotropic agents regulate the expression of osteoclast differentiation factor and osteoprotegerin in osteoblastic stromal cells. Endocrinology 4743–6.

62. Hsu H, Lacey DL, Dunstan CR, Solovyev I, Colombero A, Timms E, et al. (1999) Tumor necrosis factor receptor family member RANK mediates osteoclast differentiation and activation induced by osteoprotegerin ligand. Proc Natl Acad Sci USA 96:3540–5.

63. Huber DM, Bendixen AC, Pathrose P, Srivastava S, Dienger KM, Shevde NK, et al. (2001) Androgens suppress osteoclast formation induced by RANKL and macrophage-colony stimulating factor. Endocrinology 142:3800–8.

64. Hughes AE, Ralston SH, Marken J, Bell C, MacPherson H, Wallace RG, et al. (2000) Mutations in TNFRSF11A, affecting the signal peptide of RANK, cause familial expansile osteolysis. Nat Genet 24:45–8.

65. Ibbotson KJ, Roodman GD, McManus LM, Mundy GR (1984) Identification and characterization of osteoclast-like cells and their progenitors in cultures of feline marrow mononuclear cells. J Cell Biol 99:471–80.

66. Ikeda T, Utsuyama M, Hirokawa K (2001) Expression profiles of receptor activator of nuclear factor kappaB ligand, receptor activator of nuclear factor kappaB, and osteoprotegerin messenger RNA in aged and ovariectomized rat bones. J Bone Miner Res 16:1416–25.

67. Ishida N, Hayashi K, Hoshijima M, Ogawa T, Koga S, Miyatake Y, et al. (2002) Large scale gene expression analysis of osteoclastogenesis in vitro and elucidation of NFAT2 as a key regulator. J Biol Chem 277:41147–56.

68. Itoh K, Udagawa N, Katagiri T, Iemura S, Ueno N, Yasuda H, et al. (2001) Bone morphogenetic protein 2 stimulates osteoclast differentiation and survival supported by receptor activator of nuclear factor-kappaB ligand. Endocrinology 142:3656–62.

69. Itoh K, Udagawa N, Matsuzaki K, Takami M, Amano H, Shinki T, et al. (2000) Importance of membrane- or matrix-associated forms of M-CSF and RANKL/ODF in osteoclastogenesis supported by SaOS-4/3 cells expressing recombinant PTH/PTHrP receptors. J Bone Miner Res 15:1766–75.

70. Jamal SA, Browner WS, Bauer DC, Cummings SR (1998) Intermittent use of nitrates increases bone mineral density: the study of osteoporotic fractures. J Bone Miner Res 13:1755–9.

71. Jamieson JC, Wayne S, Belo RS, Wright JA, Spearman MA (1992) The importance of N-linked glycoproteins and dolichyl phosphate synthesis for fusion of L6 myoblasts. Biochem Cell Biol 70:408–12.

72. Jimi E, Akiyama S, Tsurukai T, Okahashi N, Kobayashi K, Udagawa N, et al. (1999) Osteoclast differentiation factor acts as a multifunctional regulator in murine osteoclast differentiation and function. J Immunol 163:434–42.

73. Jochum W, David JP, Elliott C, Wutz A, Plenk H, Jr., Matsuo K, et al. (2000) Increased bone formation and osteosclerosis in mice overexpressing the transcription factor Fra-1. Nat Med 6:980–4.

74. Junttila I, Bourette RP, Rohrschneider LR, Silvennoinen O (2003) M-CSF induced differentiation of myeloid precursor cells involves activation of PKC-delta and expression of Pkare. J Leukoc Biol 73:281–8.

75. Kahn AJ, Simmons DJ (1975) Investigation of cell lineage in bone using a chimaera of chick and quial embryonic tissue. Nature 258:325–7.

76. Kanematsu M, Yoshimura K, Takaoki M, Sato A (2002) Vector-averaged gravity regulates gene expression of receptor activator of NF-kappaB (RANK) ligand and osteoprotegerin in bone marrow stromal cells via cyclic AMP/protein kinase A pathway. Bone 30:553–8.

77. Kasten TP, Collin-Osdoby P, Patel N, Osdoby P, Krukowski M, Misko TP, et al. (1994) Potentiation of osteoclast bone-resorption activity by inhibition of nitric oxide synthase. Proc Natl Acad Sci USA 91: 3569–73.

78. Khosla S, Arrighi HM, Melton LJ, 3rd, Atkinson EJ, O'Fallon WM, Dunstan C, et al. (2002) Correlates of osteoprotegerin levels in women and men. Osteoporos Int 13:394–9.

79. Khosla S, Atkinson EJ, Dunstan CR, O'Fallon WM (2002) Effect of estrogen versus testosterone on circulating osteoprotegerin and other cytokine levels in normal elderly men. J Clin Endocrinol Metab 87: 1550–4.

80. Kim N, Takami M, Rho J, Josien R, Choi Y (2002) A novel member of the leukocyte receptor complex regulates osteoclast differentiation. J Exp Med 195:201–9.

81. Kimble RB, Srivastava S, Ross FP, Matayoshi A, Pacifici R (1996) Estrogen deficiency increases the ability of stromal cells to support murine osteoclastogenesis via an interleukin-1and tumor necrosis factor-mediated stimulation of macrophage colony-stimulating factor production. J Biol Chem 271:28890–7.

82. Kitazawa R, Kitazawa S, Maeda S (1999) Promoter structure of mouse RANKL/TRANCE/OPGL/ODF gene. Biochim Biophys Acta 1445:134–41.

83. Kobayashi K, Takahashi N, Jimi E, Udagawa N, Takami M, Kotake S, et al. (2000) Tumor necrosis factor alpha stimulates osteoclast differentiation by a mechanism independent of the ODF/RANKL-RANK interaction. J Exp Med 191:275–86.

84. Kobayashi N, Kadono Y, Naito A, Matsumoto K, Yamamoto T, Tanaka S, et al. (2001) Segregation of TRAF6-mediated signaling pathways clarifies its role in osteoclastogenesis. EMBO J 20:1271–80.

85. Kodaira K, Mizuno A, Yasuda H, Shima N, Murakami A, Ueda M, et al. (1999) Cloning and characterization

of the gene encoding mouse osteoclast differentiation factor. Gene 230:121–7.

86. Kodama H, Nose M, Niida S, Yamasaki A (1991) Essential role of macrophage colony-stimulating factor in the osteoclast differentiation supported by stromal cells. J Exp Med 173:1291–4.

87. Kolliker A. (1873) Die normale Resorption des Knochengewebes und ihre Bedeutung für die Entstehung der typischen Knochenformen, edn. In: Vogel F, editor Leipzig.

88. Kondo M, Weissman IL, Akashi K (1997) Identification of clonogenic common lymphoid progenitors in mouse bone marrow. Cell 91:661–72.

89. Kong YY, Feige U, Sarosi I, Bolon B, Tafuri A, Morony S, et al. (1999) Activated T cells regulate bone loss and joint destruction in adjuvant arthritis through osteoprotegerin ligand. Nature 402:304–9.

90. Kong YY, Yoshida H, Sarosi I, Tan HL, Timms E, Capparelli C, et al. (1999) OPGL is a key regulator of osteoclastogenesis, lymphocyte development and lymph-node organogenesis. Nature 397:315–23.

91. Kukita A, Chenu C, McManus LM, Mundy GR, Roodman GD (1990) Atypical multinucleated cells form in long-term marrow cultures from patients with Paget's disease. J Clin Invest 85:1280–6.

92. Kurachi T, Morita I, Oki T, Ueki T, Sakaguchi K, Enomoto S, et al. (1994) Expression on outer membranes of mannose residues, which are involved in osteoclast formation via cellular fusion events. J Biol Chem 269:17572 6.

93. Kurihara N, Chenu C, Miller M, Civin C, Roodman GD (1990) Identification of committed mononuclear precursors for osteoclast-like cells formed in long term human marrow cultures. Endocrinology 126:2733–41.

94. Kurihara N, Gluck S, Roodman GD (1990) Sequential expression of phenotype markers for osteoclasts during differentiation of precursors for multinucleated cells formed in long-term human marrow cultures. Endocrinology 127:3215–21.

95. Kurihara N, Suda T, Miura Y, Nakauchi H, Kodama H, Hiura K, et al. (1989) Generation of osteoclasts from isolated hematopoietic progenitor cells. Blood 74:1295–302.

96. Lacey DL, Tan HL, Lu J, Kaufman S, Van G, Qiu W, et al. (2000) Osteoprotegerin ligand modulates murine osteoclast survival in vitro and in vivo. Am J Pathol 157:435–48.

97. Lacey DL, Timms E, Tan HL, Kelley MJ, Dunstan CR, Burgess T, et al. (1998) Osteoprotegerin ligand is a cytokine that regulates osteoclast differentiation and activation. Cell 93:165–76.

98. Lam J, Nelson CA, Ross FP, Teitelbaum SL, Fremont DH (2001) Crystal structure of the TRANCE/RANKL cytokine reveals determinants of receptor-ligand specificity. J Clin Invest 108:971–9.

99. Lam J, Takeshita S, Barker JE, Kanagawa O, Ross FP, Teitelbaum SL (2000) TNF-alpha induces osteoclastogenesis by direct stimulation of macrophages exposed to permissive levels of RANK ligand. J Clin Invest 106:1481–8.

100. Lean JM, Fuller K, Chambers TJ (2001) FLT3 ligand can substitute for macrophage colony-stimulating factor in support of osteoclast differentiation and function. Blood 98:2707–13.

101. Lean JM, Matsuo K, Fox SW, Fuller K, Gibson FM, Draycott G, et al. (2000) Osteoclast lineage commitment of bone marrow precursors through expression of membrane-bound TRANCE. Bone 27:29–40.

102. Lee MY, Lottsfeldt JL, Fevold KL (1992) Identification and characterization of osteoclast progenitors by clonal analysis of hematopoietic cells. Blood 80:1710–16.

103. Lee SK, Goldring SR, Lorenzo JA (1995) Expression of the calcitonin receptor in bone marrow cell cultures and in bone: a specific marker of the differentiated osteoclast that is regulated by calcitonin. Endocrinology 136:4572–81.

104. Lee SK, Lorenzo JA (1999) Parathyroid hormone stimulates TRANCE and inhibits osteoprotegerin messenger ribonucleic acid expression in murine bone marrow cultures: correlation with osteoclast-like cell formation. Endocrinology 140:3552–61.

105. Lee SK, Lorenzo JA (2002) Regulation of receptor activator of nuclear factor-kappa B ligand and osteoprotegerin mRNA expression by parathyroid hormone is predominantly mediated by the protein kinase a pathway in murine bone marrow cultures. Bone 31:252–9.

106. Lomaga MA, Yeh WC, Sarosi I, Duncan GS, Furlonger C, Ho A, et al. (1999) TRAF6 deficiency results in osteopetrosis and defective interleukin-1, CD40, and LPS signaling. Genes Dev 13:1015–24.

107. Lowik C, Nibberin PH, van de Ruit M, Papapoulos SE (1994) Inducible produciton of nitric oxide in osteoblast-like cells and in fetal mouse bone explants is associated with suppression of osteoclastic bone resorption. J Clin Invest 93:1465–72.

108. Luchin A, Purdom G, Murphy K, Clark MY, Angel N, Cassady AI, et al. (2000) The microphthalmia transcription factor regulates expression of the tartrate-resistant acid phosphatase gene during terminal differentiation of osteoclasts. J Bone Miner Res 15:451–60.

109. Luchin A, Suchting S, Merson T, Rosol TJ, Hume DA, Cassady AI, et al. (2001) Genetic and physical interactions between Microphthalmia transcription factor and PU.1 are necessary for osteoclast gene expression and differentiation. J Biol Chem 276:36703–10.

110. Lum L, Wong BR, Josien R, Becherer JD, Erdjument-Bromage H, Schlondorff J, et al. (1999) Evidence for a role of a tumor necrosis factor-alpha (TNF-alpha)-converting enzyme-like protease in shedding of TRANCE, a TNF family member involved in osteoclastogenesis and dendritic cell survival. J Biol Chem 274:13613–8.

111. Ma YL, Cain RL, Halladay DL, Yang X, Zeng Q, Miles RR, et al. (2001) Catabolic effects of continuous human pth (1–38) in vivo is associated with sustained stimulation of rankl and inhibition of osteoprotegerin and gene-associated bone formation. Endocrinology 142:4047–54.

112. MacDonald BR, Mundy GR, Clark S, Wang EA, Kuehl TJ, Stanley ER, et al. (1986) Effects of human recombinant CSF-GM and highly purified CSF-1 on the formation of multinucleated cells with osteoclast characteristics in long-term bone marrow cultures. J Bone Miner Res 1:227–33.

113. Mansky K, Sankar U, Han J, Ostrowski M (2002) Microphthalmia transcription factor is a target of the p38 MAPK pathway in response to receptor activator of NF-kappa B ligand signaling. J Biol Chem 277:11077–83.

114. Massey HM, Scopes J, Horton MA, Flanagan AM (2001) Transforming growth factor-beta1 (TGF-beta) stimulates the osteoclast-forming potential of peripheral blood hematopoietic precursors in a lymphocyte-rich microenvironment. Bone 28:577–82.

115. Matsuo K, Owens JM, Tonko M, Elliott C, Chambers TJ, Wagner EF (2000) Fosl1 is a transcriptional target of c-Fos during osteoclast differentiation. Nat Genet 24:184–7.

116. Mbalaviele G, Chen H, Boyce BF, Mundy GR, Yoneda T (1995) The role of cadherin in the generation of multinucleated osteoclasts from mononuclear precursors in murine marrow. J Clin Invest 95:2757–65.

117. McCauley LK, Koh AJ, Beecher CA, Rosol TJ (1997) Proto-oncogene c-fos is transcriptionally regulated by parathyroid hormone (PTH) and PTH-related protein in a cyclic adenosine monophosphate-dependent manner in osteoblastic cells. Endocrinology 138:5427–33.

118. McHugh KP, Hodivala-Dilke K, Zheng MH, Namba N, Lam J, Novack D, et al. (2000) Mice lacking beta3 integrins are osteosclerotic because of dysfunctional osteoclasts. J Clin Invest 105:433–40.

119. Menaa C, Devlin RD, Reddy SV, Gazitt Y, Choi SJ, Roodman GD (1999) Annexin II increases osteoclast formation by stimulating the proliferation of osteoclast precursors in human marrow cultures. J Clin Invest 103:1605–13.

120. Menaa C, Reddy SV, Kurihara N, Maeda H, Anderson D, Cundy T, et al. (2000) Enhanced RANK ligand expression and responsivity of bone marrow cells in Paget's disease of bone. J Clin Invest 105:1833–8.

121. Min H, Morony S, Sarosi I, Dunstan CR, Capparelli C, Scully S, et al. (2000) Osteoprotegerin reverses osteoporosis by inhibiting endosteal osteoclasts and prevents vascular calcification by blocking a process resembling osteoclastogenesis. J Exp Med 192:463–74.

122. Miyauchi A, Kuroki Y, Fukase M, Fujita T, Chihara K, Shiozawa S (1994) Persistent expression of proto-oncogene c-fos stimulates osteoclast differentiation. Biochem Biophys Res Commun 205:1547–55.

123. Mochizuki H, Hakeda Y, Wakatsuki N, Usui N, Akashi S, Sato T, et al. (1992) Insulin-like growth factor-I supports formation and activation of osteoclasts. Endocrinology 131:1075–80.

124. Mori K, Nishimura M, Tsurudome M, Ito M, Nishio M, Kawano M, et al. (2003) The functional interaction between CD98 and CD147 in regulation of virus-induced cell fusion and osteoclast formation. Med Microbiol Immunol (Berl).

125. Morishima S, Morita I, Tokushima T, Kawashima H, Miyasaka M, Omura K, et al. (2003) Expression and role of mannose receptor/terminal high-mannose type oligosaccharide on osteoclast precursors during osteoclast formation. J Endocrinol 176:285–92.

126. Motyckova G, Weilbaecher KN, Horstmann M, Rieman DJ, Fisher DZ, Fisher DE (2001) Linking osteopetrosis and pycnodysostosis: regulation of cathepsin K expression by the microphthalmia transcription factor family. Proc Natl Acad Sci USA 98:5798–803.

127. Nakamura I, Tanaka H, Rodan GA, Duong LT (1998) Echistatin inhibits the migration of murine prefusion osteoclasts and the formation of multinucleated osteoclast-like cells. Endocrinology 139:5182–93.

128. Nakano H, Oshima H, Chung W, Williams-Abbott L, Ware C, Yagita H, et al. (1996) TRAF5, an activator of NF-kappaB and putative signal transducer for the lymphotoxin-beta receptor. J Biol Chem 271:14661–4.

129. Nakashima T, Kobayashi Y, Yamasaki S, Kawakami A, Eguchi K, Sasaki H, et al. (2000) Protein Expression and Functional Difference of Membrane-Bound and Soluble Receptor Activator of NF-kappaB Ligand: Modulation of the Expression by Osteotropic Factors and Cytokines. Biochem Biophys Res Commun 275:768–775.

130. Nakashima T, Kobayashi Y, Yamasaki S, Kawakami A, Eguchi K, Sasaki H, et al. (2000) Protein expression and functional difference of membrane-bound and soluble receptor activator of NF-kappaB ligand: modulation of the expression by osteotropic factors and cytokines. Biochem Biophys Res Commun 275:768–75.

131. Niida S, Kaku M, Amano H, Yoshida H, Kataoka H, Nishikawa S, et al. (1999) Vascular endothelial growth factor can substitute for macrophage colony-stimulating factor in the support of osteoclastic bone resorption. J Exp Med 190:293–8.

132. Nutt SL, Heavey B, Rolink AG, Busslinger M (1999) Commitment to the B-lymphoid lineage depends on the transcription factor Pax5. Nature 401:556–62.

133. O'Brien CA, Kern B, Gubrij I, Karsenty G, Manolagas SC (2002) Cbfa1 does not regulate RANKL gene activity in stromal/osteoblastic cells. Bone 30:453–62.

134. Okada Y, Montero A, Zhang X, Sobue T, Lorenzo J, Doetschman T, et al. (2003) Impaired osteoclast formation in bone marrow cultures of Fgf2 null mice in response to parathyroid hormone. J Biol Chem 278:21258–66.

135. Osawa M, Hanada K, Hamada H, Nakauchi H (1996) Long-term lymphohematopoietic reconstitution by a single CD34-low/negative hematopoietic stem cell. Science 273:242–5.

136. Perkins S, Kling S (1995) Local concentrations of MCSF mediate osteoclastic differentiation. Amer J Physiol 269:E1024–30.

137. Povolny BT, Lee MY (1993) The role of recombinant human M-CSF, IL-3, GM-CSF and calcitriol in clonal development of osteoclast precursors in primate bone marrow. Exp Hematol 21:532–7.

138. Ragab AA, Lavish SA, Banks MA, Goldberg VM, Greenfield EM (1998) Osteoclast differentiation requires ascorbic acid. J Bone Miner Res 13:970–7.

139. Ragab AA, Nalepka JL, Bi Y, Greenfield EM (2002) Cytokines synergistically induce osteoclast differentiation: support by immortalized or normal calvarial cells. Am J Physiol Cell Physiol 283:C679–87.

140. Roggia C, Gao Y, Cenci S, Weitzmann MN, Toraldo G, Isaia G, et al. (2001) Up-regulation of TNF-producing T cells in the bone marrow: a key mechanism by which estrogen deficiency induces bone loss in vivo. Proc Natl Acad Sci USA 98:13960–5.

141. Roodman GD, Ibbotson KJ, MacDonald BR, Kuehl TJ, Mundy GR (1985) 1,25-Dihydroxyvitamin D3 causes formation of multinucleated cells with several osteoclast characteristics in cultures of primate marrow. Proc Natl Acad Sci USA 82:8213–17.

142. Rubin C, Gross T, Qin YX, Fritton S, Guilak F, McLeod K (1996) Differentiation of the bone-tissue remodeling response to axial and torsional loading in the turkey ulna. J Bone Joint Surg Am 78:1523–33.

143. Rubin C, Lanyon L (1984) Regulation of bone formation by applied dynamic loads. J Bone Joint Surgery 66A:397–402.

144. Rubin J, Ackert-Bicknell C, Zhu L, Fan X, Murphy T, Nanes M, et al. (2002) Insulin Like Growth Factor-I (IGF-I) regulates osteoprotegerin (OPG) and RANK Ligand (RANKL) in vitro and osteoprotogerin in vivo. Journal of Clinical Endocrinology and Metabolism 87:4273–9.

145. Rubin J, Fan X, Thornton D, Bryant R, Biskobing D (1996) Regulation of murine osteoblast macrophage colony-stimulating factor production by 1,25(OH)2D3. Calcified Tissue 59:291–6.

146. Rubin J, Murphy T, Fan X, Goldschmidt M, Taylor W (2002) Mechanical strain inhibits RANKL expression through activation of ERK1/2 in bone marrow stromal cells. J Bone Miner Res 17:1452–60.

147. Rubin J, Murphy T, Nanes MS, Fan X (2000) Mechanical strain inhibits expression of osteoclast differentiation factor by murine stromal cells. Am J Physiol Cell Physiol 278:C1126–32.

148. Rubin J, Titus L, Nanes MS (1992) cAMP promotion of osteoclast-like cell development from mouse bone marrow cells requires a permissive action of 1,25-(OH)2D3. J Bone Miner Res 7:611–17.

149. Ruther U, Komitowski D, Schubert FR, Wagner EF (1989) c-fos expression induces bone tumors in transgenic mice. Oncogene 4:861–5.

150. Saika M, Inoue D, Kido S, Matsumoto T (2001) 17beta-estradiol stimulates expression of osteoprotegerin by a mouse stromal cell line, ST-2, via estrogen receptor-alpha. Endocrinology 142:2205–12.

151. Sato T, Morita I, Murota S (1998) Involvement of cholesterol in osteoclast-like cell formation via cellular fusion. Bone 23:135–40.

152. Sells Galvin RJ, Gatlin CL, Horn JW, Fuson TR (1999) TGF-beta enhances osteoclast differentiation in hematopoietic cell cultures stimulated with RANKL and M-CSF. Biochem Biophys Res Commun 265:233–9.

153. Sherr CJ (1990) Colony-stimulating factor-1 receptor. Blood 75:1–12.

154. Sherr CJ (1990) The colony-stimulating factor 1 receptor: pleiotropy of signal-response coupling. Lymphokine Res 9:543–8.

155. Sherr CJ (1991) Mitogenic response to colony-stimulating factor 1. Trends Genet 7:398–402.

156. Shevde NK, Bendixen AC, Dienger KM, Pike JW (2000) Estrogens suppress RANK ligand-induced osteoclast differentiation via a stromal cell independent mechanism involving c-Jun repression. Proc Natl Acad Sci USA 97:7829–34.

157. Simonet WS, Lacey DL, Dunstan CR, Kelley M, Chang MS, Luthy R, et al. (1997) Osteoprotegerin: a novel secreted protein involved in the regulation of bone density. Cell 89:309–19.

158. Soriano P, Montgomery C, Geske R, Bradley A (1991) Targeted disruption of the c-src proto-oncogene leads to osteopetrosis in mice. Cell 64:693–702.

159. Spangrude GJ, Heimfeld S, Weissman IL (1988) Purification and characterization of mouse hematopoietic stem cells. Science 241:58–62.

160. Stanley ER, ed.: Thomson A (1994) Colony stimulating factor-1 (Macrophage colony stimulating factor). The Cytokine Handbook. 387–418, Academic Press, London.

161. Steinbeck MJ, Kim JK, Trudeau MJ, Hauschka PV, Karnovsky MJ (1998) Involvement of hydrogen peroxide in the differentiation of clonal HD-11EM cells into osteoclast-like cells J Cell Physiol 176:574–87.

162. Suda T, Suda J, Kajigaya S, Nagata S, Asano S, Saito M, et al (1987) Effects of recombinant murine granulocyte colony-stimulating factor on granulocyte-macrophage and blast colony formation Exp Hematol 15:958–65.

163. Suda T, Takahashi N, Martin J (1992) Modulation of osteoclast differentiation. Endocrine Rev 13:66–80.

164. Suda T, Takahashi N, Udagawa N, Jimi E, Gillespie MT, Martin TJ (1999) Modulation of osteoclast differentiation and function by the new members of the tumor necrosis factor receptor and ligand families. Endocr Rev 20:345–57.

165. Suda T, Udagawa N, Nakamura I, Miyaura C, Takahashi N (1995) Modulation of osteoclast differentiation by local factors. Bone 17:87S–91S.

166. Szulc P, Hofbauer LC, Heufelder AE, Roth S, Delmas PD (2001) Osteoprotegerin serum levels in men: correlation with age, estrogen, and testosterone status. J Clin Endocrinol Metab 86:3162–5.

167. Takahashi N, Udagawa N, Akatsu T, Tanaka H, Shionome M, Suda T (1991) Role of colony-stimulating factors in osteoclast development. J Bone Miner Res 6:977–85.

168. Takahashi N, Yamana H, Yoshiki S, Roodman GD, Mundy GR, Jones SJ, et al. (1988) Osteoclast-like cell formation and its regulation by osteotropic hormones in mouse bone marrow cultures. Endocrinology 122:1373–82.

169. Takahashi S, Reddy SV, Chirgwin JM, Devlin R, Haipek C, Anderson J, et al. (1994) Cloning and identification of annexin II as an autocrine/paracrine factor that increases osteoclast formation and bone resorption. J Biol Chem 269:28696–701.

170. Takai H, Kanematsu M, Yano K, Tsuda E, Higashio K, Ikeda K, et al. (1998) Transforming growth factor-beta stimulates the production of osteoprotegerin/osteoclastogenesis inhibitory factor by bone marrow stromal cells. J Biol Chem 273:27091–6.

171. Takayanagi H, Kim S, Koga T, Nishina H, Isshiki M, Yoshida H, et al. (2002) Induction and activation of the transcription factor NFATc1 (NFAT2) integrate RANKL signaling in terminal differentiation of osteoclasts. Dev Cell 3:889–901.

172. Takayanagi H, Kim S, Matsuo K, Suzuki H, Suzuki T, Sato K, et al. (2002) RANKL maintains bone homeostasis through c-Fos-dependent induction of interferon-beta. Nature 416:744–9.

173. Takayanagi H, Ogasawara K, Hida S, Chiba T, Murata S, Sato K, et al. (2000) T-cell-mediated regulation of osteoclastogenesis by signalling cross-talk between RANKL and IFN-gamma. Nature 408:600–5.

174. Takeshita S, Namba N, Zhao JJ, Jiang Y, Genant HK, Silva MJ, et al. (2002) SHIP-deficient mice are severely osteoporotic due to increased numbers of hyper-resorptive osteoclasts. Nat Med 8:943–9.

175. Tanaka S, Takahashi N, Udagawa N, Tamura T, Akatsu T, Stanley E, et al. (1993) Macrophage colony stimulating factor is indispensable for both proliferation and differentiation of osteoclast progenitors. J Clin Invest 92:257–63.

176. Thesingh CW, Scherft JP (1985) Fusion disability of embryonic osteoclast precursor cells and macrophages in the microphthalmic osteopetrotic mouse. Bone 6:43–52.

177. Thirunavukkarasu K, Halladay D, Miles R, Yang X, Galvin R, Chandrasekhar S, et al. (2000) The osteoblast-specific transcription factor Cbfa1 con-

tributes to the expression of osteoprotegerin, a potent inhibitor of osteoclast differentiation and function. J Biol Chem 276:25163–72.

178. Thomas GP, Baker SU, Eisman JA, Gardiner EM (2001) Changing RANKL/OPG mRNA expression in differentiating murine primary osteoblasts. J Endocrinol 170: 451–60.

179. Tondravi MM, McKercher SR, Anderson K, Erdmann JM, Quiroz M, Maki R, et al. (1997) Osteopetrosis in mice lacking haematopoietic transcription factor PU.1. Nature 386:81–4.

180. Toraldo G, Roggia C, Qian WP, Pacifici R, Weitzmann MN (2003) IL-7 induces bone loss in vivo by induction of receptor activator of nuclear factor kappa B ligand and tumor necrosis factor alpha from T cells. Proc Natl Acad Sci USA 100:125–30.

181. Udagawa N, Takahashi N, Jimi E, Matsuzaki K, Tsurukai T, Itoh K, et al. (1999) Osteoblasts/stromal cells stimulate osteoclast activation through expression of osteoclast differentiation factor/RANKL but not macrophage colony-stimulating factor: receptor activator of NF-kappaB ligand. Bone 25:517–23.

182. Udagawa N, Takahashi N, Katagiri T, Tamura T, Wada S, Findlay DM, et al. (1995) Interleukin (IL)-6 induction of osteoclast differentiation depends on IL-6 receptors expressed on osteoblastic cells but not on osteoclast progenitors. J Exp Med 182:1461–8.

183. Udagawa N, Takahashi N, Yasuda H, Mizuno A, Itoh K, Ueno Y, et al. (2000) Osteoprotegerin produced by osteoblasts is an important regulator in osteoclast development and function. Endocrinology 141:3478–84.

184. Underwood J (1984) From where comes the osteoclast? J Pathol 144:225–6.

185. van de Wijngaert FP, Tas MC, Burger EH (1987) Characteristics of osteoclast precursor-like cells grown from mouse bone marrow. Bone Miner 3:111–23.

186. Van Wesenbeeck L, Odgren PR, MacKay CA, D'Angelo M, Safadi FF, Popoff SN, et al. (2002) The osteopetrotic mutation toothless (tl) is a loss-of-function frameshift mutation in the rat Csf1 gene: Evidence of a crucial role for CSF-1 in osteoclastogenesis and endochondral ossification. Proc Natl Acad Sci USA 99:14303–8.

187. Walker DG (1975) Bone resorption restored in osteopetrotic mice by transplants of normal bone marrow and spleen cells. Science 190:784–5.

188. Wani MR, Fuller K, Kim NS, Choi Y, Chambers T (1999) Prostaglandin E2 cooperates with TRANCE in osteoclast induction from hemopoietic precursors: synergistic activation of differentiation, cell spreading, and fusion. Endocrinology 140:1927–35.

189. Weilbaecher KN, Motyckova G, Huber WE, Takemoto CM, Hemesath TJ, Xu Y, et al. (2001) Linkage of M-CSF signaling to Mitf, TFE3, and the osteoclast defect in Mitf(mi/mi) mice. Mol Cell 8:749–58.

190. Weir E, Lowik C, Paliwal I, Insogna K (1996) Colony stimulating factor-1 plays a role in osteoclast formation and function in bone resorption induced by parathyroid hormone and parathyroid hormone-related protein. J Bone Miner Res 11:1474–81.

191. Weitzmann MN, Cenci S, Rifas L, Haug J, Dipersio J, Pacifici R (2001) T cell activation induces human osteoclast formation via receptor activator of nuclear factor kappaB ligand-dependent and -independent mechanisms. J Bone Miner Res 16:328–37.

192. Whyte MP, Obrecht SE, Finnegan PM, Jones JL, Podgornik MN, McAlister WH, et al. (2002) Osteoprotegerin deficiency and juvenile Paget's disease. N Engl J Med 347:175–84.

193. Wiktor-Jedrzejczak W, Bartocci A, Ferrante AJ, Ahmed-Ansari A, Sell K, Pollard J, et al. (1990) Total absence of colony-stimulating factor 1 in the macrophage-deficient osteopetrotic (op/op) mouse. Proc Natl Acad Sci USA 87:4828–32.

194. Wimalawansa S, Chapa T, Fang L, Yallampalli C, Simmons D (2000) Frequency-dependent effect of nitric oxide donor nitroglycerin on bone. J Bone Miner Res 15:1119–25.

195. Wimalawansa SJ (2000) Nitroglycerin therapy is as efficacious as standard estrogen replacement therapy (Premarin) in prevention of oophorectomy-induced bone loss: a human pilot clinical study. J Bone Miner Res 15:2240–4.

196. Wong BR, Besser D, Kim N, Arron JR, Vologodskaia M, Hanafusa H, et al. (1999) TRANCE, a TNF family member, activates Akt/PKB through a signaling complex involving TRAF6 and c-Src. Mol Cell 4:1041–9.

197. Wong BR, Josien R, Lee SY, Sauter B, Li HL, Steinman RM, et al. (1997) TRANCE (tumor necrosis factor [TNF]-related activation-induced cytokine), a new TNF family member predominantly expressed in T cells, is a dendritic cell-specific survival factor. J Exp Med 186:2075–80.

198. Wong BR, Josien R, Lee SY, Vologodskaia M, Steinman RM, Choi Y (1998) The TRAF family of signal transducers mediates NF-kappaB activation by the TRANCE receptor. J Biol Chem 273:28355–9.

199. Yagami-Hiromasa T, Sato T, Kurisaki T, Kamijo K, Nabeshima Y, Fujisawa-Sehara A (1995) A metalloprotease-disintegrin participating in myoblast fusion. Nature 377:652–6.

200. Yakar S, Rosen CJ (2003) From mouse to man: redefining the role of insulin-like growth factor-I in the acquisition of bone mass. Exp Biol Med (Maywood) 228: 245–52.

201. Yakar S, Rosen CJ, Beamer WG, Ackert-Bicknell CL, Wu Y, Liu JL, et al. (2002) Circulating levels of IGF-1 directly regulate bone growth and density. J Clin Invest 110:771–81.

202. Yamane T, Kunisada T, Yamazaki H, Nakano T, Orkin SH, Hayashi SI (2000) Sequential requirements for SCL/tal-1, GATA-2, macrophage colony-stimulating factor, and osteoclast differentiation factor/osteoprotegerin ligand in osteoclast development. Exp Hematol 28:833–40.

203. Yamashita T, Asano K, Takahashi N, Akatsu T, Udagawa N, Sasaki T, et al. (1990) Cloning of an osteoblastic cell line involved in the formation of osteoclast-like cells. J Cell Physiol 145:587–95.

204. Yao GQ, Sun B, Hammond EE, Spencer EN, Horowitz MC, Insogna KL, et al. (1998) The cell-surface form of colony-stimulating factor-1 is regulated by osteotropic agents and supports formation of multinucleated osteoclast- like cells. J Biol Chem 273:4119–28.

205. Yao GQ, Wu JJ, Sun BH, Troiano N, Mitnick MA, Insogna K (2003) The cell surface form of colony-stimulating factor-1 is biologically active in bone in vivo. Endocrinology 144:3677–82.

206. Yasuda H, Shima N, Nakagawa N, Yamaguchi K, Kinosaki M, Mochizuki S, et al. (1998) Osteoclast differentiation factor is a ligand for osteoprotegerin/

osteoclastogenesis-inhibitory factor and is identical to TRANCE/RANKL. Proc Natl Acad Sci USA 95:3597–602.

207. Yeh W, Shahinian A, Speiser D, Kraunus J, Billia F, Wakeham A, et al. (1997) Early lethality, functional NF-kappaB activation, and increased sensitivity to TNF-induced cell death in TRAF2-deficient mice. Immunity 7:715–25.

208. Yoshida H, Hayashi S, Kunisada T, Ogawa M, Nishikawa S, Okamura H, et al. (1990) The murine mutation osteopetrosis is in the coding region of the macrophage colony stimulating factor gene. Nature 345:442–4.

209. Yu C, Shen K, Lin M, Chen P, Lin C, Chang GD, et al. (2002) GCMa regulates the syncytin-mediated trophoblastic fusion. J Biol Chem 277:50062–8.

210. Zhang J, Dai J, Qi Y, Lin DL, Smith P, Strayhorn C, et al. (2001) Osteoprotegerin inhibits prostate cancer-induced osteoclastogenesis and prevents prostate tumor growth in the bone. J Clin Invest 107:1235–44.

2.

Osteolytic Enzymes of Osteoclasts

Merry Jo Oursler

Introduction

Ninety percent of the protein in bone is type I collagen in the form of a cross-linked triple helical structure, making it more resistant to proteolysis and enzymatic cleavage. The stability that this structure confers means that specific proteases are required for effective degradation [112, 113]. Bone also contains minerals in the form of hydroxyapatite crystals. Thus, for bone resorption to occur both the mineral and the protein components of this matrix must be removed. Osteoclasts are unique in that they create an external acidic hemivacuole adjacent to the bone surface as an early step in bone resorption [4]. This compartment is created when osteoclasts attach to bone. After attachment, osteoclasts transport lysosomes to the portion of the plasma membrane that is juxtaposed to the area of the bone that is to be resorbed. The vesicles fuse with the plasma membrane and thereby increase the plasma membrane surface area in this restricted region. Lysosome membranes also contain membrane tartrate-resistant acid phosphatase (TRAP) and high levels of a hydrogen pump. Both of these enzymes are retained in the plasma membrane after fusion. Lysosome contents are discharged into this compartment as the vesicles fuse with the plasma membrane and this is followed by hydrogen pump-mediated acidification of the hemivacuole. The combined action of enzymes from the lysosomes (such as TRAP and cathepsins), the matrix metalloproteases (MMPs), and the reduction in pH together cause bone to be resorbed. It has therefore been of great interest to discover the identity and nature of the enzymes that execute bone resorption in the hope of targeting these enzymes to regulate rates of bone loss. The osteolytic roles of TRAP, cathepsins, and MMPs are discussed in the remainder of this chapter.

Tartrate-Resistant Acid Phosphatase (TRAP)

TRAP, expressed mainly in osteoclasts and related monohistiocytic cells, has the capacity to hydrolyze phosphoproteins, ATP and other nucleotide triphosphates, and arylphosphates [73]. Although it has been known for many years that osteoclasts express this membrane enzyme, its role in osteoclast activity has remained elusive. The porcine homolog, uteroferrin, may have as its function the delivery of iron that is secreted by the endometrium in utero [29]. However, there is no indication that the enzyme fills this potential role in osteoclasts. Although there is only limited sequence similarity between the kidney bean purple acid phosphatase and TRAP, the fact that the conformation of what is thought to be the active site of TRAP resembles that of the known catalytic domain of the bean phosphatase strengthens the inference that the presumed site in TRAP is in fact the active site [111]. The crystal structure of TRAP also revealed a protease sensitive surface loop near the active site [111]. This explains the need for proteolytic activation of the enzyme.

Targeted TRAP disruption in mice resulted in altered epiphyseal growth plate development [55]. This is consistent with a disruption in chondro/osteoclast activity. In these animals, moreover, early onset osteopetrosis was observed. Since osteoclast differentiation levels seemed normal, the osteopetrosis probably resulted from reduced osteoclast activity. Given that osteoclasts in these mice contain high numbers of cytoplasmic vesicles near the ruffled border, the question arose whether TRAP in the lysosomal vesicle membrane was involved in transport to or fusion with the plasma membrane. Osteoclasts from these mice secreted normal levels of cathepsin K, leading to the conclusion that the accumulating vesicles were not lysosomal vesicles that fail to merge with the plasma membrane [55]. Microphthalmia-associated transcription factor (MITF) and PU.1 are two transcription factors that synergistically activate TRAP gene expression [79]. Mice that are heterozygous for mutant MITF and a PU.1 null allele exhibit early-onset osteopetrosis with osteoclasts of normal size and number [79]. The above studies support the concept that TRAP is involved in osteoclast activity, but its precise role has remained unresolved. Recent data document that cathepsin K is a physiological activator of TRAP and that TRAP can dephosphorylate osteopontin [3]. Osteopontin is involved in stimulating osteoclast activity by promoting adhesion, migration, and resorption [13, 14, 30, 39, 57, 59, 82, 93, 96]. Razzouk et al. [93] have investigated the importance of osteopontin phosphorylation in these roles and their data support that osteopontin phosphorylation may be involved in promoting resorption, but not attachment or actin ring formation. Thus, TRAP-mediated osteopontin dephosphorylation would repress bone resorption.

TRAP is expressed in osteoclasts, some tissue macrophages, dendritic cells, parenchymal liver cells, glomerular mesangial kidney cells, and pancreatic acinar cells [115]. In many cases, there are different RNAs expressed by these different cell types as the 5' untranslated regions of the mRNAs differ due to altered first exons. Walsh et al. [115] have identified an osteoclast-specific transcription initiation site and further documented that there are four different promoter regions that are restricted in a tissue- and cell-specific manner. Since TRAP has long been considered a pivotal marker for osteoclasts, attempts have been made to correlate serum TRAP levels with resorption rates *in vivo*. This has met with little success. Attempts have recently been made to measure type 5b TRAP, whose expression is thought to be restricted osteoclasts [60].

Cathepsins

Many studies have linked these lysosomal cysteine proteases to osteoclast-mediated bone resorption. Much of the evidence indicates that cysteine protease inhibition can block bone resorption *in vitro* and *in vivo* [17, 19, 20, 22, 36, 46, 47, 53, 69, 72, 87, 90, 95, 99]. This includes studies where the activities of cathepsin B and cathepsin L were inhibited and resorption was slowed or stopped [22, 46, 47, 69, 87, 90, 95, 99]. In some studies, however, inhibition of either protease had only a modest or no effect on resorption [52, 64, 95, 110, 111, 118]. This has led to a search for alternate proteases responsible for osteoclast-mediated bone resorption. Cathepsin K (also referred to as O or X) was first identified by differential screening of a rabbit osteoclast cDNA library and both human and mouse homologs have subsequently been cloned [61, 92, 109]. Mice with cathepsin K knocked out exhibited osteopetrosis, abnormal joint morphology, increased bone volume, greater trabecular thickness, and more trabeculae [48]. Differentiated osteoclasts were found in association with demineralized bone. This suggests that osteoclasts deficient in cathepsin K can demineralize the matrix but cannot degrade it. In other studies of cathepsin K null mice, osteopetrosis was observed even though the osteoclast numbers were normal, suggesting impaired osteoclast activity [97, 98]. In addition, the resorption surface was broadly demineralized, but there was undigested collagen present. The absence of cathepsin K and the presence of undigested collagen suggest that cathepsin K is involved in collagen degradation. Cultured osteoclasts from these mice also had impaired resorption activity [98]. Studies of human cathepsin K using giant cell tumors of the bone and bone tissues show that cathepsin K was highly expressed in osteoclasts, with no detectable cathepsin B or L expression [28]. From these studies it appears that other tissues do not express cathepsin K. However, the failure to detect cathepsins B and L may simply be due to an insufficiently sensitive assay, inasmuch as in other reports these enzymes are detected in osteoclasts [22, 46, 47, 69, 87, 90, 95, 99]. Indeed, although the above study suggested that cathepsin K might be exclusively expressed by osteoclasts, it is clear from other data that cathepsin K expression is not restricted to osteoclasts [10–12, 15, 25, 26, 49–51, 68, 74, 78, 83, 84, 91, 92, 107].

The human disease pycnodysostosis is a lysosome disease that manifests itself as an inherited sclerosing skeletal dysplasia. Gelb et al. [44] have shown that patients with this disease have nonsense, missense, or stop codon mutations in their cathepsin K genes. Similar to mouse models lacking cathepsin K, pycnodysostotic osteoclasts can demineralize bone matrix but cannot degrade the matrix. These data support that cathepsin K is involved in human osteoclast-mediated bone resorption. In mice, Rantakokko et al. [92] observed cathepsin K in both osteoclasts and hypertrophic chondrocytes. This observation adds support to the hypothesis that cathepsin K plays a role in matrix degradation as well.

An interesting study by Dodds et al. [27] has examined the patterns of inactive and active cathepsin K protein in osteoclasts. In osteoclasts that are not involved in bone resorption, most of the cathepsin K was present as an inactive zymogen. In osteoclasts that were located closer to the bone matrix, active cathepsin K appeared restricted to the osteoclast area closest to the bone. When osteoclasts were actively resorbing bone, they contained only active cathepsin K that was localized at the bone surface in the ruffled membrane. Thus, local factors present in the immediate vicinity of the bone seem to be important in stimulating cathepsin K activation.

Early studies of the ability of cathepsin K to degrade bone proteins suggested that it was not very effective against collagen or fibronectin, but readily degraded osteonectin [9]. It has since been documented that optimal cathepsin K activity toward collagen requires a complex of the cathepsin molecule and soluble glycosaminoglycans [58]. Intriguingly, Hou et al. [58] have shown that cathepsin K cleaved aggrecan aggregates at two specific sites, thereby generating the soluble glycosaminoglycans required for formation of the active complex themselves. Most cathepsins typically target collagen nonhelical regions or the destabilized helical region once collagenase has cleaved the structure [94]. Unlike other cathepsins, cathepsin K cleaves both helical and telopeptide regions of collagen [43]. Thus, typical of cathepsins, cathepsin K can cleave outside of the helical region. In addition, it can also act inside the helical region, i.e., the region that is usually attacked by the MMPs and neutral elastase [2, 6, 65, 75, 76, 88]. This dual ability to target both collagen regions is unique among the mammalian collagenases and is reminiscent of bacterial collagenase. A confirmation of the critical role played by cathepsin K in collagen digestion in humans comes from a study in which fibroblasts in pycnodysostotic embryos accumulate undigested collagen in lysosomal vacuoles [37]. Thus, cathepsin K can degrade the stable collagen triple helical structure and is therefore likely to be a reasonable target for pharmacologic intervention to block bone resorption (reviewed in [117]). As noted above, another role for cathepsin K in bone resorption may be to activate TRAP, causing osteopontin dephosphorylation and thereby inhibiting bone resorption.

Cathepsin K inhibition by antisense or small molecules has been used to assess its role in osteoclast-mediated bone resorption. Pharmacological inhibitors of cathepsin K that span the active site inhibit resorption both *in vivo* and *in vitro* [71, 106, 110]. Blocking cathepsin K with antisense repressed bone resorption as well [62]. In an *in vivo* study using SB-357114 to block bone resorption, the inhibitor blocked both cathepsin K and cathepsin L activity [106]. Since these osteoclasts expressed much more cathepsin K than cathepsin L, cathepsin K may be the likely inhibition target, but this has not been directly tested. Independent of the molecular target of this inhibitor, resorption was blocked, raising hope that targeted disruption of cathepsins may become an effective antiresorptive therapy.

This returns us to the issue of the conflicting data of the potential roles of different cathepsins in osteoclast-mediated bone resorption. An interesting study by Furuyama et al. [42] may help resolve this issue. Using calvarial organ cultures, they were able to detect trace levels of cathepsin L in untreated osteoclasts. When the cultures were treated with 1,25-dihydroxyvitamin D_3, parathyroid hormone, interleukin-1α, interleukin-6, or tumor necrosis factor-α – all known to stimulate bone loss – the cathepsin L levels increased. In contrast, cathepsin K was abundant under basal conditions and its concentration was unchanged following treatment with these stimulatory agents. Under basal conditions, resorption was blocked when cathepsin K was inhibited, but not when cathepsin L was inhibited. However, when the calvaria were treated with stimulatory factors, inhibition of either cathepsin K or cathepsin L partially inhibited resorption, with inhibition becoming additive when both inhibitors were used. These findings demonstrate that cathepsin K is important in basal bone resorption. Cathepsin L, on the other hand, may be involved in bone loss under pathological conditions when its expression is elevated.

Matrix Metalloproteases (MMPs)

Studies of patients with pycnodysostosis have shown that, for the typical bone phenotype to become evident, there must be complete loss of cathepsin K activity [44]. However, even in cases with complete loss, whether in patients or mice, the calvaria appear normal. It would therefore seem that some bone resorption is taking place [16]. The collagenolytic mechanisms in these cases remain unknown, but may involve overexpression of other cathepsins, perhaps in conjunction with MMPs.

Individual MMPs are known by a variety of names and their substrates are as varied as their names. We will discuss MMP1, 3, 9, 12, 13, and 14 and their potential roles in osteoclast-mediated bone resorption. MMP1 also is known as collagenase-I. Its matrix substrates include intact collagen types I, II, III, VII, VIII, X [104]. MMP3 also is known as stromelysin and its substrates include osteopontin [1], decorin, proteoglycan, fibronectin, laminin, and type IV collagen, but not interstitial type I collagen [116]. MMP9 also is known as gelatinase B and its substrates include aggrecans, denatured type I collagen [40], and collagens IV, V, VIII, X, and XIV [104]. MMP12 also is known as macrophage metalloelastase. Its substrate is elastin and it has no collagen substrates [104]. MMP13 is also known as collagenase-3 and MMP14 is also known as MTI-MMP. Their substrates include type I collagen, other collagens, and additional extracellular matrix proteins [104]. Other non-matrix targets also exist for each MMP [104].

In bone, osteoblasts are a major source of MMP production. However, MMP13 in bone is produced by osteocytes or mononuclear cells located near osteoclasts [23, 41, 102, 103]. Osteoclasts also produce some MMPs. Lin et al. [77] found that rat osteoclasts expressed MMP1 mRNA. Further, rabbit osteoclasts express MMP9 mRNA and MMP1 and 9 mRNAs were present in human neonatal rib osteoclasts [7, 108]. Intriguingly, MMP1 and MMP9 mRNAs also were seen in a subset of osteoclasts situated at resorption sites, and MMP9 mRNA was expressed in human giant cell tumors with the degree of expression correlating with the severity of the osteolysis [8, 70]. Moreover, osteoclast MMP1 and 9 production is regulated by IL-1, a cytokine that promotes bone resorption *in vivo* [54]. These data suggest a role for MMPs 1 and 9 in osteoclast-mediated bone degradation.

All MMPs require zinc for activity and, compared to MMP1, MMP3 has a deeper S_1-specificity pocket, which is distinctly different from the active site of MMP1 [24]. This could explain why it has proven possible to develop specific inhibitors that differentiate between these two enzymes. X-ray structure comparisons of MMPs 1 and 3 indicate there are two clusters of regions of differences between these two MMPs in regions that form the entrances to the active sites [24]. Differences in substrate specificity may be attributed to these structural differences [24].

Given that MMPs can destroy tissues, their enzymatic activity must be tightly regulated [104]. MMP activity can be controlled by modulating the gene expression level, by stimulating or inhibiting proenzyme activation, or with the aid of inhibitory molecules such as the tissue inhibitors of metalloproteinases (TIMPs) [105]. Expression stimulators include the membrane-anchored reversion-inducing cysteine-rich protein with Kazal motifs (RECK) and alpha2-macroglobulin [81, 85, 86]. MMPs are synthesized with a pro-domain that blocks activity by means of an unpaired cysteine in the carboxy terminus. X-ray analysis has shown that, by inserting the pro-domains of MMP3 and 9 into their respective clefts, activity is blocked [5, 31]. The unpaired cysteine acts as a fourth inactivating ligand for the zinc atom that is present in the active site. Activation can be by either proteolysis, so as to remove the pro-domain, or by a conformational change that releases the zinc atom from the cysteine. In that situation, the thiol group is replaced by water and the enzyme is thus enabled to remove the pro-domain. In most cases, MMP activation takes place outside of the cell. Given that MMPs reside in bone as latent enzymes, MMP family members not synthesized by osteoclasts can be activated by osteoclastic proteolytic activity and then participate in bone degradation. Inactivation mechanisms include expression of TIMPs, which interact with the active site of MMPs, and thus block activity [45]. In normal human bone, TIMP1 is highly expressed in osteoclasts derived from neonatal bone, but was absent in osteoclasts from pathological tissues (osteophytic and heterotopic bone – both having poorly organized bone formation) [7]. TIMP1 expression may therefore be important in the regulation of normal bone remodeling in the course of development.

Selective MMP inhibition studies have shown that the functional importance of a given MMP varies with the type of bone [38]. Moreover, the presence of inflammatory cytokines may alter MMP levels. Hill et al. [54] have documented that MMP9 inhibition did not inhibit basal osteoclast activity *in vitro*, but did inhibit IL-1-stimulated calvarial explant bone resorption. Consequently, MMP9 may play a role in inflammatory cytokine-stimulated bone loss. Thus the specific function of MMPs in bone resorption seems to depend on the bone and/or the type of resorption stimulus.

Inhibition of either cathepsin or MMP decreased bone resorption, but inhibiting both was not additive [34, 36]. Even though cathepsins and MMPs thus appear to have similar functions and may be able to substitute for each other, MMPs act later in the resorption process than cathepsins do [38]. In view of the fact that these two enzyme classes act on different resorption steps, their actions may not be additive.

MMP13, synthesized by osteocytes but not by osteoclasts, has been detected in the resorption pits of cathepsin K null mice [35]. This observation raises the possibility that osteocytes may participate in osteoclast-mediated bone resorption by synthesizing and secreting MMP13. Everts et al. [35] have proposed that the role of MMP13 is to "mop up" after cathepsin K-mediated bone resorption is completed.

Studies of mice lacking a given MMP provide insight into specific functions of the various family members. Bone resorption rates were normal in mice lacking MMP9, MMP12, and MMP14 [16]. However, mice lacking MMP13 had reduced bone resorption rates. This finding again supports a role for MMP13 in bone resorption. Although there was no apparent impact of MMP9 knock-out on bone resorption, the bones from these mice had lengthened growth plates [114]. Since introduction of normal marrow restored development to normal, it was apparent that the defect was in the chondroclasts [114]. MMP9 knockout mice exhibited delayed osteoclast recruitment [32]. In patients with vanishing bone syndrome, there is severe bone degradation, mainly in the hands and the feet; this is due to the loss of the MMP2 gene [80]. The reasons that loss of an MMP causes bone destruction are unknown, but possibilities include a compensatory overproduction of other MMPs or a loss of coupling between osteoclasts and osteoblasts. Mice lacking MMP2 do not exhibit the same phenotype. This is another indication why reliance on mouse genetics may mislead in understanding human disease.

MMPs also facilitate other aspects of osteoclast function. Inhibition of MMPs blocked osteoclast migration through collagen gel in an *in vitro* assay [16]. Osteoclasts deficient in MMPs 9, 12, and 14 have been examined for their migratory patterns [16]. MMP12-deficient osteoclasts migrated at normal rates, whereas osteoclasts deficient in MMP9 or MMP14 had slower migration patterns. The MMPs can be found in podosomes, the osteoclast-bone attachment structure, and at the leading edges of normal migrating osteoclasts [63, 100]. Further supporting a MMP role in migration, MMP inhibition increased the lifespan of a podosome; this in turn will decrease migration[100]. Another function of MMPs may be to stimulate osteoclast recruitment [16].

One hypothesis is that MMP13-generated collagen fragments initiate bone resorption by activating osteoclasts [56]. In addition, MMP9 activity released transforming growth factor-β from bone matrix, where transforming growth factor-ß is stored in significant amounts [66]. TGF-ß causes cell retraction, thus leading to greater bone surface exposure, increasing osteoclast precursor attraction to the bone surface [66]. MMP14 causes membrane receptor activator of NFkappaB ligand (RANKL) release, thereby perhaps influencing osteoclast differentiation and/or activation [67, 101]. Thus, MMPs most likely coordinate matrix degradation and recruitment and differentiation of osteoclasts and chondroclasts and may be an important component of bone metabolism [89].

Conclusions

In light of the above information, cooperation among proteases is likely to be important in osteoclast-mediated bone resorption [18, 19, 21, 33, 36, 112, 113]. Although much more now is known about the enzymatic mechanisms by which bone is resorbed, it is equally clear that many gaps in our knowledge remain. The role of TRAP in bone resorption remains unresolved, as do the respective roles of cathepsins and MMPs. Furthermore, the mechanisms by which resorption occurs in the course of bone development are likely to differ from those involved in bone turnover in the process of pathological bone loss. Changes in bone mass such as those that occur during menopause or as a result of anti-inflammatory therapies may involve a different set of enzymes. Similarly, bone loss induced by inflammatory cytokines may involve mechanisms that differ from those in other conditions of bone resorption. It seems reasonable to hope that future studies of osteolytic enzymes will improve our knowledge of this important aspect of bone metabolism.

Acknowledgments

Dr. Oursler is supported by the Department of the Army Grant DAMD17-00-1-0346 and the National Institutes of Health Grant DE14680.

References

1. Agnihotri R, Crawford HC, Haro H, Matrisian LM, Havrda MC, Liaw L (2001) Osteopontin, a novel substrate for matrix metalloproteinase-3 (stromelysin-1) and matrix metalloproteinase-7 (matrilysin). J Biol Chem 276:28261–7.
2. Aimes RT, Quigley JP (1995) Matrix metalloproteinase-2 is an interstitial collagenase. Inhibitor-free enzyme catalyzes the cleavage of collagen fibrils and soluble native type I collagen generating the specific 3/4- and 1/4-length fragments. J Biol Chem 270:5872–6.
3. Andersson G, Ek-Rylander B, Hollberg K, Ljusberg-Sjolander J, Lang P, Norgard M, et al. (2003) TRACP as an osteopontin phosphatase. J Bone Miner Res 18: 1912–15.
4. Baron R, Neff L, Louvard D, Courtoy PJ (1985) Cell-mediated extracellular acidification and bone resorption: Evidence for a low pH in resorbing lacunae and localization of a 100-kDa lysosomal membrane protein at the osteoclast ruffled border. J Cell Biol 101:2210–22.
5. Becker JW, Marcy AI, Rokosz LL, Axel MG, Burbaum JJ, Fitzgerald PM, et al. (1995) Stromelysin-1: three-dimensional structure of the inhibited catalytic domain and of the C-truncated proenzyme. Protein Sci 4:1966–76.
6. Birkedal-Hansen H, Moore WG, Bodden MK, Windsor LJ, Birkedal-Hansen B, DeCarlo A, et al. (1993) Matrix metalloproteinases: a review. Crit Rev Oral Biol Med 4:197–250.
7. Bord S, Horner A, Beeton CA, Hembry RM, Compston JE (1999) Tissue inhibitor of matrix metalloproteinase-1 (TIMP-1) distribution in normal and pathological human bone. Bone 24:229–35.
8. Bord S, Horner A, Hembry RM, Reynolds JJ, Compston JE (1997) Distribution of matrix metalloproteinases and their inhibitor, TIMP-1, in developing human osteophytic bone. J Anat 191(Pt 1):39–48.
9. Bossard MJ, Tomaszek TA, Thompson SK, Amegadzie BY, Hanning CR, Jones C, et al. (1996) Proteolytic activity of human osteoclast cathepsin K. Expression, purification, activation, and substrate identification. J Biol Chem 271:12517–24.
10. Brubaker KD, Vessella RL, True LD, Thomas R, Corey E (2003) Cathepsin K mRNA and protein expression in prostate cancer progression. J Bone Miner Res 18:222–30.
11. Buhling F, Reisenauer A, Gerber A, Kruger S, Weber E, Bromme D, et al. (2001) Cathepsin K – a marker of macrophage differentiation? J Pathol 195:375–82.
12. Buhling F, Waldburg N, Gerber A, Hackel C, Kruger S, Reinhold D, et al. (2000) Cathepsin K expression in human lung. Adv Exp Med Biol 477:281–6.
13. Chellaiah MA, Hruska KA (2003) The integrin alpha(v)beta(3) and CD44 regulate the actions of osteopontin on osteoclast motility. Calcif Tissue Int 72:197–205.
14. Chellaiah MA, Kizer N, Biswas R, Alvarez U, Strauss-Schoenberger J, Rifas L, et al. (2003) Osteopontin deficiency produces osteoclast dysfunction due to reduced CD44 surface expression. Mol Biol Cell 14: 173–89.
15. Chiellini C, Costa M, Novelli SE, Amri EZ, Benzi L, Bertacca A, et al. (2003) Identification of cathepsin K as a novel marker of adiposity in white adipose tissue. J Cell Physiol 195:309–21.
16. Delaisse JM, Andersen TL, Engsig MT, Henriksen K, Troen T, Blavier L (2003) Matrix metalloproteinases (MMP) and cathepsin K contribute differently to osteoclastic activities. Microsc Res Tech 61:504–13.
17. Delaisse JM, Boyde A, Maconnachie E, Ali NN, Sear CH, Eeckhout Y, et al. (1987) The effects of inhibitors of cysteine-proteinases and collagenase on the resorptive activity of isolated osteoclasts. Bone 8:305–13.
18. Delaisse JM, Eeckhout Y, Sear C, Galloway A, McCullagh K, Vaes G (1985) A new synthetic inhibitor of mammalian tissue collagenase inhibits bone resorp-

tion in culture. Biochem Biophys Res Commun 133: 483–90.

19. Delaisse JM, Eeckhout Y, Vaes G (1980) Inhibition of bone resorption in culture by inhibitors of thiol proteinases. Biochem J 192:365–8.

20. Delaisse JM, Eeckhout Y, Vaes G (1984) In vivo and in vitro evidence for the involvement of cysteine proteinases in bone resorption. Biochem Biophys Res Commun 125:441–7.

21. Delaisse JM, Eeckhout Y, Vaes G (1985) Bisphosphonates and bone resorption: effects on collagenase and lysosomal enzyme excretion. Life Sci 37:2291–6.

22. Delaisse JM, Ledent P, Vaes G (1991) Collagenolytic cysteine proteinases of bone tissue. Cathepsin B, (pro)cathepsin L and a cathepsin L-like 70 kDa proteinase. Biochem J 279(Pt 1):167–74.

23. Dew G, Murphy G, Stanton H, Vallon R, Angel P, Reynolds JJ, et al. (2000) Localisation of matrix metalloproteinases and TIMP-2 in resorbing mouse bone. Cell Tissue Res 299:385–94.

24. Dhanaraj V, Ye QZ, Johnson LL, Hupe DJ, Ortwine DF, Dunbar JB, Jr., et al. (1996) X-ray structure of a hydroxamate inhibitor complex of stromelysin catalytic domain and its comparison with members of the zinc metalloproteinase superfamily. Structure 4:375–86.

25. Diaz A, Willis AC, Sim RB (2000) Expression of the proteinase specialized in bone resorption, cathepsin K, in granulomatous inflammation. Mol Med 6:648–59.

26. Diaz A, Willis AC, Sim RB (2002) Cathepsin K expression in epithelioid and multinucleated giant cells. J Pathol 197:690; author reply 691.

27. Dodds RA, James IE, Rieman D, Ahern R, Hwang SM, Connor JR, et al. (2001) Human osteoclast cathepsin K is processed intracellularly prior to attachment and bone resorption. J Bone Miner Res 16:478–86.

28. Drake FH, Dodds RA, James IE, Connor JR, Debouck C, Richardson S, et al. (1996) Cathepsin K, but not cathepsins B, L, or S is abundantly expressed in human osteoclasts. Journal of Biological Chemistry 271: 12511–16.

29. Ducsay CA, Buhi WC, Bazer FW, Roberts RM, Combs GE (1984) Role of uteroferrin in placental iron transport: effect of maternal iron treatment on fetal iron and uteroferrin content and neonatal hemoglobin. J Anim Sci 59:1303–8.

30. Ek-Rylander B, Flores M, Wendel M, Heinegard D, Andersson G (1994) Dephosphorylation of osteopontin and bone sialoprotein by osteoclastic tartrate-resistant acid phosphatase. Modulation of osteoclast adhesion in vitro. J Biol Chem 269:14853–6.

31. Elkins PA, Ho YS, Smith WW, Janson CA, D'Alessio KJ, McQueney MS, et al. (2002) Structure of the C-terminally truncated human ProMMP9, a gelatin-binding matrix metalloproteinase. Acta Crystallogr D Biol Crystallogr 58:1182–92.

32. Engsig MT, Chen QJ, Vu TH, Pedersen AC, Therkidsen B, Lund LR, et al. (2000) Matrix metalloproteinase 9 and vascular endothelial growth factor are essential for osteoclast recruitment into developing long bones. J Cell Biol 151:879–89.

33. Etherington DJ, Birkedahl-Hansen H (1987) The influence of dissolved calcium salts on the degradation of hard-tissue collagens by lysosomal cathepsins. Coll Relat Res 7:185–99.

34. Everts V, Delaisse JM, Korper W, Beertsen W (1998) Cysteine proteinases and matrix metalloproteinases play distinct roles in the subosteoclastic resorption zone. J Bone Miner Res 13:1420–30.

35. Everts V, Delaisse JM, Korper W, Jansen DC, Tigchelaar-Gutter W, Saftig P, et al. (2002) The bone lining cell: its role in cleaning Howship's lacunae and initiating bone formation. J Bone Miner Res 17:77–90.

36. Everts V, Delaisse JM, Korper W, Niehof A, Vaes G, Beertsen W (1992) Degradation of collagen in the bone-resorbing compartment underlying the osteoclast involves both cysteine-proteinases and matrix metalloproteinases. J Cell Physiol 150:221–31.

37. Everts V, Hou WS, Rialland X, Tigchelaar W, Saftig P, Bromme D, et al. (2003) Cathepsin K Deficiency in Pycnodysostosis Results in Accumulation of Non-Digested Phagocytosed Collagen in Fibroblasts. Calcif Tissue Int 73:380–86.

38. Everts V, Korper W, Jansen DC, Steinfort J, Lammerse I, Heera S, et al. (1999) Functional heterogeneity of osteoclasts: matrix metalloproteinases participate in osteoclastic resorption of calvarial bone but not in resorption of long bone. Faseb J 13:1219–30.

39. Faccio R, Grano M, Colucci S, Zallone AZ, Quaranta V, Pelletier AJ (1998) Activation of alphav beta3 integrin on human osteoclast-like cells stimulates adhesion and migration in response to osteopontin. Biochem Biophys Res Commun 249:522–5.

40. Fosang AJ, Last K, Knauper V, Neame PJ, Murphy G, Hardingham TE, et al. (1993) Fibroblast and neutrophil collagenases cleave at two sites in the cartilage aggrecan interglobular domain. Biochem J 295(Pt 1):273–6.

41. Fuller K, Chambers TJ (1995) Localisation of mRNA for collagenase in osteocytic, bone surface and chondrocytic cells but not osteoclasts. J Cell Sci 108(Pt 6): 2221–30.

42. Furuyama N, Fujisawa Y (2000) Distinct roles of cathepsin K and cathepsin L in osteoclastic bone resorption. Endocr Res 26:189–204.

43. Garnero P, Borel O, Byrjalsen I, Ferreras M, Drake FH, McQueney MS, et al. (1998) The collagenolytic activity of cathepsin K is unique among mammalian proteinases. J Biol Chem 273:32347–52.

44. Gelb BD, Shi GP, Chapman HA, Desnick RJ (1996) Pycnodysostosis, a lysosomal disease caused by cathepsin K deficiency. Science 273:1236–8.

45. Gomis-Ruth FX, Maskos K, Betz M, Bergner A, Huber R, Suzuki K, et al. (1997) Mechanism of inhibition of the human matrix metalloproteinase stromelysin-1 by TIMP-1. Nature 389:77–81.

46. Goto T, Kiyoshima T, Moroi R, Tsukuba T, Nishimura Y, Himeno M, et al. (1994) Localization of cathepsins B, D, and L in the rat osteoclast by immuno-light and -electron microscopy. Histochemistry 101:33–40.

47. Goto T, Tsukuba T, Ayasaka N, Yamamoto K, Tanaka T (1992) Immunocytochemical localization of cathepsin D in the rat osteoclast. Histochemistry 97:13–18.

48. Gowen M, Lazner F, Dodds R, Kapadia R, Feild J, Tavaria M, et al. (1999) Cathepsin K knockout mice develop osteopetrosis due to a deficit in matrix degradation but not demineralization. J Bone Miner Res 14: 1654–63.

49. Haeckel C, Krueger S, Buehling F, Broemme D, Franke K, Schuetze A, et al. (1999) Expression of cathepsin K in the human embryo and fetus. Dev Dyn 216:89–95.

50. Haeckel C, Krueger S, Kuester D, Ostertag H, Samii M, Buehling F, et al. (2000) Expression of cathepsin K in chordoma. Hum Pathol 31:834–40.

51. Hansen T, Unger RE, Gaumann A, Hundorf I, Maurer J, Kirkpatrick CJ, et al. (2001) Expression of matrix-degrading cysteine proteinase cathepsin K in cholesteatoma. Mod Pathol 14:1226–31.

52. Hayman AR, Cox TM (1994) Purple acid phosphatase of the human macrophage and osteoclast. Characterization, molecular properties, and crystallization of the recombinant di-iron-oxo protein secreted by baculovirus-infected insect cells. J Biol Chem 269:1294–300.

53. Hill PA, Buttle DJ, Jones SJ, Boyde A, Murata M, Reynolds JJ, et al. (1994) Inhibition of bone resorption by selective inactivators of cysteine proteinases. J Cell Biochem 56:118–30.

54. Hill PA, Murphy G, Docherty AJ, Hembry RM, Millican TA, Reynolds JJ, et al. (1994) The effects of selective inhibitors of matrix metalloproteinases (MMPs) on bone resorption and the identification of MMPs and TIMP-1 in isolated osteoclasts. J Cell Sci 107(Pt 11): 3055–64.

55. Hollberg K, Hultenby K, Hayman A, Cox T, Andersson G (2002) Osteoclasts from mice deficient in tartrate-resistant acid phosphatase have altered ruffled borders and disturbed intracellular vesicular transport. Exp Cell Res 279:227–38.

56. Holliday LS, Welgus HG, Fliszar CJ, Veith GM, Jeffrey JJ, Gluck SL (1997) Initiation of osteoclast bone resorption by interstitial collagenase. J Biol Chem 272: 22053–8.

57. Horton MA, Nesbit MA, Helfrich MH (1995) Interaction of osteopontin with osteoclast integrins. Ann N Y Acad Sci 760:190–200.

58. Hou WS, Li Z, Buttner FH, Bartnik E, Bromme D (2003) Cleavage site specificity of cathepsin K toward cartilage proteoglycans and protease complex formation. Biol Chem 384:891–7.

59. Hultenby K, Reinholt FP, Heinegard D, Andersson G, Marks SC, Jr. (1995) Osteopontin: a ligand for the alpha v beta 3 integrin of the osteoclast clear zone in osteopetrotic (ia/ia) rats. Ann N Y Acad Sci 760: 315–18.

60. Igarashi Y, Lee MY, Matsuzaki S (2002) Acid phosphatases as markers of bone metabolism. J Chromatogr B Analyt Technol Biomed Life Sci 781:345–58.

61. Inaoka T, Bilbe G, Ishibashi O, Tezuka K, Kumegawa M, Kokubo T (1995) Molecular cloning of human cDNA for cathepsin K: novel cysteine proteinase predominantly expressed in bone. Biochem Biophys Res Commun 206:89–96.

62. Inui T, Ishibashi O, Inaoka T, Origane Y, Kumegawa M, Kokubo T, et al. (1997) Cathepsin K antisense oligodeoxynucleotide inhibits osteoclastic bone resorption. J Biol Chem 272:8109–12.

63. Irie K, Tsuruga E, Sakakura Y, Muto T, Yajima T (2001) Immunohistochemical localization of membrane type 1-matrix metalloproteinase (MT1-MMP) in osteoclasts in vivo. Tissue Cell 33:478–82.

64. James IE, Marquis RW, Blake SM, Hwang SM, Gress CJ, Ru Y, et al. (2001) Potent and selective cathepsin L inhibitors do not inhibit human osteoclast resorption in vitro. J Biol Chem 276:11507–11.

65. Kafienah W, Buttle DJ, Burnett D, Hollander AP (1998) Cleavage of native type I collagen by human neutrophil elastase. Biochem J 330(Pt 2):897–902.

66. Karsdal MA, Fjording MS, Foged NT, Delaisse JM, Lochter A (2001) Transforming growth factor-beta-induced osteoblast elongation regulates osteoclastic bone resorption through a p38 mitogen-activated protein kinase- and matrix metalloproteinase-dependent pathway. J Biol Chem 276:39350–8.

67. Khosla S (2001) Minireview: the OPG/RANKL/RANK system. Endocrinology 142:5050–5.

68. Konttinen YT, Mandelin J, Li TF, Salo J, Lassus J, Liljestrom M, et al. (2002) Acidic cysteine endoproteinase cathepsin K in the degeneration of the superficial articular hyaline cartilage in osteoarthritis. Arthritis Rheum 46:953–60.

69. Kremer M, Judd J, Rifkin B, Auszmann J, Oursler MJ (1995) Estrogen Modulation of Osteoclast Lysosomal Enzyme Secretion. J Cell Biochem 57:271–79.

70. Kumta SM, Huang L, Cheng YY, Chow LT, Lee KM, Zheng MH (2003) Expression of VEGF and MMP-9 in giant cell tumor of bone and other osteolytic lesions. Life Sci 73:1427–36.

71. Lark MW, Stroup GB, James IE, Dodds RA, Hwang SM, Blake SM, et al. (2002) A potent small molecule, non-peptide inhibitor of cathepsin K (SB 331750) prevents bone matrix resorption in the ovariectomized rat. Bone 30:746–53.

72. Lerner UH, Grubb A (1992) Human cystatin C, a cysteine proteinase inhibitor, inhibits bone resorption in vitro stimulated by parathyroid hormone and parathyroid hormone-related peptide of malignancy. J Bone Miner Res 7:433–40.

73. Li CY, Yam LT, Lam KW (1970) Acid phosphatase isoenzyme in human leukocytes in normal and pathologic conditions. J Histochem Cytochem 18:473–81.

74. Li YP, Chen W (1999) Characterization of mouse cathepsin K gene, the gene promoter, and the gene expression. J Bone Miner Res 14:487–99.

75. Li Z, Hou WS, Bromme D (2000) Collagenolytic activity of cathepsin K is specifically modulated by cartilage-resident chondroitin sulfates. Biochemistry 39: 529–36.

76. Li Z, Hou WS, Escalante-Torres CR, Gelb BD, Bromme D (2002) Collagenase activity of cathepsin K depends on complex formation with chondroitin sulfate. J Biol Chem 277:28669–76.

77. Lin SK, Kok SH, Kuo MY, Wang TJ, Wang JT, Yeh FT, et al. (2002) Sequential expressions of MMP-1, TIMP-1, IL-6, and COX-2 genes in induced periapical lesions in rats. Eur J Oral Sci 110:246–53.

78. Littlewood-Evans AJ, Bilbe G, Bowler WB, Farley D, Wlodarski B, Kokubo T, et al. (1997) The osteoclast-associated protease cathepsin K is expressed in human breast carcinoma. Cancer Res 57:5386–90.

79. Luchin A, Suchting S, Merson T, Rosol TJ, Hume DA, Cassady AI, et al. (2001) Genetic and physical interactions between Microphthalmia transcription factor and PU.1 are necessary for osteoclast gene expression and differentiation. J Biol Chem 276:36703–10.

80. Martignetti JA, Aqeel AA, Sewairi WA, Boumah CE, Kambouris M, Mayouf SA, et al. (2001) Mutation of the matrix metalloproteinase 2 gene (MMP2) causes a multicentric osteolysis and arthritis syndrome. Nat Genet 28:261–5.

81. Migita K, Eguchi K, Tominaga M, Origuchi T, Kawabe Y, Nagataki S (1997) Beta 2-microglobulin induces stromelysin production by human synovial fibroblasts. Biochem Biophys Res Commun 239:621–5.

82. Miyauchi A, Alvarez J, Greenfield EM, Teti A, Grano M, Colucci S, et al. (1993) Binding of osteopontin to the

osteoclast integrin alpha v beta 3. Osteoporos Int. 3 Suppl 1:132–5.

83. Muir P, Hayashi K, Manley PA, Colopy SA, Hao Z (2002) Evaluation of tartrate-resistant acid phosphatase and cathepsin K in ruptured cranial cruciate ligaments in dogs. Am J Vet Res 63:1279–84.

84. Nakase T, Takeuchi E, Sugamoto K, Kaneko M, Tomita T, Myoui A, et al. (2000) Involvement of multinucleated giant cells synthesizing cathepsin K in calcified tendinitis of the rotator cuff tendons. Rheumatology (Oxford) 39:1074–7.

85. Noda M, Oh J, Takahashi R, Kondo S, Kitayama H, Takahashi C (2003) RECK: a novel suppressor of malignancy linking oncogenic signaling to extracellular matrix remodeling. Cancer Metastasis Rev 22:167–75.

86. Oh J, Takahashi R, Kondo S, Mizoguchi A, Adachi E, Sasahara RM, et al. (2001) The membrane-anchored MMP inhibitor RECK is a key regulator of extracellular matrix integrity and angiogenesis. Cell 107:789–800.

87. Ohsawa Y, Nitatori T, Higuchi S, Kominami E, Uchiyama Y (1993) Lysosomal cysteine and aspartic proteinases, acid phosphatase, and an endogenous cysteine proteinase inhibitor, cystatin-beta, in rat osteoclasts. J Histochem Cytochem 41:1075–83.

88. Ohuchi E, Imai K, Fujii Y, Sato H, Seiki M, Okada Y (1997) Membrane type 1 matrix metalloproteinase digests interstitial collagens and other extracellular matrix macromolecules. J Biol Chem 272:2446–51.

89. Ortega N, Behonick D, Stickens D, Werb Z (2003) How proteases regulate bone morphogenesis. Ann N Y Acad Sci 995:109–16.

90. Page AE, Warburton MJ, Chambers TJ, Pringle JA, Hayman AR (1992) Human osteoclastomas contain multiple forms of cathepsin B. Biochim Biophys Acta 1116:57–66.

91. Punturieri A, Filippov S, Allen E, Caras I, Murray R, Reddy V, et al. (2000) Regulation of elastinolytic cysteine proteinase activity in normal and cathepsin K-deficient human macrophages. J Exp Med 192:789–99.

92. Rantakokko J, Aro HT, Savontaus M, Vuorio E (1996) Mouse cathepsin K: cDNA cloning and predominant expression of the gene in osteoclasts, and in some hypertrophying chondrocytes during mouse development. FEBS Lett 393:307–13.

93. Razzouk S, Brunn JC, Qin C, Tye CE, Goldberg HA, Butler WT (2002) Osteopontin posttranslational modifications, possibly phosphorylation, are required for in vitro bone resorption but not osteoclast adhesion. Bone 30:40–7.

94. Reynolds JJ (1970) Degradation processes in bone and cartilage. Calcif Tissue Res Suppl 1:52–56.

95. Rifkin BR, Vernillo AT, Kleckner AP, Auszmann JM, Rosenberg LR, Zimmerman M (1991) Cathepsin B and L activities in isolated osteoclasts. Biochem Biophys Res Commun 179:63–69.

96. Ross FP, Chappel J, Alvarez JI, Sander D, Butler WT, Farach-Carson MC, et al. (1993) Interactions between the bone matrix proteins osteopontin and bone sialoprotein and the osteoclast integrin alpha v beta 3 potentiate bone resorption. J Biol Chem 268:9901–7.

97. Saftig P, Hunziker E, Everts V, Jones S, Boyde A, Wehmeyer O, et al. (2000) Functions of cathepsin K in bone resorption. Lessons from cathepsin K deficient mice. Adv Exp Med Biol 477:293–303.

98. Saftig P, Hunziker E, Wehmeyer O, Jones S, Boyde A, Rommerskirch W, et al. (1998) Impaired osteoclastic bone resorption leads to osteopetrosis in cathepsin-K-deficient mice. Proc Natl Acad Sci USA 95:13453–8.

99. Sasaki T, Ueno-Matsuda E (1993) Cysteine-proteinase localization in osteoclasts: an immunocytochemical study. Cell Tissue Res 271:177–9.

100. Sato T, del Carmen Ovejero M, Hou P, Heegaard AM, Kumegawa M, Foged NT, et al. (1997) Identification of the membrane-type matrix metalloproteinase MT1-MMP in osteoclasts. J Cell Sci 110(Pt 5):589–96.

101. Schlondorff J, Lum L, Blobel CP (2001) Biochemical and pharmacological criteria define two shedding activities for TRANCE/OPGL that are distinct from the tumor necrosis factor alpha convertase. J Biol Chem 276:14665–74.

102. Shimizu H, Sakamoto M, Sakamoto S (1990) Bone resorption by isolated osteoclasts in living versus devitalized bone: differences in mode and extent and the effects of human recombinant tissue inhibitor of metalloproteinases. J Bone Miner Res 5:411–18.

103. Sodek J, Overall CM (1992) Matrix metalloproteinases in periodontal tissue remodelling. Matrix Suppl 1:352–62.

104. Somerville RP, Oblander SA, Apte SS (2003) Matrix metalloproteinases: old dogs with new tricks. Genome Biol 4:216.

105. Stamenkovic I (2003) Extracellular matrix remodelling: the role of matrix metalloproteinases. J Pathol 200:448–64.

106. Stroup GB, Lark MW, Veber DF, Bhattacharyya A, Blake S, Dare LC, et al. (2001) Potent and selective inhibition of human cathepsin K leads to inhibition of bone resorption in vivo in a nonhuman primate. J Bone Miner Res 16:1739–46.

107. Tepel C, Bromme D, Herzog V, Brix K (2000) Cathepsin K in thyroid epithelial cells: sequence, localization and possible function in extracellular proteolysis of thyroglobulin. J Cell Sci 113 Pt 24:4487–98.

108. Tezuka K, Nemoto K, Tezuka Y, Sato T, Ikeda Y, Kobori M, et al. (1994) Identification of matrix metalloproteinase 9 in rabbit osteoclasts. J Biol Chem 269:15006–9.

109. Tezuka K, Tezuka Y, Maejima A, Sato T, Nemoto K, Kamioka H, et al. (1994) Molecular cloning of a possible cysteine proteinase predominantly expressed in osteoclasts. J Biol Chem 269:1106–9.

110. Thompson SK, Halbert SM, Bossard MJ, Tomaszek TA, Levy MA, Zhao B, et al. (1997) Design of potent and selective human cathepsin K inhibitors that span the active site. Proc Natl Acad Sci USA 94:14249–54.

111. Uppenberg J, Lindqvist F, Svensson C, Ek-Rylander B, Andersson G (1999) Crystal structure of a mammalian purple acid phosphatase. J Mol Biol 290:201–11.

112. Vaes G (1988) Cellular biology and biochemical mechanism of bone resorption. A review of recent developments on the formation, activation, and mode of action of osteoclasts. Clin Orthop 239–71.

113. Vaes G, Delaisse JM, Eeckhout Y (1992) Relative roles of collagenase and lysosomal cysteine-proteinases in bone resorption. Matrix Suppl 1:383–8.

114. Vu TH, Shipley JM, Bergers G, Berger JE, Helms JA, Hanahan D, et al. (1998) MMP-9/gelatinase B is a key regulator of growth plate angiogenesis and apoptosis of hypertrophic chondrocytes. Cell 93:411–22.

115. Walsh NC, Cahill M, Carninci P, Kawai J, Okazaki Y, Hayashizaki Y, et al. (2003) Multiple tissue-specific promoters control expression of the murine tartrate-resistant acid phosphatase gene. Gene 307:111–23.

116. Wilhelm SM, Collier IE, Kronberger A, Eisen AZ, Marmer BL, Grant GA, et al. (1987) Human skin fibroblast stromelysin: structure, glycosylation, substrate specificity, and differential expression in normal and tumorigenic cells. Proc Natl Acad Sci USA 84:6725–9.

117. Yamashita DS, Dodds RA (2000) Cathepsin K and the design of inhibitors of cathepsin K. Curr Pharm Des 6:1–24.

118. Zaidi M, Troen B, Moonga BS, Abe E (2001) Cathepsin K, osteoclastic resorption, and osteoporosis therapy. J Bone Miner Res 16:1747–9.

3.

Regulation of Osteoclast Activity

Roland Baron and William C. Horne

Introduction

The maintenance of normal bone mass during adult life depends on a balance between osteoblastic bone formation and osteoclastic bone destruction. Bone resorption is primarily carried out by osteoclasts. The overall rate of osteoclastic bone resorption is regulated at two main levels: 1) determining the number of osteoclasts through the regulation of the osteoclast precursor pool and their rate of differentiation, i.e., regulating osteoclastogenesis (see Chapter 1); and 2) determining the bone resorbing activity of individual osteoclasts through the regulation of their key functional features.

In both cases, it now is apparent that activation of RANK (receptor activator of NFκB) signaling by its extracellular ligand RANKL (RANK ligand) plays a central role, as does osteoprotegerin (OPG), a decoy RANK. Indeed, many of the previously known regulators of bone resorption, such as parathyroid hormone (PTH), 1,25-$(OH)_2D_3$, or several interleukins, affect osteoclast differentiation and/or function through their impact on RANKL or OPG production by stromal cells or osteoblasts and not, as initially thought, by a direct action on the osteoclast or its precursors [16]. RANKL binds to its receptor RANK, which is expressed at the surface of osteoclast progenitors as well as in mature osteoclasts, and activates several intracellular signaling pathways. The specific individual role of each is currently being unraveled. OPG modulates RANK activation by competing with RANK for binding to RANKL.

The activation of RANK by RANKL is required for osteoclast differentiation and also regulates osteoclast activity, but the stimulation of myelomonocytic precursors also requires M-CSF to induce the formation of osteoclasts. [138, 161].

Because Chapter 1 is devoted to the regulation of osteoclast differentiation, the aim of this chapter is to focus specifically on the regulation of osteoclast activity.

The Molecular Mechanisms of Bone Resorption: Identification of the Main Effectors

The understanding of the mechanisms by which the activity of the osteoclast is regulated requires a clear comprehension of the mechanisms of bone resorption, thereby identifying the various levers through which the cell can effectively be activated or inhibited. In other words, we need to understand the effectors of bone resorption in order to understand the mechanisms by which they are regulated.

The main functional features (Figure 3.1) that define the activity of an osteoclast are 1) its adhesion to the bone surface; 2) its ability to synthesize and directionally secrete enzymes; 3) its ability to acidify the subosteoclastic bone resorbing compartment; 4) its ability efficiently to internalize the material generated by the

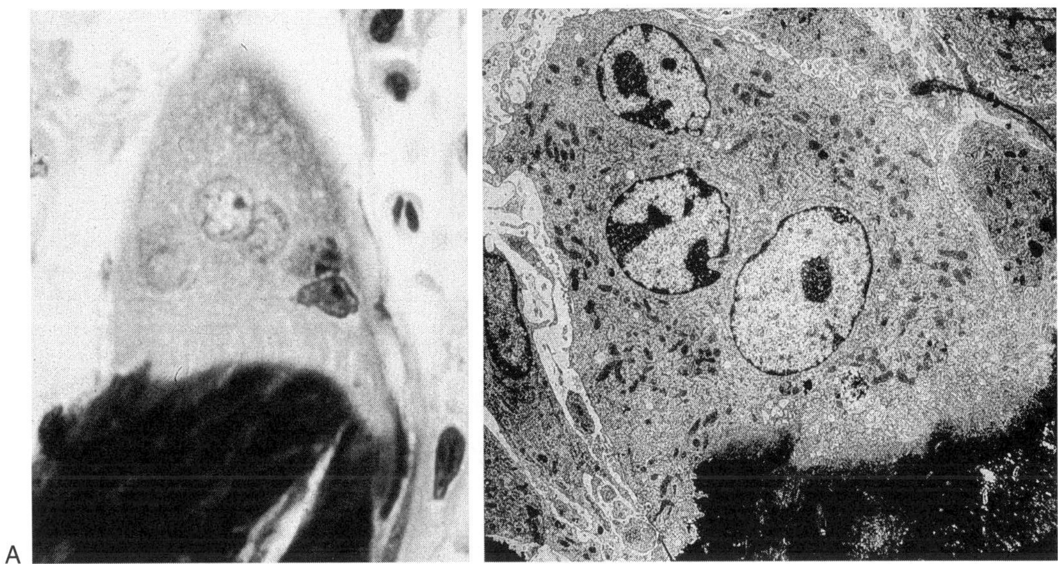

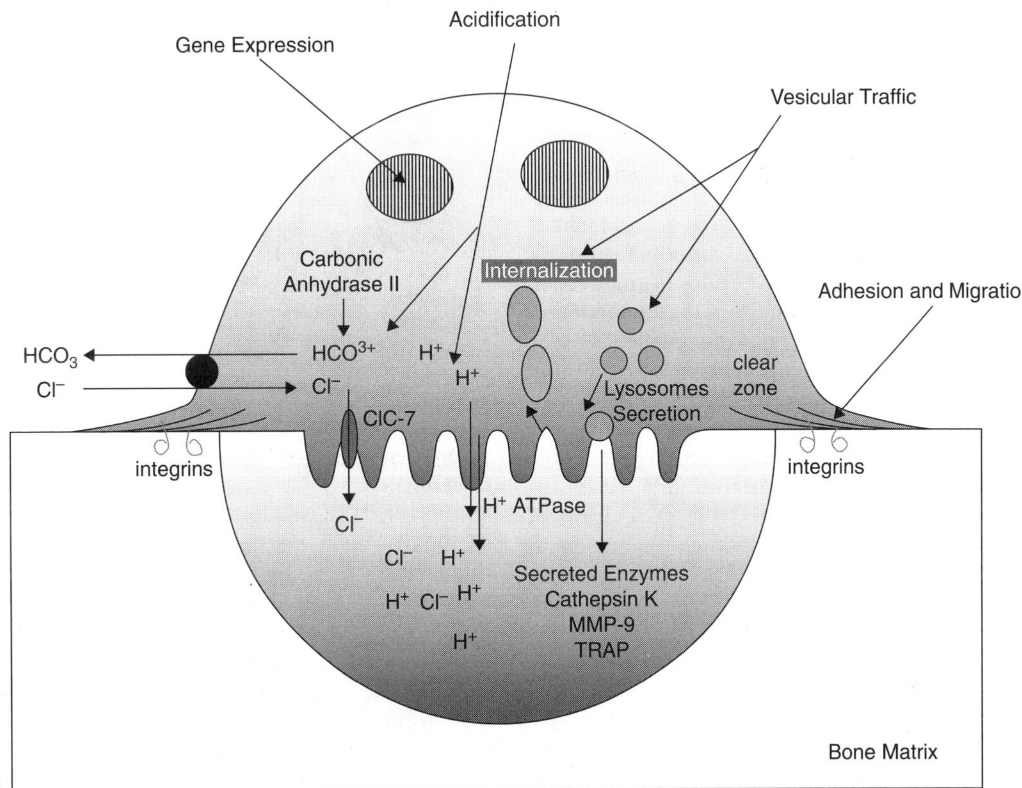

Figure 3.1 (A) The osteoclast contains multiple nuclei, an endoplasmic reticulum where lysosomal enzymes are synthesized, and prominent Golgi stacks around each nucleus. The cell is attached to bone matrix (bottom) and forms a separate compartment underneath itself, limited by the sealing zone. The plasma membrane of the cell facing this compartment is extensively folded and forms the ruffled border. Vesicles in the cytoplasm transport enzymes toward the bone matrix and internalize partially digested bone matrix. (B) Schematic representation of a polarized active osteoclast including the main molecular effectors of the process of bone resorption (see text)

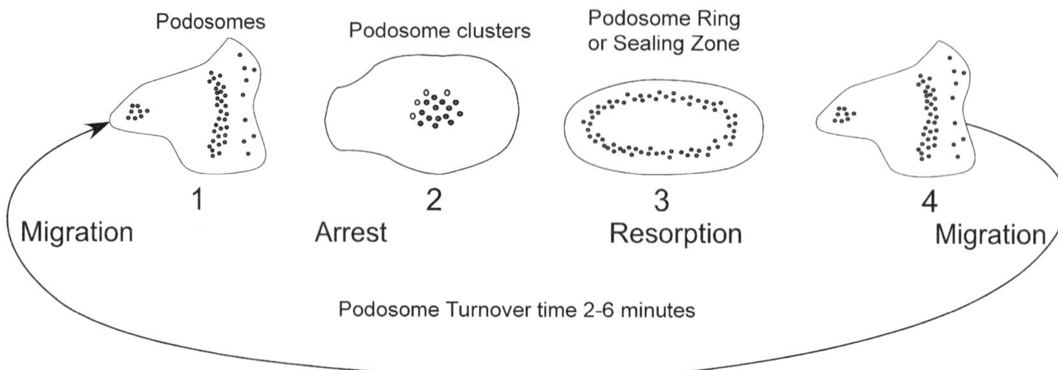

Figure 3.2   Steps in the attachment, resorption, and migration of the osteoclast: dynamics of podosomes: podosomes, or points of adhesion, are turning over every 2–6 minutes, allowing plasticity of the cell attachment and cell migration. A dense ring of podosomes, or reorganized actin, forms the sealing zone around resorption pits.

extracellular degradation of the bone matrix; and 5) its ability to migrate efficiently toward and along the bone surfaces.

Adhesion and **migration** depend essentially on adhesion receptors and their ability to regulate the cytoskeleton, particularly the rapid assembly and disassembly of cytoskeletal proteins at sites of adhesion (podosomes, Figure 3.2). **Secretion** depends essentially on vesicular transport, the directional fission-fusion of transport vesicles from the endoplasmic reticulum to the Golgi and from the Golgi to the secretory pole of the cell, i.e. the ruffled border (Figure 3.3). **Internalization** also depends upon vesicular transport, but in a retrograde manner, i.e., from the ruffled border to endosomes and lysosomes or through the cell to the basal pole in transcytosis (Figure 3.3). Finally, **acidification** depends essentially on the generation of protons by the enzyme carbonic anhydrase and their transport across the plasma membrane by the apical vacuolar proton ATPase (V-ATPase), in parallel with the extrusion of chloride ions through the ClC-7 chloride channel as well as homeostatic ion transport at the basolateral membrane (Figure 3.4).

The importance of these five key functional effectors (Figure 3.1B) in the regulation of osteoclastic activity is readily demonstrated by the fact that specific genetic alterations of these molecules or pathways all lead to altered bone resorption and osteopetrosis. Defects in adhesion receptor signaling or cytoskeletal proteins and their associated tyrosine kinases, affecting cell adhesion and cell migration, are observed in

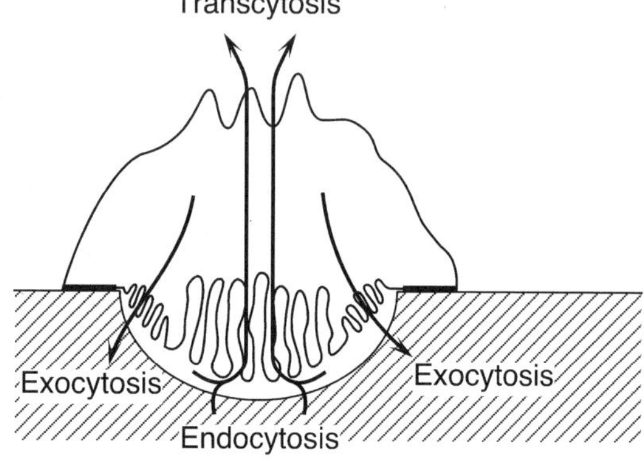

Figure 3.3   The main vesicular traffic pathways in an osteoclast: secretion via exocytosis and internalization via endocytosis and transcytosis are effected by different membrane domains.

vitronectin receptor knockout mice [116], Src and Pyk2 [143] as well as gelsolin [25] -deficient mice. Altered synthesis of key enzymes such as cathepsin K lead to osteopetrosis in mice [140] and occur in humans afflicted by pycnodysostosis [57]. A defect in vesicular traffic is the most likely cause of osteopetrosis in the gray-lethal mutation mouse [20, 139]. Finally, mutations in the V-ATPase [54, 92, 105, 149], the ClC-7 chloride channel [91], or the enzyme carbonic anhydrase II [159], essential components of the acidification process, lead to osteopetrosis in mice and in humans. These examples illustrate unequivocally the importance of these various

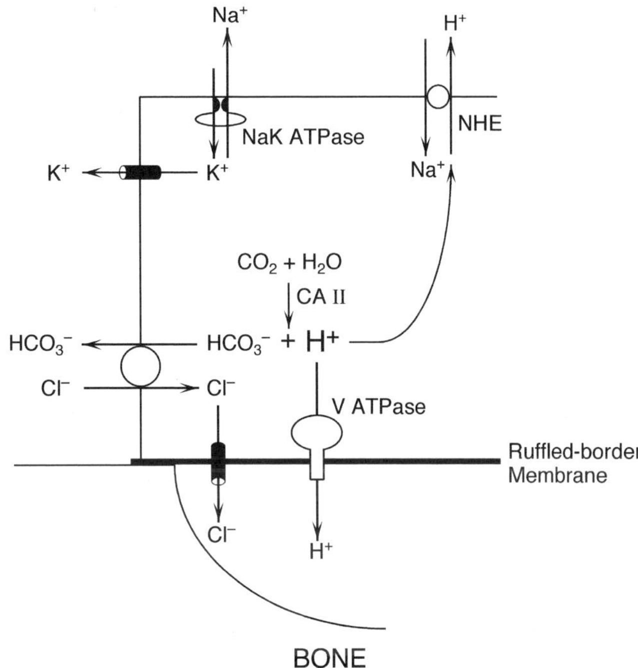

Figure 3.4 The osteoclast ion transport systems in the apical ruffled-border and the basolateral membranes allow efficient extrusion of protons via the ruffled-border vacuolar ATPase in parallel with a chloride conductance. Basolateral transport systems avoid changes in pH and/or in membrane polarization of the cell. Carbonic anhydrase generates protons and mitochondriae generate ATP.

pathways in the regulation of the activity of the osteoclast, thereby defining and validating novel targets for therapeutic intervention. Genetic mutations aside from those affecting osteoclast activity decrease bone resorption, whether in humans or in mutant or genetically altered mice, through alterations in the differentiation of osteoclast lineage rather than through modulation of the activity of the mature osteoclast.

These key functional effectors define the most prominent morphological features of the osteoclast (Figure 3.1). Besides its multinucleation, these are deep foldings of the plasma membrane in the area facing the bone matrix, i.e., the ruffled border, which is formed as a result of directional insertion of vesicles required for active secretion of protons and lysosomal enzymes toward the bone surface, as well as directional endocytic activity from the bone resorbing compartment [8, 9, 181]. This central area of the interface between the cell and the bone surface is surrounded by a ring of contractile proteins (sealing zone) that serve to attach the cell to the bone surface while ensuring its continued ability to migrate. This attachment ring seals off the subosteoclastic bone-resorbing compartment, sandwiched between the ruffled border plasma membrane and the surface of the bone matrix undergoing

bone resorption. The attachment of the cell to the matrix is performed via integrin receptors (mostly $\alpha_v\beta_3$, $\alpha_v\beta_5$, and $\alpha_2\beta_1$), which bind to specific sequences in matrix proteins, and activate a specific signaling cascade requiring several now identified signaling molecules to ensure adhesion and cell motility (c-Src, Pyk2, Cbl, Gelsolin). The plasma membrane in the ruffled border area contains proteins that also are found at the limiting membrane of endosomes and related organelles, and a specific type of electrogenic proton ATPase as well as a specific chloride channel (ClC-7) responsible for acidification of the extracellular bone resorbing compartment. The basolateral plasma membrane (Figures 3.4 and 3.5) of the osteoclast is highly and specifically enriched in Na⁺K⁺-ATPase (sodium-potassium pump), HCO_3/Cl-exchangers, and Na⁺/H⁺ exchangers, as well as several ion channels. This membrane also expresses RANK, the receptor for RANK ligand, and the M-CSF receptor, both of which are responsible for osteoclast differentiation, as well as the calcitonin receptor, which is capable of rapidly inactivating the osteoclast.

Lysosomal enzymes (for example, tartrate resistant acid phosphatase, cathepsin K) are actively synthesized by the osteoclast and are found in the endoplasmic reticulum, as well as

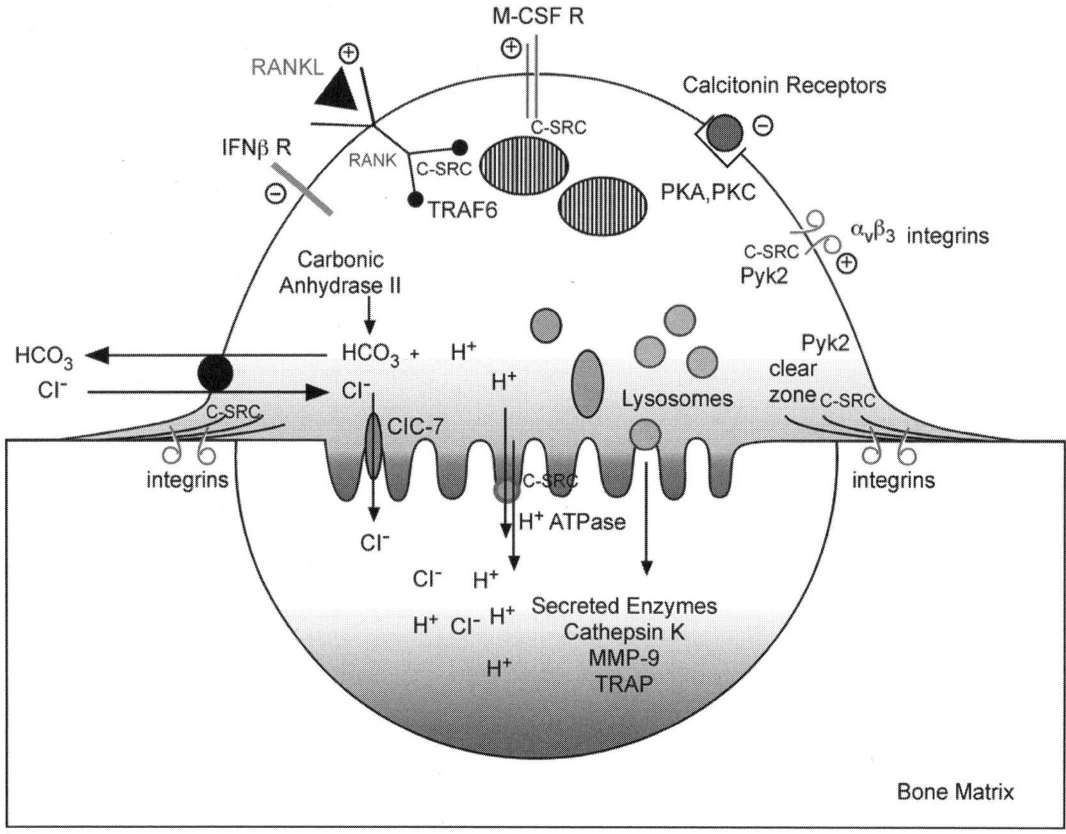

Figure 3.5   The main receptors regulating osteoclast activity target the cytoskeleton, affecting adhesion and migration, vesicular traffic, secretion and internalization, ion transport, acidification, or – on a longer-term basis – gene expression, affecting all aspects of osteoclast function.

in the Golgi apparatus. The osteoclast typically contains multiple copies of the Golgi complex, organized as rings surrounding each nucleus [8], and many readily identifiable transport vesicles moving directionally toward the ruffled border membrane [8, 9]. The enzymes are secreted, via the ruffled border, into the extracellular bone-resorbing compartment where they reach a sufficiently high extracellular concentration that allows extracellular degradation of the bone matrix, within the sealed compartment. The transport and targeting of these secreted enzymes at the apical pole of the osteoclast involves mannose-6-phosphate receptors [8]. Furthermore, the cell secretes several metalloproteases, including collagenase and gelatinase [37].

The osteoclast acidifies the extracellular compartment [9] by secreting protons across the ruffled-border membrane (Figure 3.4), a process that involves the transporting activity of vacuolar proton pumps [12, 180]. Recent genetic evidence demonstrates that the electrogenic proton-pump ATPase is related to, but different from, the pump of kidney-tubule-acidifying cells or lysosomes [54, 105, 149]. The protons are provided to the pumps by carbonic anhydrase, an enzyme that is highly concentrated in the cytosol of the osteoclast. ATP and CO_2 are provided by the mitochondria, which are characteristically found in very high numbers in the osteoclast. Apical chloride channels (ClC-7) are also found in the ruffled border membrane [92], where they serve to prevent the hyperpolarization created by the massive extrusion of positively charged protons by the V-ATPase. The basolateral membrane actively exchanges bicarbonate for chloride, thereby avoiding an alkalinization of the cytosol and providing chloride for the ruffled-border channels [67, 185]. The basolateral sodium pumps [10] might be involved in secondary active transport of calcium and/or protons in association with a Na^+/Ca^{2+} exchanger and/or a Na^+/H^+ antiport. This cell thus appears to function in a manner similar to that of kidney tubule or gastric parietal cells, which also acidify their respective lumens.

The extracellular bone-resorbing compartment is the functional equivalent of a lysosome, with (i) a low pH, (ii) lysosomal enzymes, and (iii) the substrate, i.e. the bone matrix. First, the hydroxyapatite crystals are mobilized by digestion of their link to collagen (the noncollagenous proteins) and dissolved by the acid environment. Then, the residual collagen fibers are digested by the specific action of cathepsin K at low pH [13], and possibly by the activation of latent collagenase [37, 190]. During active resorption, the degraded bone matrix is processed extracellularly, after which some products are endocytosed into the osteoclast and degraded within secondary lysosomes, and others are transported through the cell by transcytosis and secreted through the basal membrane [130, 141]. The degraded products from the bone matrix probably also are released into the local microenvironment during periods of relapse of the sealing zone, possibly induced by a calcium sensor that responds to the rise of extracellular calcium in the bone-resorbing compartment (mM). Furthermore, degradation products are left behind at the bone surface upon migration of the osteoclast away from the resorption lacuna, and may play an essential role in the coupling to bone formation during the remodeling cycle.

The various components of the osteoclast bone resorbing machinery are therefore the levers (Figure 3.1B) by which the endocrine, paracrine, or endocrine ligands found in the osteoclast microenvironment exert their positive or negative regulatory action on the bone-resorbing capacity of individual osteoclasts. Indeed, some molecules such as RANKL, OPG, and M-CSF influence both differentiation and activity of osteoclasts, whereas others, such as calcitonin or integrin ligands, appear to regulate only osteoclast activity.

Regulation of Osteoclast Activity and Bone Resorption

Integrin Signaling (Figure 3.6)

Integrins are a superfamily of heterodimeric (α and β) transmembrane receptors which mediate cell-matrix interactions. Integrin-mediated adhesion and signaling regulate a variety of cell processes [30, 146]. In addition to cell adhesion, integrin receptor assembly also organizes extracellular matrices, modulates cell shape changes, and participates in cell spreading and motility [186, 189].

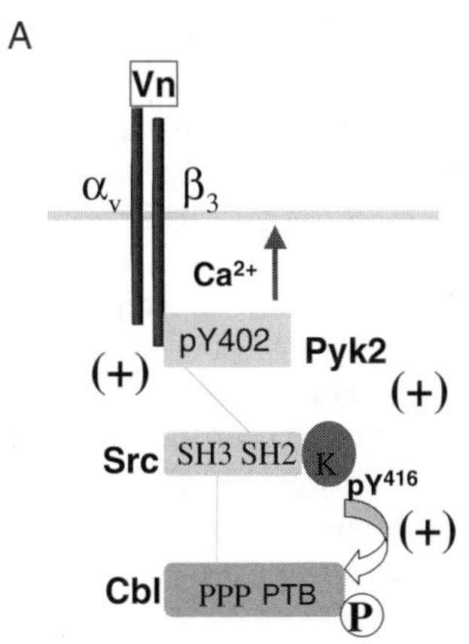

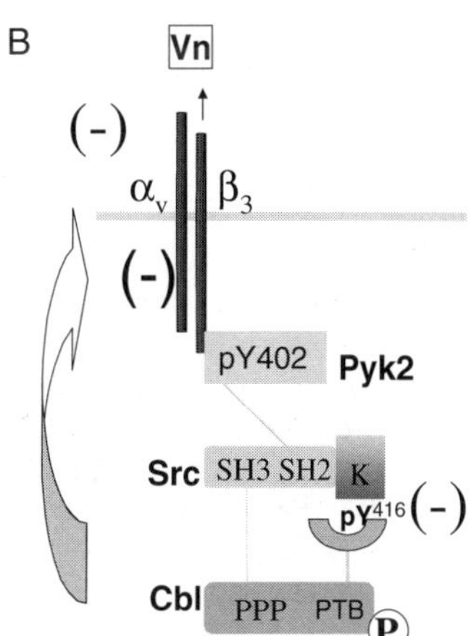

Figure 3.6 Integrin signaling controls adhesion and migration: (A) Binding of the vitronectin receptor to extracellular matrix proteins activates calcium entry into the osteoclast. This leads to Pyk2 autophosphorylation, recruitment of Src and Cbl to podosomes and Cbl (as well as several cytoskeletal proteins) becoming phosphorylated on tyrosine residues. (B) Phosphorylation of Cbl leads to Src kinase down-regulation and to loss of integrin adhesion to the substratum, allowing cell migration.

Upon ligand binding, integrins undergo receptor clustering, leading to the formation of adhesion contacts where these receptors are linked to intracellular cytoskeletal complexes, including bundles of actin filaments and signaling molecules. Indeed, the short cytoplasmic domains of the α and β integrin subunits can recruit a variety of cytoskeletal and signaling molecules. Integrin-mediated signaling changes phosphoinositide metabolism, raises intracellular calcium, and induces tyrosine or serine phosphorylation of signaling molecules [58, 146].

Adhesion of osteoclasts to the bone surface involves the interaction of integrins with extracellular matrix proteins within bone. Bone consists mainly of type I collagen (>90%) and of noncollagenous proteins interacting with a mineral phase of hydroxyapatite. Osteoclasts express very high levels of the integrin $\alpha_v\beta_3$ [75]. Mammalian osteoclasts also express lower levels of the collagen/laminin receptor $\alpha_2\beta_1$ and the vitronectin/fibronectin receptor $\alpha_v\beta_1$. Rat osteoclasts adhere in an $\alpha_v\beta_3$-dependent manner to extracellular matrix proteins containing arginine-glycine-aspartic acid (RGD) sequences, including vitronectin, osteopontin, bone sialoprotein, and a cryptic RGD-site in denatured collagen type I [51]. More recently, it was reported that rat osteoclasts adhere to native collagen type I using $\alpha_2\beta_1$ integrin, surprisingly in an RGD-dependent manner [72]. Moreover, osteoclastic bone resorption is partially inhibited by both anti-α_2 and anti-β_1 antibodies [124]. The first evidence that $\alpha_v\beta_3$ plays an important role in osteoclast function was obtained when a monoclonal antibody raised against osteoclasts inhibited bone resorption *in vitro* [21]; the antigen was later identified to be the $\alpha_v\beta_3$ integrin [35]. Furthermore, osteoclastic bone resorption *in vitro* can be inhibited by RGD-containing peptides and disintegrins or by blocking antibodies to $\alpha_v\beta_3$ [76, 87, 144].

Inhibition of $\alpha_v\beta_3$ integrins can also block bone resorption *in vivo*. In the thyroparathyroidectomized (TPTX) model, co-infusion of disintegrins such as echistatin or kinstrin and PTH completely blocked the PTH-induced increase in serum calcium [50, 87]. Echistatin was also shown to inhibit bone loss in hyperparathyroid mice maintained on a low calcium diet. In the bones of these animals, echistatin co-localizes with $\alpha_v\beta_3$ integrins in osteoclasts [111].

Additional *in vivo* studies demonstrated that echistatin or RGD-peptidomimetics inhibit bone resorption in ovariectomized rodents by blocking the function of $\alpha_v\beta_3$ integrins [47, 194]. Moreover, infusion of anti-rat β_3 integrin subunit antibody blocked the effect of PTH on serum calcium in TPTX rats [31]. Further compelling evidence for the role of $\alpha_v\beta_3$ integrin in osteoclast function was recently provided by the targeted disruption of β_3 integrin subunit in mice, which induces late onset osteopetrosis, 3 to 6 months after birth [116].

Recognition of extracellular matrix components by osteoclasts is an important step in initiating osteoclast function. Several studies have demonstrated that integrin-mediated cell adhesion to vitronectin, fibronectin or collagen induces cell spreading and actin rearrangement in osteoclasts. $\alpha_v\beta_3$ integrin plays a role in the adhesion and spreading of osteoclasts on bone [97, 129]. Expression of $\alpha_v\beta_3$ integrin is detected in mononucleated osteoclast precursors, where it mediates the adhesion and migration necessary for their fusion during osteoclast differentiation in culture [126]. Furthermore, $\alpha_v\beta_3$ integrin plays a role in the regulation of two processes required for effective osteoclastic bone resorption: cell migration and maintenance of the sealing zone [123].

Targeted disruption of β_3 integrin subunit results in an osteopetrotic phenotype [116]. Osteoclasts isolated from these mice fail to spread, do not form actin rings, have abnormal ruffled membranes, and exhibit reduced bone resorption activity *in vitro*. Thus, $\alpha_v\beta_3$ plays a pivotal role in the resorptive process, through its functions in cell adhesion-dependent signal transduction and in cell motility. Indeed, $\alpha_v\beta_3$ transmits bone matrix-derived signals, ultimately activating intracellular events that regulate cytoskeletal organization essential for osteoclast migration and polarization. Recent research interests have been focused on identifying the hierarchy of the $\alpha_v\beta_3$-regulated cascade of signaling and structural proteins required for this cytoskeletal organization. One of the earliest events initiated by integrin-ligand engagement is elevation of intracellular calcium. In rat, mouse, and human osteoclasts, RGD-containing peptides trigger a transient increase in intracellular calcium that seems to be mobilized from intracellular stores [135, 205]. This event is independent of the presence or activation of c-Src [143].

A Role for Tyrosine Kinases

c-Src Regulates $\alpha_v\beta_3$ Integrin-mediated Cytoskeletal Organization and Cell Motility

Src kinases play important roles in cell adhesion and migration, in cell cycle control, and in cell proliferation and differentiation [175]. Moreover, novel roles for Src kinases in the control of cell survival and angiogenesis have recently emerged [147]. In bone, the tyrosine kinase c-Src was found to be essential for osteoclast polarization, resorbing activity, and/or motility. Targeted disruption of c-Src in mice induces osteopetrosis due to loss of osteoclast function, and occurs without a reduction in osteoclast number [160]. Morphologically, osteoclasts in $Src^{-/-}$ mice are not able to form ruffled borders, but do form sealing zones on bone surfaces [15]. Src is highly expressed in osteoclasts, along with at least four other Src family members (Hck, Fyn, Lyn, and Yes) [74, 108]. Hck partly compensates for the absence of Src, since the double mutant $Src^{-/-}/Hck^{-/-}$ mouse is more severely osteopetrotic than the $Src^{-/-}$ mouse, despite the fact that the single mutant $Hck^{-/-}$ mouse is not obviously osteopetrotic [108]. On the other hand, transgenic expression of kinase-deficient Src in $Src^{-/-}$ mice partially rescued osteoclast function, indicating that full Src tyrosine kinase activity is not absolutely required for mediating osteoclast function. Its role as an adaptor protein to recruit downstream signaling molecules [148] is also essential to its function in osteoclasts [143].

c-Src is associated with the plasma membrane and multiple intracellular organelles [74, 167]. It is concentrated in the actin ring and the cell periphery [143], regions that are involved in osteoclast attachment and migration. This suggests that the absence of Src might compromise these aspects of osteoclast function. Indeed, $Src^{-/-}$ osteoclasts generated *in vitro* do not resorb bone and exhibit profound defects in cell adhesion and spreading on vitronectin, suggesting that c-Src plays an important role in the adhesion-dependent cytoskeletal organization in osteoclasts [96, 122]. Although $\alpha_v\beta_3$ integrin expression and ligand binding affinity are not altered in $Src^{-/-}$ osteoclasts, the lack of c-Src results in pronounced aggregation in the basal surface of resorbing osteoclasts of $\alpha_v\beta_3$ integrins and their downstream effectors, including Pyk2, p130^{Cas} and paxillin [96]. Thus, c-Src might not be important for the initial recruitment of $\alpha_v\beta_3$-dependent downstream effectors, but may mediate the turnover of the integrin-associated complex of signaling and cytoskeletal molecules. Recently, this hypothesis has been supported strongly by the finding that indeed $Src^{-/-}$ osteoclasts demonstrate significant decreases in their ability to migrate over a substrate, at least *in vitro* [143]. It is conceivable therefore, that most of the decreased bone resorption in $Src^{-/-}$ osteoclasts is attributable to low cell motility.

Pyk2 and c-Src Co-regulate $\alpha_v\beta_3$ Integrin-mediated Signals

Pyk2 was recently identified as a major adhesion-dependent tyrosine kinase in osteoclasts, both *in vivo* and *in vitro* [42] (Figure 3.6). Pyk2 is a member of the focal adhesion kinase (FAK) family that is highly expressed in cells of the central nervous system and in haematopoietic lineage [146]. Pyk2 and FAK share about 45% overall amino acid identity and have a high degree of sequence conservation surrounding binding sites of SH2- and SH3-domain-containing proteins. Although the presence of FAK has been reported in osteoclasts [11, 168], Pyk2 is expressed at much higher levels than FAK in osteoclasts [42]. Ligation of $\alpha_v\beta_3$ integrins either by ligand binding or by antibody-mediated clustering results in an increase in Pyk2 tyrosine phosphorylation [42]. Moreover, Pyk2 colocalizes with F-actin, paxillin, and vinculin in podosomes and in sealing zones of resorbing osteoclasts on bone [42]. These observations strongly implicate Pyk2 as a downstream effector in the $\alpha_v\beta_3$-dependent signaling, mediating the cytoskeletal organization associated with osteoclast adhesion, spreading, migration, and sealing zone formation.

More recently, it has been shown that osteoclasts infected with adenovirus expressing Pyk2 antisense oligonucleotides have significantly reduced levels of Pyk2 [43]. Like $Src^{-/-}$ osteoclasts, these cells do not resorb bone and exhibit defects in cell adhesion, spreading, and sealing zone organization, suggesting that Pyk2 is also important for cytoskeletal organization in osteoclasts [43]. Consistent with this, mice that lack Pyk2 develop osteopetrosis at an age similar to $\beta_3^{-/-}$ mice [158]. Furthermore, mice that lack both Src and Pyk2 are more severely osteopetrotic than either of the single mutants [158], indicating that these two proteins might interact during normal osteoclast functioning.

Tyrosine phosphorylation and kinase activity of Pyk2 have been reported to be markedly reduced in pre-osteoclasts derived from Src$^{-/-}$ mice [42]. This contrasts findings reported by Sanjay et al. [143], who reported that, upon adhesion, Src$^{-/-}$ osteoclasts demonstrated levels of Pyk2 phosphorylation comparable to those found in wild-type osteoclasts. The reasons for this discrepancy are not known, but it should be noted that the cells used in these two studies represent different stages of differentiation. Moreover, in adherent osteoclasts, Pyk2 is tightly associated with c-Src via its SH2-domain. An increase in intracellular calcium that results from the engagement or cross-linking of the $\alpha_v\beta_3$ integrin may activate Pyk2 by inducing autophosphorylation of Tyr402. This phosphorylated residue binds to the Src SH2-domain [40], displacing the inhibitory Src phosphotyrosine 527 and activating Src, leading to further recruitment and activation of Src-mediated downstream signals. At the same time, activation of Pyk2 following integrin-ligand engagement results in the recruitment of cytoskeletal proteins in a manner similar to FAK [146]. The N-terminal domain of FAK was shown to interact with the cytoplasmic domain of the β integrin subunit. Besides binding to Src, the autophosphorylation sites in FAK and Pyk2 can bind to SH2-domains of phospholipase C-γ [122, 146, 202]. Furthermore, the C-terminal domain of FAK and Pyk2 contain binding sites for Grb-2, p130^{Cas}, and paxillin [146]. The association and activation of c-Src and Pyk2 could initiate a cascade of activation and recruitment of additional signaling and structural molecules to the $\alpha_v\beta_3$ integrin-associated protein complex that together modulate the actin cytoskeleton in osteoclasts.

Association of Pyk2 with Src and c-Cbl Downstream of Integrins

Engagement of $\alpha_v\beta_3$ integrin induces the formation of a signaling complex that contains not only Src andPyk2, but also c-Cbl [143] (Figure 3.6). The product of the proto-oncogene c-Cbl is a 120 kDa adaptor protein which is tyrosine-phosphorylated in response to the activation of various signaling pathways, including M-CSF stimulation in monocytes and v-Src transformation, EGF, or PDGF activation in fibroblasts [168]. Tanaka and colleagues reported that the level of tyrosine phosphorylation of c-Cbl immunoprecipitated from Src$^{-/-}$ osteoclasts is markedly reduced, compared with levels in wild-type osteoclasts [167]. Furthermore, c-Src is found to associate and co-localize with c-Cbl in the membranes of intracellular vesicles in osteoclasts [167]. c-Cbl is a negative regulator of several receptor and non-receptor tyrosine kinases [142, 174]. Consistent with this function, overexpression of Cbl results in decreased Src kinase activity. Interestingly, inhibitory effects are seen with any fragment of Cbl that contains the N-terminal phosphotyrosine-binding (PTB) domain, regardless of whether the Src-binding proline-rich region is present [143]. The inhibition of Src kinase activity, and the binding to Src of v-Cbl (which lacks the proline-rich domain of Cbl and therefore will not bind to the Src SH3-domain) requires the presence of phosphorylated Src Tyr416, the autophosphorylation site of Src on the activation loop of the kinase domain [143].

In HEK293 cells, overexpression of the Cbl constructs inhibits cell adhesion in parallel with decreases in Src kinase activity. Thus, c-Cbl and fragments of Cbl that contain the PTB domain reduce cell adhesion, while the C-terminal half of Cbl, which contains the Src SH3-binding proline-rich region, but not the PTB domain, does not [143]. Interestingly, the absence of either c-Src or c-Cbl decreases both cell motility (the rapid extension and retraction of lamellipodia) and directional migration of authentic osteoclasts isolated from Src$^{-/-}$ or Cbl$^{-/-}$ mice, and freshly plated osteoclasts from Src$^{-/-}$ mice fail to disassemble podosomes efficiently as the cell spreads [143], suggesting that the Pyk2/Src/Cbl complex is required for the disassembly of attachment structures. Increased stability of podosomes could well explain the decreased motility of the Src$^{-/-}$ and Cbl$^{-/-}$ osteoclasts.

Another recently described function of c-Cbl could contribute to the regulation and stability of podosomes in osteoclasts. It has been recently shown that Cbl acts as a ubiquitin ligase, targeting ubiquitin conjugating enzymes to the kinases that Cbl binds and down-regulates, with the result that the kinases are ubiquitinated and degraded by the proteosome [82, 101, 199]. Since active, but not inactive, Src is ubiquitinated and degraded at this location [65], it could be that once Cbl is bound to the Pyk2/Src complex, it recruits the ubiquitinating system to the podosome. This would lead to the ubiquitination and degradation of the other components of the complex, and thereby participating in the turnover of podosome components that are required to ensure cell motility.

Recruitment of Other Cytoskeletal Proteins

Another integrin-dependent signaling adaptor recently characterized in osteoclasts is p130^{Cas} (Cas, Crk-associated substrate). In a number of different cell types, p130^{Cas} has been shown to serve as a substrate for either FAK, Pyk2, Src kinase, or Abl [146]. In osteoclasts, p130^{Cas} can directly associate with the proline-rich motifs in the C-terminal domains of FAK and Pyk2 via its SH3-domain. Similar to Pyk2, p130^{Cas} localizes to the actin ring formed in osteoclasts on glass, to the sealing zone on bone, and is highly tyrosine phosphorylated upon osteoclast adhesion to extracellular matrix proteins [95, 121]. In adherent osteoclasts, p130^{Cas} constitutively associates with Pyk2, suggesting that this adapter molecule participates in the integrin-PYK2-signaling pathway [95].

Much less is known about the signals that are generated by phosphorylation of the p130^{Cas} adaptor protein. In fibroblasts, integrin-stimulated tyrosine phosphorylation of p130^{Cas} promotes binding to the SH2-domain of either Crk [182] or Nck [145]. More recently, expression of SH3-domain of p130^{Cas} inhibited FAK-mediated cell motility [17], while overexpression of Crk was shown to promote cell migration in a Rac-dependent and Ras-independent manner [88]. Moreover, the downstream components of this Rac-mediated migration pathway appear to involve phosphatidyl inositol 3-kinase (PI3-kinase) [150]. In osteoclasts, the PI3-kinase dependent target was found to be the cytoskeletal-associated protein gelsolin [24].

$\alpha_v\beta_3$ Integrin-Dependent Activation of PI3-Kinase

In avian osteoclasts, $\alpha_v\beta_3$ is associated with the signaling molecule PI3-kinase and c-Src [78]. Interaction of $\alpha_v\beta_3$ with osteopontin resulted in increased PI3-kinase activity and association with Triton-insoluble gelsolin [24]. In murine osteoclasts formed in culture, PI3-kinase was found to translocate into the cytoskeleton upon osteoclast attachment to the bone surface [98]. In addition, potent inhibitors of PI3-kinase, such as wortmannin, inhibit mammalian osteoclastic bone resorption *in vitro* and *in vivo* [125].

Gelsolin, an actin-binding protein, regulates the length of F-actin *in vitro*, and thus cell shape and motility [32]. More recently, gelsolin-deficient mice were generated that express mild defects during hemostasis, inflammation, and possibly skin remodeling [187]. Gelsolin$^{-/-}$ mice have normal tooth eruption and bone development, with only modestly thickened calcified cartilage trabeculae attributed to delayed cartilage resorption along with a mild osteopetrosis [25]. However, osteoclasts isolated from gelsolin$^{-/-}$ mice lack podosomes and actin rings, and display reduced cell motility [25].

In conclusion, there is little doubt that the integrins that are present in the osteoclast membrane and particularly in the $\alpha_v\beta_3$ vitronectin receptor play critical roles in osteoclast biology. This involves not only adhesion, but also the regulation of "outside-in" signaling, which ensures the proper organization of the cytoskeleton, and of "inside-out" signaling, which ensures modulation of the affinity of the receptors for their substrate. These two regulatory modes ensure the assembly and disassembly of the attachment structures (podosomes), a cyclic process necessary for efficient cell motility.

A Role for Tyrosine Phosphatases

Reversible phosphorylation of tyrosine residues in proteins is a central regulator of cellular functions, and is controlled by the opposing actions of protein tyrosine kinases (PTKs) and tyrosine phosphatases (PTPs) [3, 80, 103, 178].

Tyrosine phosphorylation plays a major role in regulating bone resorption, as discussed above, and one may consequently expect that dysregulation of PTPs also will produce bone abnormalities. Indeed, aberrant tyrosine phosphorylation also can be caused by changes in PTP activity. Inhibition of the receptor-type phosphatase PTP-OC in cultured rabbit osteoclasts reduces their resorption activity [162, 191], while inhibition of OST-PTP abrogates differentiation of cultured osteoblasts [28, 114, 115]. In addition, as discussed below, mice lacking SHP-1 are osteopenic as a consequence of increased osteoclast function [4, 179], indicating that this PTP is a negative regulator of osteoclasts. Mice lacking PTPε show a decrease in osteoclast activity, indicating that it can be a positive regulator.

SHP1 Down-regulates Osteoclast Function

Many signaling pathways in osteoclasts crucially depend on tyrosine phosphorylation, and defective signaling by one or another tyrosine kinase is implicated in several of the currently known osteopetrotic mice (i.e., the M-CSF receptor, c-Src). The normal function of these signaling mechanisms requires that the tyrosine phosphorylation of signaling effectors be limited, both in terms of time and amplitude, by dephosphorylation catalyzed by protein tyrosine phosphatases (PTPs), and, in fact, several PTPs have recently been identified to play important roles in the modulation of osteoclast signaling.

One such PTP is the Src homology 2-domain-containing phosphatase 1 (SHP-1) [1] (also known as PTP1c [151], SHPTP-1 [136], HCP [198] or PTPN6 [137]) that functions as a cytosolic protein-tyrosine phosphatase (PTP) and is predominantly expressed in hematopoietic cells [113, 137, 151, 198]. In various cell types, SHP-1 associates with tyrosine phosphorylated receptors, including those for EGF [151, 177], interleukin (IL)-3, IL-4 and IL-13 [69, 197], c-Kit [196], erythropoietin [89], platelet-derived growth factor [200], and M-CSF [26], raising the possibility that SHP-1 might terminate signals generating from activation of these receptors.

Spontaneous homozygous mutations of the gene encoding SHP-1 (*Hcph* [153]) give rise to the "motheaten" phenotype in mice, characterized by immunodefeciency, systemic autoimmunity and premature death [62]. One mutation

(*Hcph^me^/Hcph^me^*; abbreviation *me/me*) results in a frame shift and premature truncation of the mRNA, producing an essentially SHP-1 null phenotype [153]. *me/me* animals die at about three weeks of age, a result of inflammatory lung disease [154]. Another mutation results in proteins that retain approximately 25% of the wild-type activity and the mutant mice are consequently viable and designated *me^v^/me^v^* [153].

Given the importance of tyrosine phosphorylation in pathways such as M-CSF receptor activation [68], integrins [143], and Src-dependent signaling [175], it was predicted that SHP-1 would play a significant role in the modulation of signaling in osteoclasts. This prediction was borne out by studies of the formation and function of osteoclasts using the milder *me^v^/me^v^* mutant mouse [4, 179]. The *me^v^/me^v^* mouse is osteopenic, exhibiting decreased trabecular thickness with increased bone resorption indices, particularly an increased number of osteoclasts. Impaired osteoblast function also may contribute to the phenotype, since the osteoid volume, mineralizing surface and osteoblast surface are decreased compared to controls. *In vivo* and *in vitro* data reveal that both osteoclast differentiation and osteoclast activity are increased in the absence of normal SHP-1, suggesting that this tyrosine phosphatase is a negative regulator of osteoclastogenesis and, possibly, of osteoclast resorbing activity. The increased osteoclastogenesis is attributable to effects of the *me^v^/me^v^* mutation in the hematopoietic precursor cells, because the osteoclastogenic potency of stromal cells is not affected. The fact that increased osteoclastogenesis is intrinsic to the hematopoietic lineage excludes the possibility that it could be a result of increased RANKL or of a decrease in OPG production by cells of the stromal lineage or osteoblasts [94, 157].

Thus, SHP-1 apparently down-regulates signaling in response to factor(s) that activate differentiation and possibly bone resorption. Indeed, M-CSF signaling, Src and NF-κB activity have all been shown to be affected by reduced SHP-1 activity. In *me/me* macrophages, where SHP-1 is totally inactive, the M-CSF receptor is hyperphosphorylated. At least some of its associated proteins are hyperactivated when the cells are treated with M-CSF [26] this indicates that SHP-1 is involved in the dephosphorylation of the M-CSF receptor and suggests that SHP-1 is a critical negative regulator of M-CSF signaling. The increase in osteoclast formation in *me^v^/me^v* mice could thus be explained as a result of the failure of SHP-1 to down-regulate M-CSF receptor signaling mechanisms. Src activity is regulated by its tyrosine phosphorylation state and the absence of SHP-1 in *me/me* thymocytes leads to the hyperactivation of Src family kinases [107]. A similar Src-related effect could be responsible for increased osteoclastic activity. A third possibility is that the lack of SHP-1 activity promotes the activation of NF-κB downstream of RANK in osteoclast precursors, as it does in both *me^v^/me^v* T and B cells [86].

PTPε Activates Osteoclast Function

The protein tyrosine phosphatase epsilon (PTPε) subfamily contains four distinct proteins, all products of a single gene. The two major forms of PTPε are the receptor-type (RPTPε) and non-receptor type (cyt-PTPε) isoforms [45, 46, 93, 127, 169]. Two other forms of PTPε are p67 and p65 PTPε; these are shorter molecules, whose production is regulated at the levels of translation and post-translational processing [60, 61]. The four PTPε forms differ only at their amino termini, resulting in their unique subcellular localization patterns and distinct physiological functions. RPTPε assists Neu-induced mouse mammary tumor cells maintain their transformed phenotype, most likely by dephosphorylating and activating Src *in vivo* [44, 46, 59]. The same form of PTPε also can down-regulate insulin receptor signaling in cultured cells [2, 120]. In some systems PTPε can down-regulate mitogenic signaling, as exemplified by its inhibition of mitogen-activated protein kinase (ERK1/2) activity [176, 183] and inhibition of Janus kinase-signal transducer and activator of transcription (JAK-STAT) signaling in M1 leukemia cells [170–172]. PTPε also has been shown to be important for proper function of macrophages [163].

In a recent study [29], mice genetically lacking PTPε were shown to have an alteration in bone remodeling, affecting primarily females. Cyt-PTPε is strongly expressed in osteoclasts, and young female mice genetically lacking PTPε exhibit increased trabecular bone mass. This phenotype is attributable to reduced bone resorption by osteoclasts, which function abnormally both *in vitro* and *in vivo*. Reduced bone resorption is most readily detected in young (<12 weeks) female mice, but markedly less so in adult female or in male mice, suggesting that lack of PTPε may affect sex hormone-related signaling pathways in osteoclasts from affected mice. At the cellular level, cultures of osteoclast-like cells from PTPε-deficient mice failed to polarize and exhibited abnormalities in the structure and localization of podosomes. Src activity, Pyk2 phosphorylation, and response to RANKL treatment were, however, normal in osteoclasts from female mice lacking PTPε, suggesting these signaling pathways are not generally affected. These results establish that PTPε is required for optimal structure and organization of podosomes in osteoclasts in the context of cell polarization, and is essential for the optimal function of these cells *in vitro* and *in vivo*.

SHIP: An Inositol Phosphatase that Down-regulates Osteoclast Function

In a recent study, Takeshita et al. [166] identified SH2-containing inositol-5-phosphatase (SHIP) as an important regular of osteoclast function. SHIP is a protein that becomes tyrosine phosphorylated and associated with Shc after activation of membrane receptors for a number of hematopoietic cytokines. SHIP has an N-terminal SH2-domain, a central inositol polyphosphate-5-phosphatase catalytic domain, and two NPXY sequences that bind phosphotyrosine binding domains when phosphorylated and a proline-rich C terminus. SHIP specifically recognizes and cleaves the 5′-phosphate group from phosphatidylinositol-3,4,5-trisphosphate (PIP3), the major product of PI3-K activity, and from inositol-1,3,4,5-tetrakisphosphate.

Signals promoting osteoclast precursor survival, differentiation, and function that are generated after engagement of M-CSF R, RANK or integrin receptors lead to activation of PI3-K. The ability of SHIP to dephosphorylate PIP3 suggested this 5′-phosphatase also may inhibit osteoclast recruitment and function, a hypothesis tested by by examining mice with a homozygous deletion of SHIP [166]. The animals did not survive after 14 weeks due to a myeloproliferative disorder, an observation that is consistent with SHIP functioning as a negative regulator of cytokine signaling. More relevant to this chapter, however, the deletion of SHIP markedly increased the sensitivity of marrow macrophages to M-CSF and RANKL, enhancing the generation of large and hyper-resorptive osteoclasts in a cell autonomous manner. As a consequence of this hyperactivity of the SHIP$^{-/-}$ osteoclasts, the mice developed a severe form of osteoporosis.

Signaling from the Calcitonin Receptor

Because of its potent inhibitory effects on osteo-clast activity, calcitonin has long been recog-nized as a potential therapeutic agent for the treatment of diseases that are characterized by increased bone resorption including osteoporo-sis, Paget's disease, and late-stage malignancies (Figure 3.7). Signaling mechanisms down-stream of the calcitonin receptor have, there-fore, been of great interest. A comprehensive discussion of calcitonin-induced signaling appears elsewhere in this volume; hence we focus here on what is known of the interaction of calcitonin-activated signaling events with attachment-related signaling.

In situ, calcitonin reduces contact of osteo-clasts with the bone surface and alters osteoclast morphology [73, 84]. Cultured *in vitro*, calci-tonin-treated osteoclasts retract and become less mobile [22, 23, 201]. These effects suggest that some of the key targets of calcitonin sig-naling are involved in cell attachment and cytoskeletal function, possibly in conjunction with the integrins and/or their signaling function.

The calcitonin receptor, a G protein-coupled receptor that has been cloned from several species and cell types, couples to multiple het-erotrimeric G proteins (G_s, $G_{i/o}$, and G_q) [19, 27, 52, 155, 156]. For technical reasons, much of the recent characterization of signaling down-stream of the calcitonin receptor has been conducted in cells other than osteoclasts, particularly cell lines that express recombinant calcitonin receptor. Because it couples to multi-ple G proteins, the proximal signaling mecha-nisms that are activated by calcitonin include many classical GPCR-activated effectors, such as adenylyl cyclase and protein kinase A (PKA); phospholipases C, D, and A$_2$; and protein kinase C (PKC). In HEK 293 cells that express the rabbit calcitonin receptor, calcitonin induces the phos-phorylation and activation of the ERK1/2 pathway via extracellular signal-regulated kinases, Erk1 and Erk2 [27, 128], via mecha-

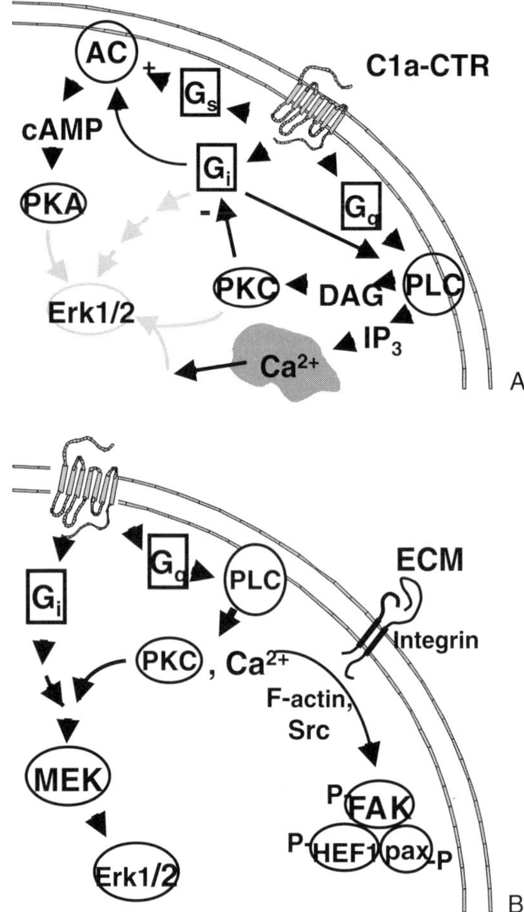

Figure 3.7 Signal transduction from the calcitonin receptor involves three different G proteins (A) and activation of PKA and PKC and PLC. (B) Cross-talk between the CTR and integrin signaling via Gi and Gq regulates the cytoskeleton.

nisms that involve the βγ subunits of pertussis toxin-sensitive G_i, as well as pertussis toxin-insensitive signaling via phospholipase C, PKC and elevated intracellular calcium, ($[Ca^{2+}]_i$).

It has been shown in the same cell line that calcitonin induces the tyrosine phosphoryla-tion and association of components of cellular adhesion complexes, including FAK, paxillin, and HEF1, a member of the p130^{Cas} family [204]. Interestingly, while these cells express both HEF1 and p130^{Cas}, only HEF1 is phosphorylated and associates with FAK and paxillin. This response to calcitonin is independent of adeny-lyl cyclase/PKA and of pertussis toxin-sensitive mechanisms and appears to be mediated by the pertussis toxin-insensitive PKC/[Ca^{2+}]$_i$ signaling pathway. The relevance of the FAK/paxillin/HEF1 phosphorylation to integrins and the actin cytoskeleton is demonstrated by its requirement for integrin attachment to the substratum and its sensitivity to agents (cytochalasin D, latrunculin A) that disrupt actin filaments [203]. The calcitonin-induced tyrosine phosphorylation of paxillin and HEF1 is enhanced by the overexpression of c-Src and strongly inhibited by the overexpression of a dominant negative kinase-dead Src, indicating that c-Src is required at some point in the coupling mechanism. Interestingly, the dominant negative Src has little effect on the calcitonin-induced phosphorylation of Erk1/2, in contrast to what has been reported for some other G protein coupled receptors [38, 39], indicating that some aspects of calcitonin-induced signaling may be significantly different from other better studied G protein-coupled receptors. These or similar events could well play important roles in mediating the calcitonin-induced changes in cell adhesion and motility in osteoclasts.

Signaling by the M-CSF Receptor (c-Fms) and RANK

These two receptors and their respective ligands, M-CSF and RANKL, have been demonstrated to be both necessary and, when co-activated, sufficient to induce the differentiation of osteoclasts precursors and to regulate the activity and survival of the mature osteoclasts [94, 138, 161]. Deletion of the genes encoding RANK, RANKL, or M-CSF lead to a block in osteoclast differentiation, producing an osteopetrotic phenotype [161, 173].

Signaling by RANK (Figure 3.8)

A number of the RANK-induced signaling pathways in osteoclasts ultimately induce the expression of several genes, including TRAP, cathepsin K, the calcitonin receptor, the $\alpha_v\beta_3$ integrin, and the transcriptional regulators mi/Mitf, myc and NFAT2. [41, 102]. Signaling is initiated by the rapid binding of TRAFs to specific domains in the cytoplasmic tail of RANK [33, 56, 79]. TRAF binding, in turn, induces at least five distinct phosphorylation cascades mediated by protein kinases: IKK, JNK, p38m Erk and Src, as well as c-fos and NFAT activation. [Six main pathways are activated downstream of RANK: TRAF6-Src, Akt, NFkB, JNK, p38, and c-fos-IFN β.] TRAF 2, 5, and 6 all have been shown to bind to RANK, and their individual docking sites have been mapped, yet only TRAF 6 inactivation results in osteopetrosis due to loss of osteoclast activity [90, 94, 106] and deletion of the membrane-proximal TRAF6 binding site specifically prevents the restoration of osteoclastogenic potential in RANK$^{-/-}$ derived hematopoietic precursors [6].

TRAF acts as a key adaptor to assemble signaling complexes that direct osteoclast-specific gene expression leading to differentiation and activation. The two best studied pathways are those leading to the activation of NFκB and AP-1 transcription factors, both of which are required for osteoclast formation [53, 64, 192]. Activation of these transcription factors is induced by phosphorylation cascades mediated by protein kinases, including IKK1/2 (NFκB), and JNK1 (AP-1) [34, 53, 64, 85, 192]. Coupling of RANK to IKK and JNK involves the ERK1/2-related TGFβ-inducible kinase, TAK1, along with the TRAF-binding adapter protein TAB2, both of which are present in activated receptor complexes [100, 119], as shown by the inhibition of RANKL-mediated activation of both IKK1/2 and JNK2 by dominant-negative mutant forms of TAK1 [193]. The ERK1/2-related kinase MKK7 also is required for JNK activation in osteoclasts.

The stress-activated protein kinase p38, apparently activated by RANK-induced phosphorylation by MKK [104, 112], also is involved in mediating key signals from RANK, coupling to the downstream activation of the transcriptional regulator mi/Mitf and the expression of TRAP and cathepsin K [110]. ERK1/2 pathway activation via the extracellular signal-regulated kinase 1 (Erk1) is also activated by RANK signaling, apparently via activation of MEK1 [77, 184]. MEK activation of Erk appears to play an important role in protecting osteoclasts from apoptosis [118].

Src binding to TRAF-6 allows RANK-mediated signaling to activate first PI3-K and consequently the Akt/PKB [188], which induce cell survival, cytoskeletal rearrangements, and motility. In dendritic cells, activated RANK recruits TRAF-6, c-Cbl, and PI3-K in a Src kinase-dependent manner [7]. TRAF-6, in turn,

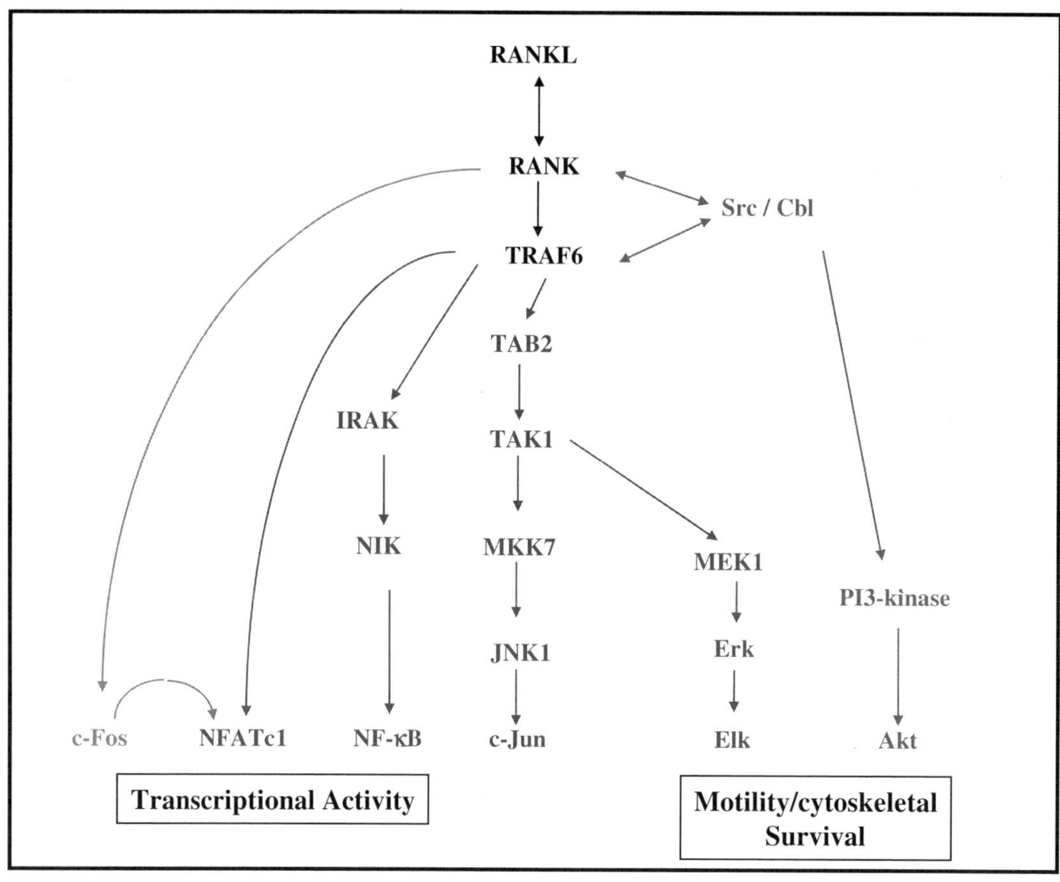

Figure 3.8 RANKL/RANK signaling activates several pathways that regulate both transcriptional activity and the cytoskeleton, as well as osteoclast survival. One such pathway involves Src and Cbl.

enhances Src kinase activity, leading to phosphorylation of downstream signaling molecules, including c-Cbl [188]. RANKL-induced activation of Akt/PKB is defective in Cbl-b$^{-/-}$ dendritic cells (but perhaps not in Cbl-b$^{-/-}$ osteoclast like cells) [7] , implicating Cbl-b as a positive modulator of RANK signaling.

RANK expression and signaling appears to be tightly controlled, with several mechanisms reported to exert positive or negative control of the pathway, thereby enhancing or inhibiting RANKL-induced osteoclastogenesis and subsequent activation. IL-1, M-CSF, TNFα, PGE2, and TGFβ all potentiate osteoclastogenesis *in vitro*, and can stimulate bone resorption *in vivo*. In contrast, inhibition of MEK1 and mTOR, its downstream target, lead to increased osteoclastogenesis *in vitro*. This suggests that activation of the Erk and Src pathways also can negatively regulate osteoclastogenesis [77, 152]. Other mechanisms switch off the RANK-signaling pathway once it has been activated. For example, RANKL induces the expression and secretion of interferon β, which is secreted and acts in an autocrine fashion to down regulate the expression of c-fos, a critical factor involved in osteoclast development [71, 164], while interferon γ promotes the degradation of TRAF 6, and inhibits *in vitro* osteoclastogenesis [165].

Signaling by c-Fms, the M-CSF Receptor

Activation of c-Fms by its ligand, M-CSF, promotes the proliferation and survival of cells of the macrophage/monocyte lineage, including osteoclasts and their precursors [48, 68]. In addition, M-CSF is required for osteoclast differentiation, at least in part by inducing the expression of RANK in osteoclast precursors, priming the cells to differentiate in response to RANKL [5]. Following M-CSF-induced dimerization, c-Fms autophosphorylates several tyrosines on its cytoplasmic tail, thereby providing binding sites for several SH2-containing proteins (c-Src, Y559; STAT 1, Y706; PI3-K, Y721; Grb 2, Y697, and Y921) that are recruited to the c-Fms-associated signaling complex. c-Cbl has been shown to interact with c-Fms via the phosphorylated tyrosine Y973. c-Cbl appears to play both positive and negative signaling roles downstream of the activated c-Fms. Once bound to c-Fms, it couples the activated receptor to several downstream signaling effectors, including PI3-K [131] and Akt/PKB, the ERK1/2s, and the JAK/STAT system (Figure 3.9). The activation of Erk 1,2 may protect osteoclasts from apoptosis [117]. At the same time, it targets the ubiquitination machinery to the activated receptor, promoting c-Fms ubiquitination and rapid endocytosis and attenuating macrophage proliferation [99].

We previously have shown that M-CSF induces Src-dependent cytoskeletal reorganiza-

tion, cell spreading, and increased migration in osteoclasts [81]. M-CSF also induces relocalization of PI3-K to the cell membrane [63, 132] and decreases bone resorption [55, 70]. Of possible relevance to our observation of elevated RANK on the surface of Cbl-b$^{-/-}$ osteoclast like cells, activating c-Fms increases the levels of RANK on the cell surface, and in addition, up-regulates other components of RANK signaling pathways [5, 109, 195].

The effect of M-CSF on the spreading of both macrophages and mature osteoclasts is brought about by cytoskeletal rearrangements, involving Src-dependent phosphorylation [81] and translocation of PI3-kinase from the cytoplasm to the cell membrane [63]. Upon ligand binding, c-Fms phosphorylates a number of proteins, including c-Cbl and ERK1/2, leading to regulation of cell cycle progression by cyclins.

Feng et al. have recently shown that of all the autophosphorylated tyrosines on the cytoplasmic domain of the activated c-Fms, only Y559 (the Src binding site) and Y807, which is the most strongly phosphorylated tyrosine whose binding partners have not yet been identified, are required for osteoclast differentiation [49]. Interestingly, Y807-dependent signaling mechanisms are not required for normal bone resorption by mature osteoclasts.

M-CSF stimulates motility and cytoplasmic spreading in mature osteoclasts and both Src and c-Cbl play important roles in these processes. In WT osteoclasts, M-CSF treatment induces rapid cytoplasmic spreading, with redistribution of F-actin from a well-delineated central attachment ring to the periphery of the cell. It simultaneously induces the phosphorylation of several cellular proteins in osteoclast-like cells, including c-Fms and c-Src, and concurrently increases Src kinase activity three-fold. More recent and unpublished studies in our laboratory have shown that treatment of RAW cells with M-CSF results in rapid phosphorylation of both c-Fms and c-Cbl, consistent with other reports of the role of c-Cbl in regulating c-Fms signaling. In other unpublished experiments, a role of c-Cbl in M-CSF-mediated signaling was demonstrated further by the decreased migration of c-Cbl$^{-/-}$ osteoclast like cells through a semipermeable membrane in response to M-CSF in a Boyden chamber assay.

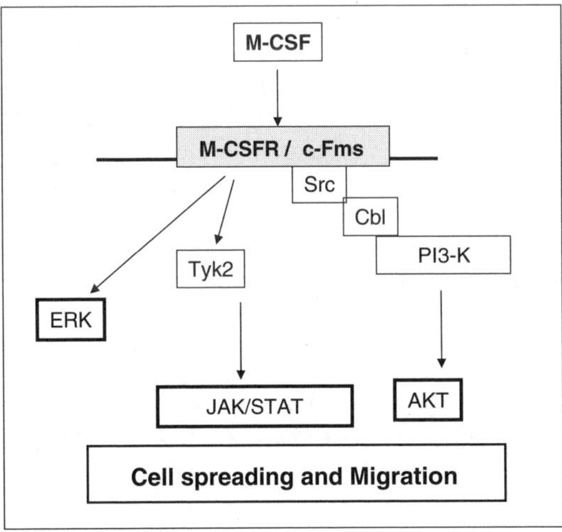

Figure 3.9 MCSF signaling activates and subsequent phosphorylation of several proteins, including Cbl. Cbl, promotes ubiquitination and endocytosis of c-Fms. PI3-kinase interacts with the receptor resulting in the activation of AKT leading to cytoskeletal reorganization and cell spreading.

DAP12 /TREM2, Co-receptors for the Immune System, Act as Key Co-receptors for RANK in the Regulation of Osteoclast Function [18, 83]

Rare TREM-2- and DAP12-deficient individuals recently have been identified [133, 134]. These individuals are affected by a genetic syndrome characterized by bone cysts and presenile dementia called Nasu-Hakola disease, or polycystic lipomembranous osteodysplasia with sclerosing leukoencephalopathy [66]. DAP12-deficient (DAP12$^{-/-}$) mice develop an increased bone mass (osteopetrosis) and a reduction of myelin (hypomyelinosis) accentuated in the thalamus. *In vitro* osteoclast induction from DAP12$^{-/-}$ bone marrow cells yielded immature cells with attenuated bone resorption activity.

In the immune system, DAP12 is expressed as a disulfide-linked homodimer that associates with various immunoreceptors, many of whose ligands are unknown, including TREM2 [14, 36]. TREMs are members of the immunoglobulin superfamily that promote myeloid cell activation by associating with DAP12. DAP12 harbors an immunoreceptor tyrosine-based activation motif (ITAM) also found in other immunoreceptor adapters such as the Fc receptor common chain. Tyrosine phosphorylation of ITAM of these immunoreceptor adapters by Src-family kinase is the primary step for generation of an activation signaling motif that functions as docking site for the protein tyrosine kinases Syk and Zap70. These kinases mediate a cascade of phosphorylation events that ultimately activate the cell. Within the TREM receptor family, TREM-2 is selectively expressed on monocyte-derived dendritic cells, promoting their migration and activation *in vitro*, suggesting that it may have a role in antigen presentation and T-cell stimulation *in vivo*. This observation suggests that the TREM-2–DAP12 complex may regulate the function of an unexpectedly vast array of myeloid cells, including osteoclasts. Indeed, TREM-2–deficient individuals have a striking defect in osteoclast development, which results in impaired bone resorption *in vitro*. TREM-2–deficient osteoclast precursors fail to fuse into multinucleated cells, do not develop podosomes, and show reduced or no expression of typical osteoclast markers such as integrin $\alpha_v\beta_3$ and calcitonin receptor. These cells demonstrate decreased activity in dentin resorption assays, potentially reflecting inefficient bone resorption *in vivo*.

Consistent with these results, defective development and resorptive function of osteoclasts have been recently observed in DAP12-deficient mice [83]. Thus, DAP12/TREM-2 may guide myeloid cell differentiation by modulating responsiveness to certain cytokines or reinforcing signaling pathways triggered by cytokine receptors or integrins [42, 121–123, 143]. The TREM-2/DAP12 signaling pathway also may play an important role in promoting actin polymerization, organization of the cytoskeleton, and ruffled border trafficking via recruitment of protein tyrosine kinases, activation of phospholipase C1, and calcium mobilization. These functions are critical for promoting cell fusion, as well as transforming osteoclast precursors into a polarized cell type capable of resorbing bone in a highly regulated fashion.

Conclusions

The last decade has brought significant progress to our understanding of the mechanisms by which osteoclasts resorb bone and of the regulation of these activities. As discussed in this chapter, the key elements of function can be summarized, beyond differentiation, as follows: 1) **Adhesion** and **migration**, via adhesion receptors and their ability to regulate the rapid assembly and disassembly of cytoskeletal proteins at sites of adhesion (podosomes). 2) **Secretion of proteolytic enzymes**, via vesicular transport to the secretory pole of the cell, i.e., the ruffled border. 3) **Internalization** also via vesicular transport, but in a retrograde manner, i.e., from the ruffled border to lysosomes or transcytosis. 4) **Acidification** via the apical vacuolar proton ATPase and the ClC-7 chloride channel at the ruffled border membrane as well as homeostatic ion transport at the basolateral membrane. The key regulatory pathways identified to date involve signaling from the adhesion receptors, particularly the integrins, signaling from the RANK and M-CSF receptors and signaling from the calcitonin receptor. These pathways converge upon both transcriptional regulation of key osteoclastic genes and upon the regulation of vesicular traffic, the cytoskeleton and ion transport systems. Most of these signaling cascades involve sequential phosphorylation and dephosphorylation events, both on tyrosines and on serine-threonines. All components of the regulatory pathways that modulate the activity of the osteoclast and bone resorption constitute valid targets for drug discovery or explain the mechanisms by which existing drugs affect the cells.

Acknowledgments

The authors are supported by NIH grants DE-04724, AR-42927, and AR-48218 to R.B. and AR-49879 to W.C.H. The authors are indebted to Archana Sanjay, Cecile Itsztein, Olivier Destaing, and Lynn Neff for help with some figures.

References

1. Adachi M, Fischer EH, Ihle J, Imai K, Jirik F, Neel B, et al. (1996) Mammalian SH2-containing protein tyrosine phosphatases. Cell. 85:15.
2. Andersen JN, Elson A, Lammers R, Romer J, Clausen JT, Moller KB, et al. (2001) Comparative study of protein tyrosine phosphatase-ε isoforms: membrane localization confers specificity in cellular signalling. Biochem J 354:581–90.
3. Andersen JN, Mortensen OH, Peters GH, Drake PG, Iversen LF, Olsen OH, et al. (2001) Structural and evolutionary relationships among protein tyrosine phosphatase domains. Mol Cell Biol 21:7117–36.
4. Aoki K, DiDomenico E, Sims NA, Mukhopadhyay K, Neff L, Houghton A, et al. (1999) The tyrosine phosphatase SHP-1 is a negative regulator of osteoclastogeneisis and osteoclast resorbing activity: increased resorption and osteopenia in me^v/me^v mutant mice. Bone 25:261–7.
5. Arai F, Miyamoto T, Ohneda O, Inada T, Sudo T, Brasel K, et al. (1999) Commitment and differentiation of osteoclast precursor cells by the sequential expression of c-Fms and receptor activator of nuclear factor κB (RANK) receptors. J Exp Med 190:1741–54.
6. Armstrong AP, Tometsko ME, Glaccum M, Sutherland CL, Cosman D, Dougall WC (2002) A RANK/TRAF6-dependent signal transduction pathway is essential for osteoclast cytoskeletal organization and resorptive function. J Biol Chem 277:44347–56.
7. Arron JR, Vologodskaia M, Wong BR, Naramura M, Kim N, Gu H, et al. (2001) A positive regulatory role for Cbl family proteins in tumor necrosis factor-related activation-induced cytokine (TRANCE) and CD40L-mediated akt activation. J Biol Chem 276:30011–17.
8. Baron R, Neff L, Brown W, Courtoy PJ, Louvard D, Farquhar MG (1988) Polarized secretion of lysosomal enzymes: co-distribution of cation- independent mannose-6-phosphate receptors and lysosomal enzymes along the osteoclast exocytic pathway. J Cell Biol 106:1863–72.
9. Baron R, Neff L, Louvard D, Courtoy PJ (1985) Cell-mediated extracellular acidification and bone resorption: evidence for a low pH in resorbing lacunae and localization of a 100-kD lysosomal membrane protein at the osteoclast ruffled border. J Cell Biol 101:2210–22.
10. Baron R, Neff L, Roy C, Boisvert A, Caplan M (1986) Evidence for a high and specific concentration of (Na^+,K^+)ATPase in the plasma membrane of the osteoclast. Cell 46:311–20.
11. Berry V, Rathod H, Pulman LB, Datta HK (1994) Immunofluorescent evidence for the abundance of focal adhesion kinase in the human and avian osteoclasts and its down regulation by calcitonin. J Endocrinol 141:R11–15.
12. Blair HC, Teitelbaum SL, Ghiselli R, Gluck S (1989) Osteoclastic bone resorption by a polarized vacuolar proton pump. Science 245:855–7.
13. Bossard MJ, Tomaszek TA, Thompson SK, Amegadzie BY, Hanning CR, Jones C, et al. (1996) Proteolytic activity of human osteoclast cathepsin K. Expression, purification, activation, and substrate identification. J Biol Chem 271:12517–24.
14. Bouchon A, Hernandez Munain C, Cella M, Colonna M (2001) A DAP12-mediated pathway regulates expression of CC chemokine receptor 7 and maturation of human dendritic cells. J Exp Med 194:1111–22.
15. Boyce BF, Yoneda T, Lowe C, Soriano P, Mundy GR (1992) Requirement of $pp60^{c-src}$ expression for osteoclasts to form ruffled borders and resorb bone in mice. J Clin Invest 90:1622–7.
16. Boyle WJ, Simonet WS, Lacey DL (2003) Osteoclast differentiation and activation. Nature 423:337–42.
17. Cary LA, Han DC, Polte TR, Hanks SK, Guan JL (1998) Identification of $p130^{Cas}$ as a mediator of focal adhesion kinase-promoted cell migration. J Cell Biol 140:211–21.
18. Cella M, Buonsanti C, Strader C, Kondo T, Salmaggi A, Colonna M (2003) Impaired differentiation of osteoclasts in TREM-2-deficient individuals. J Exp Med 198:645–51.
19. Chabre O, Conklin BR, Lin HY, Lodish HF, Wilson E, Ives HE, et al. (1992) A recombinant calcitonin receptor independently stimulates 3′,5′-cyclic adenosine monophosphate and Ca^{2+}/inositol phosphate signaling pathways. Mol Endocrinol 6:551–6.
20. Chalhoub N, Benachenhou N, Rajapurohitam V, Pata M, Ferron M, Frattini A, et al. (2003) Grey-lethal mutation induces severe malignant autosomal recessive osteopetrosis in mouse and human. Nat Med 9:399–406.
21. Chambers TJ, Fuller K, Darby JA, Pringle JA, Horton MA (1986) Monoclonal antibodies against osteoclasts inhibit bone resorption in vitro. Bone Miner 1:127–35.
22. Chambers TJ, Magnus CJ (1982) Calcitonin alters behaviour of isolated osteoclasts. J Pathol 136:27–39.
23. Chambers TJ, Revell PA, Fuller K, Athanasou NA (1984) Resorption of bone by isolated rabbit osteoclasts. J Cell Sci 66:383–99.

24. Chellaiah M, Fitzgerald C, Alvarez U, Hruska K (1998) c-Src is required for stimulation of gelsolin-associated phosphatidylinositol 3-kinase. J Biol Chem 273:11908–16.

25. Chellaiah M, Kizer N, Silva M, Alvarez U, Kwiatkowski D, Hruska KA (2000) Gelsolin deficiency blocks podosome assembly and produces increased bone mass and strength. J Cell Biol 148:665–78.

26. Chen HE, Chang S, Trub T, Neel BG (1996) Regulation of colony-stimulating factor 1 receptor signaling by the SH2 domain-containing tyrosine phosphatase SHPTP1. Mol Cell Biol 16:3685–97.

27. Chen Y, Shyu J-F, Santhanagopal A, Inoue D, David J-P, Dixon SJ, et al. (1998) The calcitonin receptor stimulates Shc tyrosine phosphorylation and Erk1/2 activation. Involvement of G_i, protein kinase C, and calcium. J Biol Chem 273:19809–16.

28. Chengalvala MV, Bapat AR, Hurlburt WW, Kostek B, Gonder DS, Mastroeni RA, et al. (2001) Biochemical characterization of osteo-testicular protein tyrosine phosphatase and its functional significance in rat primary osteoblasts. Biochemistry 40:814–21.

29. Chiusaroli R, Knobler H, Luxenburg C, Sanjay A, Granot-Attas S, Tiran Z, et al. (2004) Tyrosine phosphatase epsilon is a positive regulator of osteoclast function in vitro and in vivo. Mol Biol Cell 15:234–44.

30. Clark EA, Brugge JS (1995) Integrins and signal transduction pathways: the road taken. Science 268:233–9.

31. Crippes BA, Engleman VW, Settle SL, Delarco J, Ornberg RL, Helfrich MH, et al. (1996) Antibody to β_3 integrin inhibits osteoclast-mediated bone resorption in the thyroparathyroidectomized rat. Endocrinology 137:918–24.

32. Cunningham CC, Stossel TP, Kwiatkowski DJ (1991) Enhanced motility in NIH 3T3 fibroblasts that overexpress gelsolin. Science 251:1233–6.

33. Darnay BG, Haridas V, Ni J, Moore PA, Aggarwal BB (1998) Characterization of the intracellular domain of receptor activator of NF-κB (RANK). Interaction with tumor necrosis factor receptor-associated factors and activation of NF-κB and c-Jun N-terminal kinase. J Biol Chem 273:20551–5.

34. David J-P, Sabapathy K, Hoffmann O, Idarraga MH, Wagner EF (2002) JNK1 modulates osteoclastogenesis through both c-Jun phosphorylation-dependent and -independent mechanisms. J Cell Sci 115:4317–25.

35. Davies J, Warwick J, Totty N, Philp R, Helfrich M, Horton M (1989) The osteoclast functional antigen, implicated in the regulation of bone resorption, is biochemically related to the vitronectin receptor. J Cell Biol 109:1817–26.

36. Daws MR, Lanier LL, Seaman WE, Ryan JC (2001) Cloning and characterization of a novel mouse myeloid DAP12-associated receptor family. Eur J Immunol 31:783–91.

37. Delaisse JM, Eeckhout Y, Neff L, Francois-Gillet C, Henriet P, Su Y, et al. (1993) (Pro)collagenase (matrix metalloproteinase-1) is present in rodent osteoclasts and in the underlying bone-resorbing compartment. J Cell Sci 106:1071–82.

38. Della Rocca GJ, Maudsley S, Daaka Y, Lefkowitz RJ, Luttrell LM (1999) Pleiotropic coupling of G protein-coupled receptors to the mitogen- activated protein kinase cascade. Role of focal adhesions and receptor tyrosine kinases. J Biol Chem 274:13978–84.

39. Della Rocca GJ, van Biesen T, Daaka Y, Luttrell DK, Luttrell LM, Lefkowitz RJ (1997) Ras-dependent mitogen-activated protein kinase activation by G protein-coupled receptors. Convergence of G_i- and G_q-mediated pathways on calcium/calmodulin, Pyk2, and Src kinase. J Biol Chem 272:19125–32.

40. Dikic I, Tokiwa G, Lev S, Courtneidge SA, Schlessinger J (1996) A role for Pyk2 and Src in linking G-protein-coupled receptors with MAP kinase activation. Nature 383:547–50.

41. Dougall WC, Glaccum M, Charrier K, Rohrbach K, Brasel K, De Smedt T, et al. (1999) RANK is essential for osteoclast and lymph node development. Genes & Dev 13:2412–24.

42. Duong LT, Lakkakorpi PT, Nakamura I, Machwate M, Nagy RM, Rodan GA (1998) PYK2 in osteoclasts is an adhesion kinase, localized in the sealing zone, activated by ligation of $\alpha_v\beta_3$ integrin, and phosphorylated by Src kinase. J Clin Invest 102:881–92.

43. Duong LT, Nakamura I, Lakkakorpi PT, Lipfert L, Bett AJ, Rodan GA (2001) Inhibition of osteoclast function by adenovirus expressing antisense protein-tyrosine kinase 2. J Biol Chem 276:7484–92.

44. Elson A (1999) Protein tyrosine phosphatase ε increases the risk of mammary hyperplasia and mammary tumors in transgenic mice. Oncogene 18: 7535–42.

45. Elson A, Leder P (1995) Identification of a cytoplasmic, phorbol ester-inducible isoform of protein tyrosine phosphatase ε. Proc Natl Acad Sci USA 92:12235–9.

46. Elson A, Leder P (1995) Protein-tyrosine phosphatase ε. An isoform specifically expressed in mouse mammary tumors initiated by v-Ha-*ras* or *neu*. J Biol Chem 270:26116–22.

47. Engleman VW, Nickols GA, Ross FP, Horton MA, Griggs DW, Settle SL, et al. (1997) A peptidomimetic antagonist of the $\alpha_v\beta_3$ integrin inhibits bone resorption in vitro and prevents osteoporosis in vivo. J Clin Invest 99:2284–892.

48. Fantl WJ, Johnson DE, Williams LT (1993) Signalling by receptor tyrosine kinases. Annu Rev Biochem 62: 453–81.

49. Feng X, Takeshita S, Namba N, Wei S, Teitelbaum SL, Ross FP (2002) Tyrosines 559 and 807 in the cytoplasmic tail of the macrophage colony-stimulating factor receptor play distinct roles in osteoclast differentiation and function. Endocrinology 143:4868–74.

50. Fisher JE, Caulfield MP, Sato M, Quartuccio HA, Gould RJ, Garsky VM, et al. (1993) Inhibition of osteoclastic bone resorption in vivo by echistatin, an "arginyl-glycyl-aspartyl" (RGD)-containing protein. Endocrinology 132:1411–13.

51. Flores ME, Heinegard D, Reinholt FP, Andersson G (1996) Bone sialoprotein coated on glass and plastic surfaces is recognized by different β3 integrins. Exp Cell Res 227:40–6.

52. Force T, Bonventre JV, Flannery MR, Gorn AH, Yamin M, Goldring SR (1992) A cloned porcine renal calcitonin receptor couples to adenylyl cyclase and phospholipase C. Am J Physiol 262:F1110–15.

53. Franzoso G, Carlson L, Xing L, Poljak L, Shores EW, Brown KD, et al. (1997) Requirement for NF-κB in osteoclast and B-cell development. Genes Dev 11: 3482–96.

54. Frattini A, Orchard PJ, Sobacchi C, Giliani S, Abinun M, Mattsson JP, et al. (2000) Defects in TCIRG1 subunit of

the vacuolar proton pump are responsible for a subset of human autosomal recessive osteopetrosis. Nat Genet 25:343–6.

55. Fuller K, Owens JM, Jagger CJ, Wilson A, Moss R, Chambers TJ (1993) Macrophage colony-stimulating factor stimulates survival and chemotactic behavior in isolated osteoclasts. J Exp Med 178:1733–44.

56. Galibert L, Tometsko ME, Anderson DM, Cosman D, Dougall WC (1998) The involvement of multiple tumor necrosis factor receptor (TNFR)-associated factors in the signaling mechanisms of receptor activator of NF-κB, a member of the TNFR superfamily. J Biol Chem 273:34120–7.

57. Gelb BD, Shi G-P, Chapman HA, Desnick RJ (1996) Pycnodysostosis, a lysosomal disease caused by cathepsin K deficiency. Science 273:1236–8.

58. Giancotti FG, Ruoslahti E (1999) Integrin signaling. Science 285:1028–33.

59. Gil-Henn H, Elson A (2003) Tyrosine phosphatase-ε activates Src and supports the transformed phenotype of Neu-induced mammary tumor cells. J Biol Chem 278:15579–86.

60. Gil-Henn H, Volohonsky G, Elson A (2001) Regulation of protein-tyrosine phosphatases α and ε by calpain-mediated proteolytic cleavage. J Biol Chem 276: 31772–9.

61. Gil-Henn H, Volohonsky G, Toledano-Katchalski H, Gandre S, Elson A (2000) Generation of novel cytoplasmic forms of protein tyrosine phosphatase epsilon by proteolytic processing and translational control. Oncogene 19:4375–84.

62. Green MC, Shultz LD (1975) Motheaten, an immunodeficient mutant of the mouse. I. Genetics and pathology. J Hered 66:250–8.

63. Grey A, Chen Y, Paliwal I, Carlberg K, Insogna K (2000) Evidence for a functional association between phosphatidylinositol 3-kinase and c-src in the spreading response of osteoclasts to colony-stimulating factor-1. Endocrinology 141:2129–38.

64. Grigoriadis AE, Wang Z-Q, Cecchini MG, Hofstetter W, Felix R, Fleisch HA, et al. (1994) c-Fos: a key regulator of osteoclast-macrophage lineage determination and bone remodeling. Science 266:443–8.

65. Hakak Y, Martin GS (1999) Ubiquitin-dependent degradation of active Src. Curr. Biol 9:1039–42.

66. Hakola HP (1972) Neuropsychiatric and genetic aspects of a new hereditary disease characterized by progressive dementia and lipomembranous polycystic osteodysplasia. Acta Psychiatr Scand Suppl 232:1–173.

67. Hall TJ, Chambers TJ (1989) Optimal bone resorption by isolated rat osteoclasts requires chloride/bicarbonate exchange. Calcif Tissue Int 45:378–80.

68. Hamilton JA (1997) CSF-1 signal transduction. J Leukoc Biol 62:145–55.

69. Haque SJ, Harbor P, Tabrizi M, Yi T, Williams BRG (1998) Protein-tyrosine phosphatase Shp-1 is a negative regulator of IL-4- and IL-13-dependent signal transduction. J Biol Chem 273:33893–6.

70. Hattersley G, Dorey E, Horton MA, Chambers TJ (1988) Human macrophage colony-stimulating factor inhibits bone resorption by osteoclasts disaggregated from rat bone. J Cell Physiol 137:199–203.

71. Hayashi T, Kaneda T, Toyama Y, Kumegawa M, Hakeda Y (2002) Regulation of receptor activator of NF-kB ligand-induced osteoclastogenesis by endogenous interferon-β (INF-β) and suppressors of cytokine signaling (SOCS). The possible counteracting role of SOCSs in IFN-β-inhibited osteoclast formation. J Biol Chem 277:27880–6.

72. Helfrich MH, Nesbitt SA, Lakkakorpi PT, Barnes MJ, Bodary SC, Shankar G, et al. (1996) β$_1$ integrins and osteoclast function: involvement in collagen recognition and bone resorption. Bone 19:317–28.

73. Holtrop ME, Raisz LG, Simmons HA (1974) The effects of parathyroid hormone, colchicine, and calcitonin on the ultrastructure and the activity of osteoclasts in organ culture. J Cell Biol 60:346–55.

74. Horne WC, Neff L, Chatterjee D, Lomri A, Levy JB, Baron R (1992) Osteoclasts express high levels of pp60^{c-src} in association with intracellular membranes. J Cell Biol 119:1003–13.

75. Horton MA (1997) The αvβ3 integrin "vitronectin receptor". Int J Biochem Cell Biol 29:721–5.

76. Horton MA, Taylor ML, Arnett TR, Helfrich MH (1991) Arg-Gly-Asp (RGD) peptides and the anti-vitronectin receptor antibody 23C6 inhibit dentine resorption and cell spreading by osteoclasts. Exp Cell Res 195:368–75.

77. Hotokezaka H, Sakai E, Kanaoka K, Saito K, Matsuo K, Kitaura H, et al. (2002) U0126 and PD98059, specific inhibitors of MEK, accelerate differentiation of RAW264.7 cells into osteoclast-like cells. J Biol Chem 277:47366–72.

78. Hruska KA, Rolnick F, Huskey M, Alvarez U, Cheresh D (1995) Engagement of the osteoclast integrin α$_v$β$_3$ by osteopontin stimulates phosphatidylinositol 3-hydroxyl kinase activity. Ann NY Acad Sci 760:151–65.

79. Hsu H, Lacey DL, Dunstan CR, Solovyev I, Colombero A, Timms E, et al. (1999) Tumor necrosis factor receptor family member RANK mediates osteoclast differentiation and activation induced by osteoprotegerin ligand. Proc Natl Acad Sci USA 96:3540–5.

80. Hunter T (1995) Protein kinases and phosphatases: the yin and yang of protein phosphorylation and signaling. Cell 80:225–36.

81. Insogna KL, Sahni M, Grey AB, Tanaka S, Horne WC, Neff L, et al. (1997) Colony-stimulating factor-1 induces cytoskeletal reorganization and c-src-dependent tyrosine phosphorylation of selected cellular proteins in rodent osteoclasts. J Clin Invest 100:2476–85.

82. Joazeiro CAP, Wing SS, Huang H-K, Leverson JD, Hunter T, Liu Y-C (1999) The tyrosine kinase negative regulator c-Cbl as a RING-type, E2- dependent ubiquitin-protein ligase. Science 286:309–12.

83. Kaifu T, Nakahara J, Inui M, Mishima K, Momiyama T, Kaji M, et al. (2003) Osteopetrosis and thalamic hypomyelinosis with synaptic degeneration in DAP12-deficient mice. J Clin Invest 111:323–32.

84. Kallio DM, Garant PR, Minkin C (1972) Ultrastructural effects of calcitonin on osteoclasts in tissue culture. J Ultrastruct Res 39:205–16.

85. Karin M, Cao Y, Greten FR, Li ZW (2002) NF-κB in cancer: from innocent bystander to major culprit. Nat Rev Cancer 2:301–10.

86. Khaled AR, Butfiloski EJ, Sobel ES, Schiffenbauer J (1998) Functional consequences of the SHP-1 defect in motheaten viable mice: role of NF-κB. Cell Immunol 185:49–58.

87. King KL, D'Anza JJ, Bodary S, Pitti R, Siegel M, Lazarus RA, et al. (1994) Effects of kistrin on bone resorption

in vitro and serum calcium in vivo. J Bone Miner Res 9:381–7.

88. Klemke RL, Leng J, Molander R, Brooks PC, Vuori K, Cheresh DA (1998) CAS/Crk coupling serves as a "molecular switch" for induction of cell migration. J Cell Biol 140:961–72.

89. Klingmuller U, Lorenz U, Cantley LC, Neel BG, Lodish HF (1995) Specific recruitment of SH-PTP1 to the erythropoietin receptor causes inactivation of JAK2 and termination of proliferative signals. Cell 80:729–38.

90. Kobayashi N, Kadono Y, Naito A, Matumoto K, Yamamoto T, Tanaka S, et al. (2001) Segregation of TRAF6-mediated signaling pathways clarifies its role in osteoclastogenesis. EMBO J 20:1271–80.

91. Kornak U, Kasper D, Bosl MR, Kaiser E, Schweizer M, Schulz A, et al. (2001) Loss of the ClC-7 chloride channel leads to osteopetrosis in mice and man. Cell 104:205–15.

92. Kornak U, Schulz A, Friedrich W, Uhlhaas S, Kremens B, Voit T, et al. (2000) Mutations in the a3 subunit of the vacuolar H(+)-ATPase cause infantile malignant osteopetrosis. Hum Mol Genet 9:2059–63.

93. Krueger NX, Streuli M, Saito H (1990) Structural diversity and evolution of human receptor-like protein tyrosine phosphatases. EMBO J 9:3241–52.

94. Lacey DL, Timms E, Tan H-L, Kelley MJ, Dunstan CR, Burgess T, et al. (1998) Osteoprotegerin ligand is a cytokine that regulates osteoclast differentiation and activation. Cell 93:165–76.

95. Lakkakorpi PT, Nakamura I, Nagy RM, Parsons JT, Rodan GA, Duong LT (1999) Stable association of PYK2 and p130^{Cas} in osteoclasts and their co-localization in the sealing zone. J Biol Chem 274:4900–7.

96. Lakkakorpi PT, Nakamura I, Young M, Lipfert L, Rodan GA, Duong LT (2001) Abnormal localisation and hyperclustering of $\alpha_V\beta_3$ integrins and associated proteins in Src-deficient or tyrphostin A9-treated osteoclasts. J Cell Sci 114:149–60.

97. Lakkakorpi PT, Vaananen HK (1991) Kinetics of the osteoclast cytoskeleton during the resorption cycle in vitro. J Bone Miner Res 6:817–26.

98. Lakkakorpi PT, Wesolowski G, Zimolo Z, Rodan GA, Rodan SB (1997) Phosphatidylinositol 3-kinase association with the osteoclast cytoskeleton, and its involvement in osteoclast attachment and spreading. Exp Cell Res 237:296–306.

99. Lee PSW, Wang Y, Dominguez MG, Yeung Y-G, Murphy MA, Bowtell DDL, et al. (1999) The Cbl protooncoprotein stimulates CSF-1 receptor multiubiquitination and endocytosis, and attenuates macrophage proliferation. EMBO J 18:3616–28.

100. Lee SW, Han SI, Kim HH, Lee ZH (2002) TAK1-dependent activation of AP-1 and c-Jun N-terminal kinase by receptor activator of NF-κB. J Biochem Mol Biol 35:371–6.

101. Levkowitz G, Waterman H, Ettenberg SA, Katz M, Tsygankov AY, Alroy I, et al. (1999) Ubiquitin ligase activity and tyrosine phosphorylation underlie suppression of growth factor signaling by c-Cbl/Sli-1. Mol Cell 4:1029–40.

102. Li J, Sarosi I, Yan X-Q, Morony S, Capparelli C, Tan H-L, et al. (2000) RANK is the intrinsic hematopoietic cell surface receptor that controls osteoclastogenesis and regulation of bone mass and calcium metabolism. Proc Natl Acad Sci USA 97:1566–71.

103. Li L, Dixon JE (2000) Form, function, and regulation of protein tyrosine phosphatases and their involvement in human diseases. Semin Immunol 12:75–84.

104. Li X, Udagawa N, Itoh K, Suda K, Murase Y, Nishihara T, et al. (2002) p38 MAPK-mediated signals are required for inducing osteoclast differentiation but not for osteoclast function. Endocrinology 143:3105–13.

105. Li Y-P, Chen W, Liang Y, Li E, Stashenko P (1999) *Atp6i*-deficient mice exhibit severe osteopetrosis due to loss of osteoclast-mediated extracellular acidification. Nat Genet 23:447–51.

106. Lomaga MA, Yeh W-C, Sarosi I, Duncan GS, Furlonger C, Ho A, et al. (1999) TRAF6 deficiency results in osteopetrosis and defective interleukin-1, CD40, and LPS signaling. Genes Dev 13:1015–24.

107. Lorenz U, Ravichandran KS, Burakoff SJ, Neel BG (1996) Lack of SHPTP1 results in *src*-family kinase hyperactivation and thymocyte hyperresponsiveness. Proc Natl Acad Sci USA 93:9624–9.

108. Lowell CA, Niwa M, Soriano P, Varmus HE (1996) Deficiency of the Hck and Src tyrosine kinases results in extreme levels of extramedullary hematopoiesis. Blood 87:1780–92.

109. Ma YL, Cain RL, Halladay DL, Yang X, Zeng Q, Miles RR, et al. (2001) Catabolic effects of continuous human PTH (1–38) *in vivo* is associated with sustained stimulation of RANKL and inhibition of osteoprotegerin and gene-associated bone formation. Endocrinology 142:4047–54.

110. Mansky KC, Sankar U, Han J, Ostrowski MC (2002) Microphthalmia transcription factor is a target of the p38 MAPK pathway in response to receptor activator of NF-κB ligand signaling. J Biol Chem 277:11077–83.

111. Masarachia P, Yamamoto M, Leu CT, Rodan G, Duong L (1998) Histomorphometric evidence for echistatin inhibition of bone resorption in mice with secondary hyperparathyroidism. Endocrinology 139:1401–10.

112. Matsumoto M, Sudo T, Saito T, Osada H, Tsujimoto M (2000) Involvement of p38 mitogen-activated protein kinase signaling pathway in osteoclastogenesis mediated by receptor activator of NF-κB ligand (RANKL). J Biol Chem 275:31155–61.

113. Matthews RJ, Bowne DB, Flores E, Thomas ML (1992) Characterization of hematopoietic intracellular protein tyrosine phosphatases: description of a phosphatase containing an SH2 domain and another enriched in proline-, glutamic acid-, serine-, and threonine-rich sequences. Mol Cell Biol 12:2396–405.

114. Mauro LJ, Olmsted EA, Davis AR, Dixon JE (1996) Parathyroid hormone regulates the expression of the receptor protein tyrosine phosphatase, OST-PTP, in rat osteoblast-like cells. Endocrinology 137:925–33.

115. Mauro LJ, Olmsted EA, Skrobacz BM, Mourey RJ, Davis AR, Dixon JE (1994) Identification of a hormonally regulated protein tyrosine phosphatase associated with bone and testicular differentiation. J Biol Chem 269:30659–67.

116. McHugh KP, Hodivala-Dilke K, Zheng M-H, Namba N, Lam J, Novack D, et al. (2000) Mice lacking β3 integrins are osteosclerotic because of dysfunctional osteoclasts. J Clin Invest 105:433–40.

117. Miyazaki T, Katagiri H, Kanegae Y, Takayanagi H, Sawada Y, Yamamoto A, et al. (2000) Reciprocal role of ERK and NF-κB pathways in survival and activation of osteoclasts. J Cell Biol 148:333–42.

118. Miyazaki T, Neff L, Tanaka S, Horne WC, Baron R (2003) Regulation of cytochrome c oxidase activity by c-Src in osteoclasts. J Cell Biol 160:709–18.

119. Mizukami J, Takaesu G, Akatsuka H, Sakurai H, Ninomiya-Tsuji J, Matsumoto K, et al. (2002) Receptor activator of NF-κB ligand (RANKL) activates TAK1 mitogen-activated protein kinase kinase kinase through a signaling complex containing RANK, TAB2, and TRAF6. Mol Cell Biol 22:992–1000.

120. Moller NPH, Moller KB, Lammers R, Kharitonenkov A, Hoppe E, Wiberg FC, et al. (1995) Selective down-regulation of the insulin receptor signal by protein-tyrosine phosphatases α and ε. J Biol Chem 270: 23126–31.

121. Nakamura I, Jimi E, Duong LT, Sasaki T, Takahashi N, Rodan GA, et al. (1998) Tyrosine phosphorylation of p130^{Cas} is involved in actin organization in osteoclasts. J Biol Chem 273:11144–9.

122. Nakamura I, Lipfert L, Rodan GA, Duong LT (2001) Convergence of α$_v$β$_3$ integrin- and macrophage colony stimulating factor-mediated signals on phospholipase Cγ in prefusion osteoclasts. J Cell Biol 152: 361–73.

123. Nakamura I, Pilkington MF, Lakkakorpi PT, Lipfert L, Sims SM, Dixon SJ, et al. (1999) Role of α$_v$β$_3$ integrin in osteoclast migration and formation of the sealing zone. J Cell Sci 112:3985–93.

124. Nakamura I, Takahashi N, Sasaki T, Jimi E, Kurokawa T, Suda T (1996) Chemical and physical properties of the extracellular matrix are required for the actin ring formation in osteoclasts. J Bone Miner Res 11:1873–9.

125. Nakamura I, Takahashi N, Sasaki T, Tanaka S, Udagawa N, Murakami H, et al. (1995) Wortmannin, a specific inhibitor of phosphatidylinositol-3 kinase, blocks osteoclastic bone resorption. FEBS Lett 361:79–84.

126. Nakamura I, Tanaka H, Rodan GA, Duong LT (1998) Echistatin inhibits the migration of murine prefusion osteoclasts and the formation of multinucleated osteoclast-like cells. Endocrinology 139:5182–93.

127. Nakamura K, Mizuno Y, Kikuchi K (1996) Molecular cloning of a novel cytoplasmic protein tyrosine phosphatase PTP ε. Biochem Biophys Res Commun 218: 726–32.

128. Naro F, Perez M, Migliaccio S, Galson DL, Orcel P, Teti A, et al. (1998) Phospholipase D- and protein kinase C isoenzyme-dependent signal transduction pathways activated by the calcitonin receptor. Endocrinology 139:3241–8.

129. Nesbitt S, Nesbit A, Helfrich M, Horton M (1993) Biochemical characterization of human osteoclast integrins. Osteoclasts express α$_v$β$_3$, α$_2$β$_1$, and α$_v$β$_1$ integrins. J Biol Chem 268:16737–45.

130. Nesbitt SA, Horton MA (1997) Trafficking of matrix collagens through bone-resorbing osteoclasts. Science 276:266–9.

131. Ota J, Sato K, Kimura F, Wakimoto N, Nakamura Y, Nagata N, et al. (2000) Association of Cbl with Fms and p85 in response to macrophage colony-stimulating factor. FEBS Lett 466:96–100.

132. Palacio S, Felix R (2001) The role of phosphoinositide 3-kinase in spreading osteoclasts induced by colony-stimulating factor-1. Eur J Endocrinol 144:431–40.

133. Paloneva J, Kestila M, Wu J, Salminen A, Bohling T, Ruotsalainen V, et al. (2000) Loss-of-function mutations in TYROBP (DAP12) result in a presenile dementia with bone cysts. Nat Genet 25:357–61.

134. Paloneva J, Manninen T, Christman G, Hovanes K, Mandelin J, Adolfsson R, et al. (2002) Mutations in two genes encoding different subunits of a receptor signaling complex result in an identical disease phenotype. Am J Hum Genet 71:656–62.

135. Paniccia R, Riccioni T, Zani BM, Zigrino P, Scotlandi K, Teti A (1995) Calcitonin down-regulates immediate cell signals induced in human osteoclast-like cells by the bone sialoprotein-IIA fragment through a postintegrin receptor mechanism. Endocrinology 136:1177–86.

136. Plutzky J, Neel BG, Rosenberg RD (1992) Isolation of a src homology 2-containing tyrosine phosphatase. Proc Natl Acad Sci USA 89:1123–7.

137. Plutzky J, Neel BG, Rosenberg RD, Eddy RL, Byers MG, Jani-Sait S, et al. (1992) Chromosomal localization of an SH2-containing tyrosine phosphatase (PTPN6). Genomics 13:869–72.

138. Quinn JMW, Elliott J, Gillespie MT, Martin TJ (1998) A combination of osteoclast differentiation factor and macrophage-colony stimulating factor is sufficient for both human and mouse osteoclast formation in vitro. Endocrinology 139:4424–7.

139. Rajapurohitam V, Chalhoub N, Benachenhou N, Neff L, Baron R, Vacher J (2001) The mouse osteopetrotic grey-lethal mutation induces a defect in osteoclast maturation/function. Bone 28:513–23.

140. Saftig P, Hunziker E, Wehmeyer O, Jones S, Boyde A, Rommerskirch W, et al. (1998) Impaired osteoclastic bone resorption leads to osteopetrosis in cathepsin-K-deficient mice. Proc Natl Acad Sci USA 95:13453–8.

141. Salo J, Lehenkari P, Mulari M, Metsikko K, Vaananen HK (1997) Removal of osteoclast bone resorption products by transcytosis. Science 276:270–3.

142. Sanjay A, Horne WC, Baron R (2001) The Cbl family: ubiquitin ligases regulating signaling by tyrosine kinases. Science's STKE. http://stke.sciencemag.org/cgi/content/full/OC_sigtrans;2001/110/pe40.

143. Sanjay A, Houghton A, Neff L, Didomenico E, Bardelay C, Antoine E, et al. (2001) Cbl associates with Pyk2 and Src to regulate Src kinase activity, α$_v$β$_3$ integrin-mediated signaling, cell adhesion, and osteoclast motility. J Cell Biol 152:181–95.

144. Sato M, Sardana MK, Grasser WA, Garsky VM, Murray JM, Gould RJ (1990) Echistatin is a potent inhibitor of bone resorption in culture. J Cell Biol 111:1713–23.

145. Schlaepfer DD, Broome MA, Hunter T (1997) Fibronectin-stimulated signaling from a focal adhesion kinase-c-Src complex: involvement of the Grb2, p130^{cas}, and Nck adaptor proteins. Mol Cell Biol 17:1702–13.

146. Schlaepfer DD, Hauck CR, Sieg DJ (1999) Signaling through focal adhesion kinase. Prog Biophys Mol Biol 71:435–378.

147. Schlessinger J (2000) New roles for Src kinases in control of cell survival and angiogenesis. Cell 100: 293–6.

148. Schwartzberg PL, Xing L, Hoffmann O, Lowell CA, Garrett L, Boyce BF, et al. (1997) Rescue of osteoclast function by transgenic expression of kinase-deficient Src in src$^{-/-}$ mutant mice. Genes Dev 11:2835–44.

149. Scimeca JC, Franchi A, Trojani C, Parrinello H, Grosgeorge J, Robert C, et al. (2000) The gene encoding the mouse homologue of the human osteoclast-

specific 116-kDa V-ATPase subunit bears a deletion in osteosclerotic (*oc/oc*) mutants. Bone 26:207–13.

150. Shaw LM, Rabinovitz I, Wang HH-F, Toker A, Mercurio AM (1997) Activation of phosphoinositide 3-OH kinase by the α6β4 integrin promotes carcinoma invasion. Cell 91:949–60.

151. Shen S-H, Bastien L, Posner BI, Chretien P (1991) A protein-tyrosine phosphatase with sequence similarity to the SH2 domain of the protein-tyrosine kinases. Nature 352:736–9.

152. Shui C, Riggs BL, Khosla S (2002) The Immunosuppressant rapamycin, alone or with transforming growth factor-β, enhances osteoclast differentiation of RAW264.7 monocyte-macrophage cells in the presence of RANK-ligand. Calcif Tissue Int 71:437–46.

153. Shultz LD, Schweitzer PA, Rajan TV, Yi T, Ihle JN, Matthews RJ, et al. (1993) Mutations at the murine motheaten locus are within the hematopoietic cell protein-tyrosine phosphatase (*Hcph*) gene. Cell 73: 1445–54.

154. Shultz LD, Sidman CL (1987) Genetically determined murine models of immunodeficiency. Annu Rev Immunol 5:367–403.

155. Shyu J-F, Inoue D, Baron R, Horne WC (1996) The deletion of 14 amino acids in the seventh transmembrane domain of a naturally occurring calcitonin receptor isoform alters ligand binding and selectively abolishes coupling to phospholipase C. J Biol Chem 271:31127–34.

156. Shyu J-F, Zhang Z, Hernandez-Lagunas L, Camerino C, Chen Y, Inoue D, et al. (1999) Protein kinase C antagonizes pertussis-toxin-sensitive coupling of the calcitonin receptor to adenylyl cyclase. Eur J Biochem 262:95–101.

157. Simonet WS, Lacey DL, Dunstan CR, Kelley M, Chang M-S, Luthy R, et al. (1997) Osteoprotegerin: a novel secreted protein involved in the regulation of bone density. Cell 89:309–19.

158. Sims NA, Aoki K, Bogdanovich Z, Maragh M, Okigaki M, Logan S, et al. (1999) Impaired osteoclast function in Pyk2 knockout mice and cumulative effects in Pyk2/Src double knockout. J Bone Miner Res 14 (Suppl. 1):S183.

159. Sly WS, Hewett-Emmett D, Whyte MP, Yu Y-S, Tashian RE (1983) Carbonic anhydrase II deficiency identified as the primary defect in the autosomal recessive syndrome of osteopetrosis with renal tubular acidosis and cerebral calcification. Proc Natl Acad Sci USA 80: 2752–6.

160. Soriano P, Montgomery C, Geske R, Bradley A (1991) Targeted disruption of the c-src proto-oncogene leads to osteopetrosis in mice. Cell 64:693–702.

161. Suda T, Takahashi N, Udagawa N, Jimi E, Gillespie MT, Martin TJ (1999) Modulation of osteoclast differentiation and function by the new members of the tumor necrosis factor receptor and ligand families. Endocr Rev 20:345–57.

162. Suhr SM, Pamula S, Baylink DJ, Lau K-HW (2001) Antisense oligodeoxynucleotide evidence that a unique osteoclastic protein-tyrosine phosphatase is essential for osteoclastic resorption. J Bone Miner Res 16: 1795–1803.

163. Sully V, Pownall S, Vincan E, Bassal S, Borowski AH, Hart PH, et al. (2001) Functional abnormalities in protein tyrosine phosphatase ε-deficient macrophages. Biochem Biophys Res Commun 286:184–8.

164. Takayanagi H, Kim S, Matsuo K, Suzuki H, Suzuki T, Sato K, et al. (2002) RANKL maintains bone homeostasis through c-Fos-dependent induction of *interferon-β*. Nature 416:744–9.

165. Takayanagi H, Ogasawara K, Hida S, Chiba T, Murata S, Sato K, et al. (2000) T-cell-mediated regulation of osteoclastogenesis by signalling cross- talk between RANKL and IFN-γ. Nature 408:600–5.

166. Takeshita S, Namba N, Zhao JJ, Jiang Y, Genant HK, Silva MJ, et al. (2002) SHIP-deficient mice are severely osteoporotic due to increased numbers of hyper-resorptive osteoclasts. Nat Med 8:943–9.

167. Tanaka S, Amling M, Neff L, Peyman A, Uhlmann E, Levy JB, et al. (1996) c-Cbl is downstream of c-Src in a signalling pathway necessary for bone resorption. Nature 383:528–31.

168. Tanaka S, Neff L, Baron R, Levy JB (1995) Tyrosine phosphorylation and translocation of the c-Cbl protein after activation of tyrosine kinase signaling pathways. J Biol Chem 270:14347–51.

169. Tanuma N, Nakamura K, Kikuchi K (1999) Distinct promoters control transmembrane and cytosolic protein tyrosine phosphatase ε expression during macrophage differentiation. Eur J Biochem 259:46–54.

170. Tanuma N, Nakamura K, Shima H, Kikuchi K (2000) Protein-tyrosine phosphatase PTPεC inhibits Jak-STAT signaling and differentiation induced by interleukin-6 and leukemia inhibitory factor in M1 leukemia cells. J Biol Chem 275:28216–21.

171. Tanuma N, Shima H, Nakamura K, Kikuchi K (2001) Protein tyrosine phosphatase εC selectively inhibits interleukin-6- and interleukin- 10-induced JAK-STAT signaling. Blood 98:3030–4.

172. Tanuma N, Shima H, Shimada S, Kikuchi K (2003) Reduced tumorigenicity of murine leukemia cells expressing protein-tyrosine phosphatase, PTPεC. Oncogene 22:1758–62.

173. Teitelbaum SL (2000) Bone resorption by osteoclasts. Science 289:1504–8.

174. Thien CBF, Langdon WY (2001) Cbl: many adaptations to regulate protein tyrosine kinases. Nat Rev Mol Cell Biol 2:294–305.

175. Thomas SM, Brugge JS (1997) Cellular functions regulated by Src family kinases. Annu. Rev Cell Dev Biol 13:513–609.

176. Toledano-Katchalski H, Kraut J, Sines T, Granot-Attas S, Shohat G, Gil-Henn H, et al. (2003) Protein tyrosine phosphatase ε inhibits signaling by mitogen-activated protein kinases. Mol Cancer Res 1:541–50.

177. Tomic S, Greiser U, Lammers R, Kharitonenkov A, Imyanitov E, Ullrich A, et al. (1995) Association of SH2 domain protein tyrosine phosphatases with the epidermal growth factor receptor in human tumor cells. Phosphatidic acid activates receptor dephosphorylation by PTP1C. J Biol Chem 270:21277–84.

178. Tonks NK, Neel BG (2001) Combinatorial control of the specificity of protein tyrosine phosphatases. Curr Opin Cell Biol 13:182–95.

179. Umeda S, Beamer WG, Takagi K, Naito M, Hayashi S-I, Yonemitsu H, et al. (1999) Deficiency of SHP-1 protein-tyrosine phosphatase activity results in heightened osteoclast function and decreased bone density. Am J Pathol 155:223–33.

180. Vaananen HK, Karhukorpi EK, Sundquist K, Roininen I, Hentunen T, Tuukkanen J, et al. (1990) Evidence for the presence of a proton pump of the vacuolar H⁺-

ATPase type in the ruffled border of osteoclasts. J Cell Biol 111:1305–11.

181. Vaananen HK, Zhao H, Mulari M, Halleen JM (2000) The cell biology of osteoclast function. J Cell Sci 113: 377–81.

182. Vuori K, Hirai H, Aizawa S, Ruoslahti E (1996) Introduction of p130^{cas} signaling complex formation upon integrin-mediated cell adhesion: a role for Src family kinases. Mol Cell Biol 16:2606–13.

183. Wabakken T, Hauge H, Finne EF, Wiedlocha A, Aasheim H (2002) Expression of human protein tyrosine phosphatase epsilon in leucocytes: a potential ERK pathway-regulating phosphatase. Scand J Immunol 56: 195–203.

184. Wei S, Wang MW-H, Teitelbaum SL, Ross FP (2002) Interleukin-4 reversibly inhibits osteoclastogenesis via inhibition of NF-κB and mitogen-activated protein kinase signaling. J Biol Chem 277:6622–30.

185. Weinreb M, Halperin D (1998) Rat osteoclast precursors in vivo express a vitronectin receptor and a chloride-bicarbonate exchanger. Connect Tissue Res 37:177–82.

186. Wennerberg K, Lohikangas L, Gullberg D, Pfaff M, Johansson S, Fassler R (1996) β1 integrin-dependent and -independent polymerization of fibronectin. J Cell Biol 132:227–38.

187. Witke W, Sharpe AH, Hartwig JH, Azuma T, Stossel TP, Kwiatkowski DJ (1995) Hemostatic, inflammatory, and fibroblast responses are blunted in mice lacking gelsolin. Cell 81:41–51.

188. Wong BR, Besser D, Kim N, Arron JR, Vologodskaia M, Hanafusa H, et al. (1999) TRANCE, a TNF family member, activates Akt/PKB through a signaling complex involving TRAF6 and c-Src. Mol Cell 4:1041–9.

189. Wu C, Hughes PE, Ginsberg MH, McDonald JA (1996) Identification of a new biological function for the integrin α$_v$β$_3$: initiation of fibronectin matrix assembly. Cell Adhes Commun 4:149–58.

190. Wu H, Byrne MH, Stacey A, Goldring MB, Birkhead JR, Jaenisch R, et al. (1990) Generation of collagenase-resistant collagen by site-directed mutagenesis of murine proα1(I) collagen gene. Proc Natl Acad Sci USA 87:5888–92.

191. Wu L-W, Baylink DJ, Lau K-H (1996) Molecular cloning and expression of a unique rabbit osteoclastic phosphotyrosyl phosphatase. Biochem J 316:515–23.

192. Xing L, Bushnell TP, Carlson L, Tai Z, Tondravi M, Siebenlist U, et al. (2002) NF-κB p50 and p52 expression is not required for RANK-expressing osteoclast progenitor formation but is essential for RANK- and cytokine-mediated osteoclastogenesis. J Bone Miner Res 17:1200–10.

193. Yamamoto A, Miyazaki T, Kadono Y, Takayanagi H, Miura T, Nishina H, et al. (2002) Possible involvement of IκB kinase 2 and MKK7 in osteoclastogenesis induced by receptor activator of nuclear factor κB ligand. J Bone Miner Res 17:612–21.

194. Yamamoto M, Fisher JE, Gentile M, Seedor JG, Leu C-T, Rodan SB, et al. (1998) The integrin ligand echistatin prevents bone loss in ovariectomized mice and rats. Endocrinology 139:1411–19.

195. Yan T, Riggs BL, Boyle WJ, Khosla S (2001) Regulation of osteoclastogenesis and RANK expression by TGF-β1. J Cell Biochem 83:320–5.

196. Yi T, Ihle JN (1993) Association of hematopoietic cell phosphatase with c-Kit after stimulation with c-Kit ligand. Mol Cell Biol 13:3350–8.

197. Yi T, Mui AL, Krystal G, Ihle JN (1993) Hematopoietic cell phosphatase associates with the interleukin-3 (IL-3) receptor beta chain and down-regulates IL-3-induced tyrosine phosphorylation and mitogenesis. Mol Cell Biol 13:7577–86.

198. Yi TL, Cleveland JL, Ihle JN (1992) Protein tyrosine phosphatase containing SH2 domains: characterization, preferential expression in hematopoietic cells, and localization to human chromosome 12p12-p13. Mol Cell Biol 12:836–46.

199. Yokouchi M, Kondo T, Houghton A, Bartkiewicz M, Horne WC, Zhang H, et al. (1999) Ligand-induced ubiquitination of the epidermal growth factor receptor involves the interaction of the c-Cbl RING finger and UbcH7. J Biol. Chem 274:31707–12.

200. Yu Z, Su L, Hoglinger O, Jaramillo ML, Banville D, Shen SH (1998) SHP-1 associates with both platelet-derived growth factor receptor and the p85 subunit of phosphatidylinositol 3-kinase. J Biol Chem 273:3687–9364.

201. Zaidi M, Datta HK, Moonga BS, MacIntyre I (1990) Evidence that the action of calcitonin on rat osteoclasts is mediated by two G proteins acting via separate postreceptor pathways. J Endocrinol 126:473–81.

202. Zhang X, Chattopadhyay A, Ji QS, Owen JD, Ruest PJ, Carpenter G, et al. (1999) Focal adhesion kinase promotes phospholipase C-γ1 activity. Proc Natl Acad Sci USA 96:9021–6.

203. Zhang Z, Baron R, Horne WC (2000) Integrin engagement, the actin cytoskeleton, and c-Src are required for the calcitonin-induced tyrosine phosphorylation of paxillin and HEF1, but not for calcitonin-induced Erk1/2 phosphorylation. J Biol Chem 275:37219–23.

204. Zhang Z, Hernandez-Lagunas L, Horne WC, Baron R (1999) Cytoskeleton-dependent tyrosine phosphorylation of the maily member HEF1 downstream of the G protein-couopled calcitonin receptor. Calcitonin induces the association of HEF1, paxillin, and focal adhesion of kinase. J Biol Chem 274:25093–8.

205. Zimolo Z, Weolowski G, Tanaka H, Hyman JL, Hoyer JR, Rodan GA (1994) Soluble α$_v$β$_3$-integrin ligands raise [Ca2+]I in rat osteoclasts and mouse-derived osteoclast-like cells. Am J Physiol 266:C376–81.

4.

Structural Aspects of Bone Resorption

Steven D. Bain and Ted S. Gross

Introduction

The skeleton is a metabolically active organ system, comprised of tissue-specific cells and an extracellular matrix that undergoes continuous removal and replacement throughout life. At a fundamental level, the removal and replacement of the extracellular matrix is necessary to establish and maintain bone mass and architecture. However, the removal and replacement of the matrix is regulated within a physiologic framework that requires the bone tissue to function simultaneously in locomotion, as support and site of muscle attachment, as a protector of vital internal organs, and as a storehouse of calcium and phosphorus ions. Interestingly, these diverse structural and metabolic functions are principally driven by the interplay between just two cell types; the bone-resorbing osteoclast and the bone-forming osteoblast. Moreover, it is recognized that the interplay between osteoclast and osteoblast must be finely balanced as even minor disturbances in the resorbing and forming activities of these cell types can lead to both structural and metabolic pathologies.

From a structural perspective, it is the osteoclast that is responsible for initiating the bone renewal process, which in the adult skeleton is termed bone remodeling. Thus, it is only by first removing preexisting bone matrix that the tissue is able to alter its shape and morphology in response to the demands engendered by locomotor and/or metabolic stimuli. The objective of this chapter is to provide an overview of the structural aspects of this process with a specific focus on the osteoclastic behaviors that modulate bone mass and architecture.

Resorption of Cortical Bone

Bone remodeling in the adult skeleton is the process whereby bone matrix is first removed by osteoclasts and then replaced by osteoblasts. The cellular basis of the remodeling cycle was first described by Frost, who named this physiologic relationship the basic multicellular unit or the BMU [26, 28]. Known also as a bone remodeling unit or BRU [70], the BMU describes the sequential activities of osteoclasts and osteoblasts that are spatially and temporally coupled to ensure that the removal of mineralized matrix is replaced by an equivalent quantity of new bone [27, 48, 69]. Thus, over innumerable remodeling cycles the collective activities of individual BMUs ensure that an organism's bone mass remains in constant balance and its skeletal architecture relatively unchanged [29, 43, 71].

It is now evident from investigations of the bone remodeling cycle that the skeleton's mass and its corresponding architecture are dependent on the coordinated activity of the BMU, which is commonly separated into four distinct phases: activation, resorption, reversal, and formation [71, 85, 93, 94]. In both cortical and cancellous bone, the BMU life cycle begins with the activation of a quiescent (i.e., resting) bone surface in response to an enabling stimulus that triggers differentiation and recruitment of osteoclast precursors, which fuse to form mature, multinucleated, bone-resorbing osteoclasts (for review see [91]). The multinucleated osteoclast then attaches to and transits over the bone surface, dissolving and resorbing the mineralized matrix. In this fashion, groups of osteoclasts are recruited to the resorption site until a discrete packet or quantum of bone matrix is removed [28, 30, 36, 40, 69, 71]. As the osteoclastic activity subsides, a resorption cavity, termed a Howship's lacunae, is formed [35].

Within this anatomic framework the structural outcomes that result from bone resorption are more difficult to assess than those arising from bone formation, simply because the osteoclast behaviors must be inferred from the anatomic changes that result from osteoclast resorption, whereas osteoblast activity creates a mineralized record that can be measured directly [16, 20, 70, 75]. This limitation not withstanding, reconstruction of the BMU in cortical bone (Figure 4.1) has provided the basis for quantifying the spatial and temporal behavior of osteoclasts in bone resorption [48, 76, 77]. Spatially, the activation of the osteoclast machinery in cortical bone populates a resorptive front that tunnels through the cortex. The apex of this structure is termed the cutting cone [44]. Data from studies in non-human primates [70, 88] and canines [39] indicate that osteoclasts are able to tunnel longitudinally at rates of 35–40 µm per day. Furthermore, as the resorption front proceeds through the cortex it expands radially at a rate of about 6–7 µm per day, which reflects the matrix resorbing capacity of the individual osteoclast [20, 70]. These data are similar to those reported in human subjects [70]. The resorptive tunnel excavated by the osteoclasts is eventually filled in by osteoblastic bone formation, producing a mature

lamellar structure that is termed a bone structural unit or BSU [36]. This structure is also known as Haversian canal or a secondary osteon.

Studies of the temporal nature of osteoclastic activity have shown that the time to complete resorption at one BMU level (i.e., the resorption sigma), is 9–15 days, depending on the species [70]. This time period is roughly equivalent to the 10–12-day life span of individual osteoclasts [38], which at a longitudinal resorption rate of 35 µm per day would burrow several hundred µm through the cortex. However, as the completed BSU is from 2–6 mm in length, it is evident that the intracortical progression of bone remodeling requires the continual recruitment and mobilization of osteoclasts. This recruitment has been substantiated by autoradiographic studies conducted in dogs which have shown that the entry of new nuclei into the osteoclast population is approximately 8% per day [37]. Thus, when the life span and resorption rates of individual osteoclasts are superimposed over the spatial construct of a cortical bone BMU it becomes possible to define a structure that travels roughly 4,000 µm through the cortex at about 20 µm per day, with a life span of 200 days [79].

When considering the impact that normal Haversian remodeling has on cortical bone structure it can be assumed that the process of bone resorption is ultimately governed by the physiologic purposes of bone remodeling [76]. Bone remodeling replaces old bone with new, a stochastic process that prevents mean bone age from exceeding an acceptable level [5, 56, 74, 79, 84], and is a directed process that removes bone matrix that is micro- or macroscopically damaged [4, 7, 25, 53, 62], or has been function-

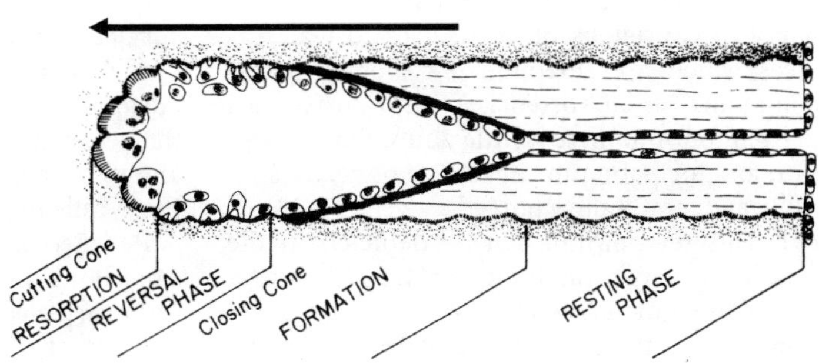

Figure 4.1 Diagram of a longitudinal section of a cortical BMU or Haversian system. The cortical BMU moves toward the left behind the resorptive front which is termed the cutting cone. By covering the upper half of the diagram it is possible to visualize the structure of the BMU in cancellous bone. (Reproduced from Baron R 2003 General Principles of Bone Biology. In Favus M (ed.) *Primer on the Metabolic Bone Diseases and Disorders of Mineral Metabolism*, 5th ed. American Society for Bone and Mineral Research, Washington DC, USA, pp. 1–8 with permission of the Amercian Society for Bone and Mineral Research)

ally suboptimal [14, 50, 51, 66, 86, 95]. Regardless of the remodeling stimuli, the amount of normal adult skeleton undergoing intracortical remodeling at any point in time is about 5% [70]. Therefore, given the evolutionary success of terrestrial vertebrates, it is likely that this underlying level of remodeling (and by inference, resorptive activity) has been genetically programmed to maintain the skeleton's structural competence [77].

Within this evolutionary context, Martin has proposed that stochastic osteoclast tunneling would have the effect of frequently replacing osteocytes so that the homeostatic function of the osteocyte network remains intact [58]. Furthermore, targeted osteoclastic resorption would not only serve to remove microdamage [6, 79], but also the new fiber-matrix structure created by the BMU. It is clear that multiple factors are involved in selecting for osteoclast behaviors that are structurally beneficial [79] and that these behaviors need not be 100% efficient to repair tissue. Indeed, Parfitt argues convincingly that most remodeling is "redundant, surplus, spare or stochastic" [78], as evidenced by the lack of harm caused by low bone turnover in hypothyroid [22] and hypoparathyroid states [49]. Conversely, it is important to note that recent experimental evidence indicates that bisphosphonates can suppress both targeted and non-targeted remodeling, which may lead to the accumulation of microdamage [54]. However, the extent to which the suppression of remodeling by therapeutic agents actually clinically compromises the skeleton's functional role remains to be elucidated.

Resorption of Cancellous Bone

Because of its solid nature, the replacement of cortical bone occurs only at sites where bone has been resorbed by osteoclasts recruited for that purpose. This physical constraint does not apply to cancellous or cortical endosteal surfaces which are surrounded by open spaces containing both osteoclast and osteoblast progenitors, but there is little doubt that resorption and formation in cancellous bone are spatially and temporally coupled as well [27–29, 68, 69]. This relationship can be depicted in the classic "up-down" or life-cycle diagram represented in Figure 4.2, which faithfully reflects the sequential nature of BMU activities at discrete two-dimensional locations.

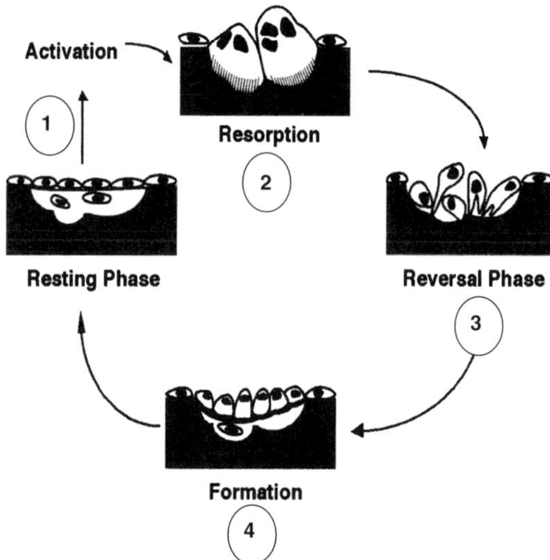

Figure 4.2   Two-dimensional representation of the life cycle stages of the BMU on a cancellous bone surface. Activation of a resting surface (1) results in the recruitment and activation of bone resorbing osteoclasts, which work in teams to resorb bone matrix (2). Osteoclastic resorption subsides during the reversal phase (3) at which time osteoblasts are recruited to refill the resorption cavity with organic matrix (4) that subsequently mineralizes, returning the remodeling site to the resting or quiescent phase. (Reproduced from Baron R 2003 General Principles of Bone Biology. In Favus M (ed.) *Primer on the Metabolic Bone Diseases and Disorders of Mineral Metabolism*, 5th ed. American Society for Bone and Mineral Research, Washington DC, USA, pp. 1–8 with permission of the Amercian Society for Bone and Mineral Research.)

However, such representations ignore the two-dimensional organization of cancellous BMUs and promote the mistaken concept that osteoclasts and osteoblasts are never present at the same BMU simultaneously [82]. In actuality, the cancellous BMU is hemi-osteonal in nature [31, 76], with the principal difference that rather than boring a cylindrical tunnel through the cortex (as depicted in Figure 4.1) the osteoclasts resorb a trench-like structure across the bone's surface (Figure 4.3) [15]. The hemi-osteonal model of the cancellous BMU has the added advantage of depicting the cellular relationships that exist within the remodeling space, which allows for a more accurate visualization of how these cells might communicate *in vivo* [76].

Reconstruction of the resorptive phase in cancellous bone has revealed at least four distinct variables associated with bone resorption: erosion depth, active erosion period, erosion rate, and bone resorption rate [20]. Of these

Figure 4.3 A diagrammatic representation of the cancellous BMU based on a histomorphometric reconstruction that shows the duration and depth of the phases of the bone remodeling sequence. (Reproduced with permission form Eriksen EF, Axelrod DW, Melsen F. Bone Histomorphometry. Lippincott Williams & Wilkins. 1994, 7.)

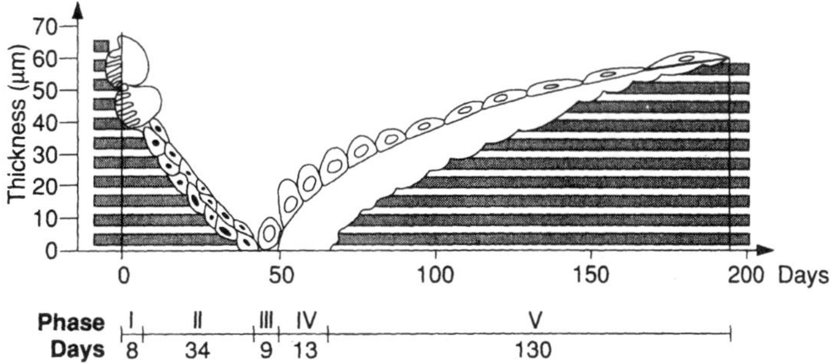

Table 4.1. Methodology for measuring cancellous bone resorption depths (i.e., erosion depth) that have been reported in the literature (modified from Compston and Croucher [9]).

Reference	Methodology	Resorption Depth (μm)
Eriksen et al. [17]	Erosion depths are measured by counting the number of eroded lamellae that are microscopically identified below a) osteoclasts, b) mononuclear cells, and c) preosteoblast-like cells. The number of lamellae is then multiplied by the lamellar thickness.	a) 19.0 b) 49.1 c) 62.6
Eriksen et al. [21]	Age-related differences in resorption depth of lacunae underlying preosteoblastic cells measured by counting lamellae in a) females and b) males	a) 57.2 b) 55.0
Palle et al. [67]	Erosion depths determined by counting lamellae but without cell characterization in a) middle-aged males (33 yr), b) elderly males (67 yr), and c) elderly females (64 yr).	a) 33.0 b) 28.9 c) 27.2
Eriksen et al. [18]	Maximum erosion depth was determined as in [17] and [21] for a) osteoporotics and b) age-matched controls	a) 55.0 b) 49.1[a]
Croucher et al. [10]	Eroded bone surface is reconstructed by fitting a smooth line connecting the bone surface on each side of a resorption cavity. The line is used as baseline to determine mean and maximum erosion depths. Values were determined for a) females and b) males.	a) 15.7[b] b) 17.0[b]
Cohen-Solal et al. [8]	Erosion depth determined at sites where resorption had been completed. The bone surface was reconstructed by drawing a line joining the adjacent quiescent surfaces, creating a smooth contour over resorption site. Orthogonal intercept lines were then drawn between this contour and closest cement line.	40.8

Values for resorption depth represent mean values, [a]median, or [b]geometric mean.

variables, erosion depth has the greatest impact on bone structure as it relates directly to the quantum (i.e., packet) of bone that must be replaced by osteoblastic bone formation [8, 9]. Consequently, if the bone formed in the resorption cavity is insufficient to replace the amount resorbed, due either to an increase in the amount resorbed, a decrease in the amount formed, or some combination of the two, a negative balance and a potentially irreversible bone loss will occur at the remodeling site.

As in cortical bone, osteoclast behaviors and their outcomes, including erosion depths, must be inferred from what has been removed. Several methods exist for measuring erosion depth and each involves reconstruction of the resorption cavity. While a detailed explanation of each method and the morphometric assumptions associated with their application is beyond the scope of this chapter, Table 4.1 summarizes the basic methodologies that have been used to assess bone resorption and the results from several prominent investigations. Perhaps not surprisingly, the values for erosion depth vary, depending on the methodology employed. However, it is instructive to note that when resorption cavities are filled with new bone, the resulting values for wall width are less variable. Indeed, the values for wall width in normal subjects are generally on the order of 40–50 μm [11, 16, 55, 61, 80, 89, 90], which indicates that erosion depth values less than 40 μm are most likely underestimating the structural impact of osteoclast resorption.

Structural Implications of Bone Resorption

Regardless of the methodological debate surrounding measurement of erosion depth, there is no argument about the importance of osteoclastic resorption in the maintenance of bone mass and tissue architecture. As discussed previously, intracortical and cancellous bone resorption are clearly initiating events in the removal of aged [5, 56, 74, 79, 84] and/or damaged bone tissue [4, 7, 25, 53, 62], which is subsequently replaced by osteoblastic bone formation. This activity serves continually to rejuvenate the bone mineral and optimizes bone architecture in response to functional loading [14, 50, 64, 66, 95]. Recent studies have also provided insight into how osteoclast resorption participates in the modification of cancellous bone structures to increase bone mass. Specifi-

cally, longitudinal tunneling of trabeculae that have been thickened by parathyroid hormone treatment has been shown to convert them into multiple trabeculae (Figure 4.5). These trabeculae have a normal thickness, but the resulting increase in trabecular number has a positive effect on cancellous bone volumes [42].

The ability of the osteoclast to modify bone structure can also be substantiated by studies that have classified resorption lacunae according to their microstructural profiles. In that regard, Gentzsch et al. [33] have used light and scanning electron microscopy to show that osteoclasts not only resorb cancellous bone in the familiar hemi-osteonal fashion (i.e., longitudinally extended resorption lacunae), but they also sculpt bone surfaces in reticulate patches. The reticulate patch morphology is particularly reminiscent of the resorption pits that have been observed when osteoclasts resorb mineralized matrices *in vitro* [45, 65].

In addition to the osteoclasts' role in maintaining and/or modifying normal bone structure, osteoclastic activities are major contributors to cancellous bone pathologies. For example, in osteoporosis, the early, rapid bone loss experienced at the menopause is the result of osteoclast hyperactivity and increased resorption depth [2, 18, 19, 81], which leads to focal trabecular perforations and subsequent loss of complete structural elements [3, 9, 73, 81]. These perforations occur either via direct tunneling through individual trabeculae [33] or by excessive lacunar resorption on trabecular surfaces [33, 63]. The net result of such activity is the conversion of the plate-like cancellous

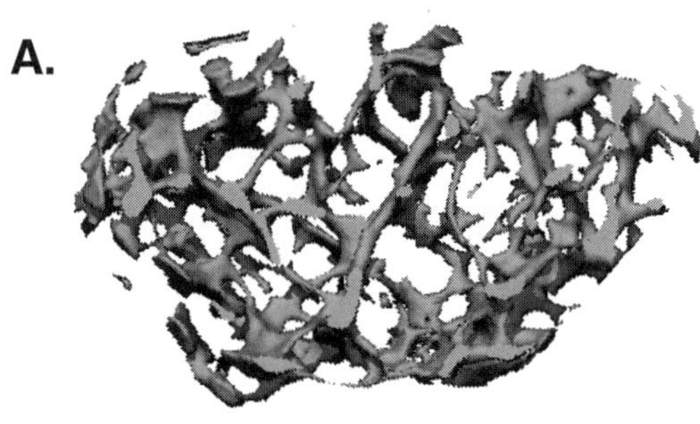

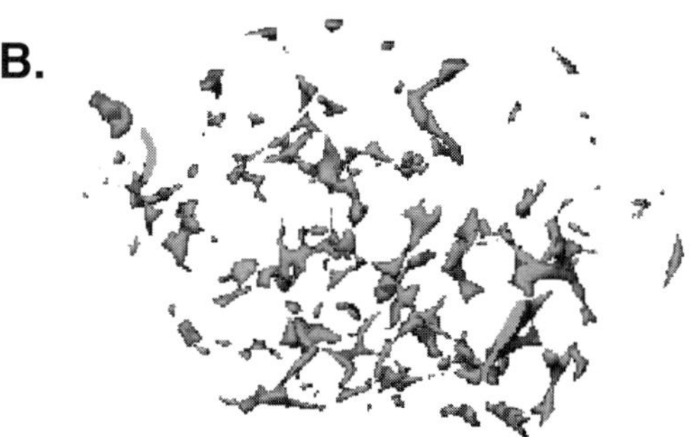

Figure 4.4 Three-dimensional micro-CT images of trabeculae from the distal femur of C57/B6 mice. The normal highly connected trabecular structure (A) is drastically eroded by just 3 weeks of limb disuse (B).

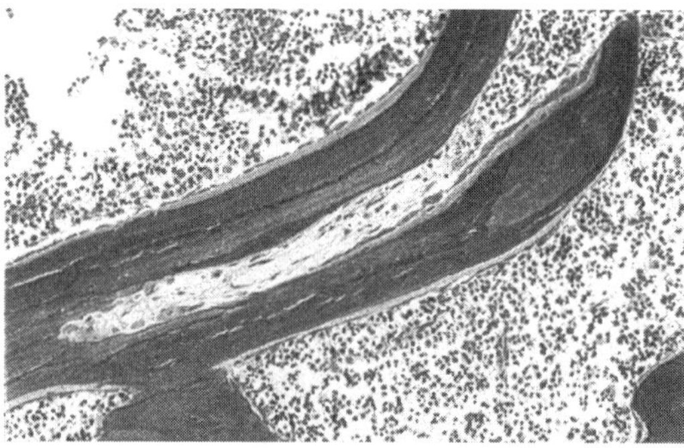

Figure 4.5 Photomicrograph of osteoclast cutting cone in cancellous bone of non-human primate treated with parathyroid hormone. The cutting cone is dividing a single, thickened trabeculae into two trabeculae of normal thickness.

structure to rods [81, 83], producing a disproportionate loss of strength due to loss of connectivity [72, 73]. This weakness in the trabecular structure is only partially compensated for by the increased thickness of the remaining trabeculae.

The structural pathologies documented by bone histomorphometry have been substantiated by Thomsen et al. [92], who have used a computer simulation model to demonstrate that the number of cancellous perforations was correlated with the final resorption depth. In addition, analysis of digital microimages of trabecular bone obtained by *in vivo* magnetic resonance imaging attributed the perforation of trabecular plates and rods to osteoclastic resorption [96]. Furthermore, microCT analyses of tibial cancellous bone have yielded three-dimensional confirmation of the age-related conversion of the cancellous bone structure from plates to rods [12]. However, it should be emphasized that even though osteoclast hyperactivity and increased erosion depth may serve as the catalyst for trabecular perforations, the incomplete filling of resorption cavities by osteoblasts still plays a major role in the structural pathologies associated with osteoporotic bone loss [18, 71, 92].

While there is an extensive literature detailing how bone structure is altered by postmenopausal estrogen depletion and aging, both pathologies result from changes in osteoclast and osteoblast function that occur over a time course of years. In contrast, changes in bone structure induced by disuse occur much more rapidly, providing a means to explore the question of how bone resorption affects bone structure without the confounding influence of systemic abnormalities and metabolic insufficiencies.

Disuse-engendered bone resorption is precipitated when the bone's normal loading environment is withdrawn or substantially diminished. Thus, disuse-induced bone loss is provoked by a variety of conditions, including extended bedrest or motor-neuron-deficiency induced paralysis [23, 47]. Distinct from bone loss induced by perturbations of systemic hormones or cytokines, disuse-induced bone loss is confined to the bones deprived of loading. The specific stimulus for disuse induced osteoclastogenesis is relatively unexplored, but it has been speculated that the loss of physical stimuli directly removes some factor inhibiting forma-

tion of osteoclasts from marrow precursors [87]. Alternately, disuse rapidly induces osteocyte hypoxia [13], and it has been observed that direct oxygen deprivation of marrow culture stimulates significant osteoclastogenesis [1].

In the context of structural adaptation in adult mammalian cortical bone, disuse rapidly precipitates substantial loss of bone mass. This bone loss is the net result of rapid and profound osteoclastic resorption on endocortical and intracortical surfaces [52]. Periosteal resorption is not evident in adult mammalian and avian models of disuse-induced bone loss [34, 41]. Endocortical resorption resulting in reduced cortical thickness is the primary contributor to disuse-induced bone loss [32], as intracortical resorption precipitated by disuse is eventually coupled with subsequent osteoblastic recruitment that aspires to fill in each excavated cone of bone. In young adults, nearly all of bone resorbed intracortically is replaced by osteoblasts, while in older adults intracortical resorption results in a net loss of intracortical bone [32].

Following an acute period of disuse, such as 4 weeks, substantial endocortical and intracortical erosion has ensued, while intracortical remodeling is incomplete, even in the young adult. Degradation in bone strength in response to acute disuse therefore arises from both endocortical expansion and heightened intracortical porosity. Although the loss of bone strength in humans due to acute disuse is obviously not directly assessable, it is possible to generate a bracketing estimate from the literature. An expanded endocortical surface diminishes bone's moment of inertia and thereby limits resistance to bending or torsion. The endocortical surface can be expected to expand 5–15% within 4 weeks following the onset of disuse, depending on species and model [34, 46, 47]. Assuming uniform endocortical erosion, a 1–10% decrease in the bone's moment of inertia about the primary axis of bending would be anticipated, depending upon the initial proportions of the cortex (e.g., a small diameter, thick cortex bone would be less affected than a large diameter, thin cortex bone). As a result, ultimate bone strength (if loaded about this axis) would be expected to decline proportionately. Elevated intracortical porosity serves to elevate local tissue strains for a given load and substantially degrades fracture toughness [97]. Intracortical porosity can be estimated to double from 5–10%

under normal conditions and 10–20% following acute disuse [24, 34, 59]. Mechanical testing data suggest that such an alteration would degrade bone strength 10–25% [60]. As a comparison, it has been estimated that cortical bone strength degrades 15–20% between the ages of 35 and 70 [57].

Conclusion

Osteoclastic resorption plays a central role in the regulation of bone mass and architecture. Moreover, osteoclast resorption is a prerequisite to maintaining the structural health of cortical and cancellous bone by removing aged tissue and by initiating the repair of bone micro-damage. Conversely, hyperactive osteoclasts and excessive bone resorption can lead to irre-versible bone loss and structurally weakened bone. From these observations we have arrived at an understanding of how osteoclast behaviors participate in both normal and pathological changes to bone structure but investigations into the regulatory cues that target osteoclasts to bone remodeling sites are only now begin-ning. Future work aimed at understanding these pathways should therefore provide a scientific basis for the design and development of therapeutic modalities that will optimize bone structure.

References

1. Arnett TR, Gibbons DC, Utting JC, Orriss IR, Hoebertz A, Rosendaal M, et al. (2003) Hypoxia is a major stimu-lator of osteoclast formation and bone resorption. J Cell Physiol 196:2–8.
2. Arnold JS (1970) Focal excessive endosteal resorption in aging and senile osteoporosis, edn. In: Barzel US, editor. Osteoporosis. Grune and Stratton, Inc., New York, 80–100.
3. Arnold JS (1981) Trabecular patterns and shapes in aging and osteoporosis, edn. In: Jee WSS, Parfitt AM, editors(eds). Bone Histomorphometry: Third Interna-tional Workshop. Armour Montagu, Paris, 297–308.
4. Bentolila V, Boyce TM, Fyhrie DP, Drumb R, Skerry TM, Schaffler MB (1998) Intracortical remodeling in adult rat long bones after fatigue loading. Bone 23:275–81.
5. Boivin G, Meunier PJ (2002) Changes in bone remodel-ing rate influence the degree of mineralization of bone. Connect Tissue Res 43:535–7.
6. Burr DB (2002) Targeted and nontargeted remodeling. Bone 30:2–4.
7. Burr DB, Martin RB, Schaffler MB, Radin EL (1985) Bone remodeling in response to in vivo fatigue micro-damage. J Biomech 18:189–200.
8. Cohen-Solal ME, Shih MS, Lundy MW, Parfitt AM (1991) A new method for measuring cancellous bone erosion depth: application to the cellular mechanisms of bone loss in postmenopausal osteoporosis. J Bone Miner Res 6:1331–8.
9. Compston JE, Croucher PI (1991) Histomorphometric assessment of trabecular bone remodelling in osteo-porosis. Bone Miner 14:91–102.
10. Croucher PI, Garrahan NJ, Mellish RW, Compston JE (1991) Age-related changes in resorption cavity char-acteristics in human trabecular bone. Osteoporos Int 1:257–61.
11. Croucher PI, Mellish RW, Vedi S, Garrahan NJ, Compston JE (1989) The relationship between resorp-tion depth and mean interstitial bone thickness: age-related changes in man. Calcif Tissue Int 45:15–19.
12. Ding M, Hvid I (2000) Quantification of age-related changes in the structure model type and trabecular thickness of human tibial cancellous bone. Bone 26:291–5.
13. Dodd JS, Raleigh JA, Gross TS (1999) Osteocyte hypoxia: a novel mechanotransduction pathway. Am J Phys Cell Phys 277:C589–602.
14. Epker BN, Frost HM (1965) Correlation of Bone Resorp-tion and Formation with the Physical Behavior of Loaded Bone. J Dent Res 44:33–41.
15. Eriksen EF (1986) Normal and pathological remodeling of human trabecular bone: three dimensional recon-struction of the remodeling sequence in normals and in metabolic bone disease. Endocr Rev 7:379–408.
16. Eriksen EF (1993) Assessment of erosion depth by lamellar counting. Bone 14:443–7.
17. Eriksen EF, Gundersen HJ, Melsen F, Mosekilde L (1984) Reconstruction of the formative site in iliac trabecular bone in 20 normal individuals employing a kinetic model for matrix and mineral apposition. Metab Bone Dis Relat Res 5:243–52.
18. Eriksen EF, Hodgson SF, Eastell R, Cedel SL, O'Fallon WM, Riggs BL (1990) Cancellous bone remodeling in type I (postmenopausal) osteoporosis: quantitative assessment of rates of formation, resorption, and bone loss at tissue and cellular levels. J Bone Miner Res 5:311–19.
19. Eriksen EF, Langdahl B, Vesterby A, Rungby J, Kassem M (1999) Hormone replacement therapy prevents osteo-clastic hyperactivity: A histomorphometric study in early postmenopausal women. J Bone Miner Res 14:1217–21.
20. Eriksen EF, Melsen F, Mosekilde L (1984) Reconstruc-tion of the resorptive site in iliac trabecular bone: a kinetic model for bone resorption in 20 normal indi-viduals. Metab Bone Dis Relat Res 5:235–42.
21. Eriksen EF, Mosekilde L, Melsen F (1985) Trabecular bone resorption depth decreases with age: differences between normal males and females. Bone 6:141–6.
22. Eriksen EF, Steiniche T, Mosekilde L, Melsen F (1989) Histomorphometric analysis of bone in metabolic bone disease. Endocrinol Metab Clin North Am 18:919–54.
23. Eser P, Frotzler A, Zehnder Y, Wick L, Knecht H, Denoth J, et al. (2004) Relationship between the duration of paralysis and bone structure: a pQCT study of spinal cord injured individuals. Bone 34:869–80.

24. Feik SA, Thomas CD, Clement JG (1997) Age-related changes in cortical porosity of the midshaft of the human femur. J Anat 191(Pt 3):407–16.
25. Frost HM (1960) Presence of microcracks in vivo in bone. Henry Ford Hosp Med J 8:25–35.
26. Frost HM (1964) Dynamics of bone remodeling, edn. In: Frost HM, editor. Bone Biodynamics. Little, Brown and Co, Boston, 315–33.
27. Frost HM (1966) Bone dynamics in osteoporosis and osteomalacia, edn. In: (ed) Series Titl. Charles C. Thomas, Springfield, IL, pp ••.
28. Frost HM (1969) Tetracycline-based histological analysis of bone remodeling. Calcif Tissue Int 3:211–37.
29. Frost HM (1973) Bone Remodeling and its Relationship to Metabolic Bone Disease, edn. In: (ed) Series Titl. Charles C. Thomas, Springfield, IL, pp ••.
30. Frost HM (1983) The skeletal intermediary organization. Metab Bone Dis Relat Res 4:281–90.
31. Frost HM (1986) Intermediary Organization of the Skeleton, edn. In: (ed) Series Title. CRC Press, Inc., Boca Raton, FL, pp ••.
32. Frost HM (1992) Perspectives: bone's mechanical usage windows. Bone Miner 19:257–71.
33. Gentzsch C, Delling G, Kaiser E (2003) Microstructural classification of resorption lacunae and perforations in human proximal femora. Calcif Tissue Int 72:698–709.
34. Gross TS, Rubin CT (1995) Uniformity of resorptive bone loss induced by disuse. J Orthop Res 13:708–14.
35. Howship J (1817) Experiments and observations in order to determine the means employed by the animal economy in the formation of bone. Transactions of the Medico-Chirurgical Society (London). 6:263–301.
36. Jaworski ZF (1984) Lamellar bone turnover system and its effector organ. Calcif Tissue Int 36(Suppl 1):S46–55.
37. Jaworski ZF, Duck B, Sekaly G (1981) Kinetics of osteoclasts and their nuclei in evolving secondary Haversian systems. J Anat 133:397–405.
38. Jaworski ZF, Hooper C (1980) Study of cell kinetics within evolving secondary Haversian systems. J Anat 131:91–102.
39. Jaworski ZF, Lok E (1972) The rate of osteoclastic bone erosion in Haversian remodeling sites of adult dog's rib. Calcif Tissue Res 10:103–12.
40. Jaworski ZFG (1981) The quantum concept of bone remodeling in adults, edn. In: Norman AM, Schaefer K, Coburn JW, DeLuca HF, Fraser D, Grigoleit HG, et al., editors(eds). Vitamin D: Biochemical, Chemical, and Clinical Aspects Related to Calcium Metabolism. Degruyter, Berlin.
41. Jaworski ZFG, Uthoff HK (1986) Reversibility of non-traumatic disuse osteoporosis during its active phase. Bone 7:431–9.
42. Jerome CP, Burr DB, Van Bibber T, Hock JM, Brommage R (2001) Treatment with human parathyroid hormone (1–34) for 18 months increases cancellous bone volume and improves trabecular architecture in ovariectomized cynomolgus monkeys (Macaca fascicularis). Bone 28:150–9.
43. Jilka RL (2003) Biology of the basic multicellular unit and the pathophysiology of osteoporosis. Med Pediatr Oncol 41:182–5.
44. Johnson LC (1964) Morphological analysis in pathology: the kinetics of disease and general biology of bone, edn. In: Frost HM, editor. Bone Biodynamics. Little Brown, Boston, 543–654.
45. Jones SJ, Boyde A, Ali NN, Maconnachie E (1986) Variation in the sizes of resorption lacunae made in vitro. Scan Electron Microsc 15:71–80.
46. Judex S, Garman R, Squire M, Busa B, Donahue LR, Rubin C (2004) Genetically linked site-specificity of disuse osteoporosis. J Bone Miner Res 19:607–13.
47. Kiratli BJ, Smith AE, Nauenberg T, Kallfelz CF, Perkash I (2000) Bone mineral and geometric changes through the femur with immobilization due to spinal cord injury. J Rehabil Res Dev 37:225–33.
48. Landeros O, Frost HM (1964) A Cell System in Which Rate and Amount of Protein Synthesis Are Separately Controlled. Science 145:1323–4.
49. Langdahl BL, Mortensen L, Vesterby A, Eriksen EF, Charles P (1996) Bone histomorphometry in hypoparathyroid patients treated with vitamin D. Bone 18:103–8.
50. Lanyon LE (1984) Functional strain as a determinant for bone remodeling. Calcif Tissue Int 36:S56–61.
51. Lanyon LE (1992) The success and failure of the adaptive response to functional load- bearing in averting bone fracture. Bone 13:S17–21.
52. Leblanc AD, Schneider VS, Evans HJ, Engelbretson DA, Krebs JM (1990) Bone mineral loss and recovery after 17 weeks of bed rest. J Bone Miner Res 5:843–50.
53. Lee TC, Staines A, Taylor D (2002) Bone adaptation to load: microdamage as a stimulus for bone remodelling. J Anat 201:437–46.
54. Li J, Mashiba T, Burr DB (2001) Bisphosphonate treatment suppresses not only stochastic remodeling but also the targeted repair of microdamage. Calcif Tissue Int 69:281–6.
55. Lips P, Courpron P, Meunier PJ (1978) Mean wall thickness of trabecular bone packets in the human iliac crest: changes with age. Calcif Tissue Res 26:13–17.
56. Martin B (1993) Aging and strength of bone as a structural material. Calcif Tissue Int 53:S34–9; discussion S39–40.
57. Martin B (1993) Aging and strength of bone as a structural material. Calcif Tissue Int 53(Suppl 1):S34–9; discussion S39–40.
58. Martin RB (2002) Is all cortical bone remodeling initiated by microdamage? Bone 30:8–13.
59. Martin RB, Pickett JC, Zinaich S (1980) Studies of skeletal remodeling in aging men. Clin Orthop 268–82.
60. McCalden RW, McGeough JA, Barker MB, Court-Brown CM (1993) Age-related changes in the tensile properties of cortical bone. The relative importance of changes in porosity, mineralization, and microstructure. J Bone Joint Surg Am 75:1193–205.
61. Meunier PJ (1983) Histomorphometry of the skeleton, edn. In: Peck WA, editor. Bone and Mineral Research. Annual 1. Excerpta Medica, Amsterdam, 191–222.
62. Mori S, Burr DB (1993) Increased intracortical remodeling following fatigue damage. Bone 14:103–9.
63. Mosekilde L (1990) Consequences of the remodelling process for vertebral trabecular bone structure: a scanning electron microscopy study (uncoupling of unloaded structures). Bone Miner 10:13–35.
64. Mosekilde L (2000) Age-related changes in bone mass, structure, and strength – effects of loading. Z Rheumatol 59(Suppl 1):1–9.
65. Murrills RJ, Shane E, Lindsay R, Dempster DW (1989) Bone resorption by isolated human osteoclasts in vitro: effects of calcitonin. J Bone Miner Res. 4:259–68.

66. Noble BS, Peet N, Stevens HY, Brabbs A, Mosley JR, Reilly GC, et al. (2003) Mechanical loading: biphasic osteocyte survival and targeting of osteoclasts for bone destruction in rat cortical bone. Am J Physiol Cell Physiol 284:C934–43.

67. Palle S, Chappard D, Vico L, Riffat G, Alexandre C (1989) Evaluation of the osteoclastic population in iliac crest biopsies from 36 normal subjects: a histoenzymologic and histomorphometric study. J Bone Miner Res 4: 501–6.

68. Parfitt AM (1979) Quantum concept of bone remodeling and turnover: implications for the pathogenesis of osteoporosis. Calcif Tissue Int 28:1–5.

69. Parfitt AM (1982) The coupling of bone formation to bone resorption: a critical analysis of the concept and of its relevance to the pathogenesis of osteoporosis. Metab Bone Dis Relat Res 4:1–6.

70. Parfitt AM (1983) The physiologic and clinical significance of bone histomorphometric data, edn. In: Recker RR, editor. Bone Histomorphometry: Techniques and Interpretation. CRC Press, Boca Raton, FL, 143–224.

71. Parfitt AM (1984) The cellular basis of bone remodeling: the quantum concept reexamined in light of recent advances in the cell biology of bone. Calcif Tissue Int 36(Suppl 1):S37–45.

72. Parfitt AM (1987) Trabecular bone architecture in the pathogenesis and prevention of fracture. Am J Med 82:68–72.

73. Parfitt AM (1992) Implications of architecture for the pathogenesis and prevention of vertebral fracture. Bone 13(Suppl 2):S41–7.

74. Parfitt AM (1993) Bone age, mineral density, and fatigue damage. Calcif Tissue Int 53(Suppl 1):S82–5; discussion S85–6.

75. Parfitt AM (1993) Morphometry of bone resorption: introduction and overview. Bone 14:435–41.

76. Parfitt AM (1994) Osteonal and hemi-osteonal remodeling: the spatial and temporal framework for signal traffic in adult human bone. J Cell Biochem 55:273–86.

77. Parfitt AM (1996) Skeletal heterogeneity and the purposes of bone remodeling, edn. In: Marcus R, Feldman B, Kelsey J, editors(eds). Osteoporosis. Academic Press, San Diego.

78. Parfitt AM (2000) BMU origination and progression: relationship to targeted and nontargeted remodeling. J Bone Mine Res 15:823.

79. Parfitt AM (2002) Targeted and nontargeted bone remodeling: relationship to basic multicellular unit origination and progression. Bone 30:5–7.

80. Parfitt AM, Foldes J (1991) The ambiguity of interstitial bone thickness: a new approach to the mechanism of trabecular thinning. Bone 12:119–22.

81. Parfitt AM, Mathews CH, Villanueva AR, Kleerekoper M, Frame B, Rao DS (1983) Relationships between surface, volume, and thickness of iliac trabecular bone in aging and in osteoporosis. Implications for the microanatomic and cellular mechanisms of bone loss. J Clin Invest 72:1396–409.

82. Parfitt AM, Mundy GR, Roodman GD, Hughes DE, Boyce BF (1996) A new model for the regulation of bone resorption, with particular reference to the effects of bisphosphonates. J Bone Miner Res 11:150–9.

83. Parisien MV, McMahon D, Pushparaj N, Dempster DW (1988) Trabecular architecture in iliac crest bone biopsies: infra-individual variability in structural parameters and changes with age. Bone 9:289–95.

84. Polig E, Jee WS (1987) Bone age and remodeling: a mathematical treatise. Calcif Tissue Int 41:130–6.

85. Raisz LG (1999) Physiology and pathophysiology of bone remodeling. Clin Chem 45:1353–8.

86. Rubin CT (1984) Skeletal strain and the functional significance of bone architecture. Calcif Tissue Int 36:S11–18.

87. Rubin J, Fan X, Biskobing DM, Taylor WR, Rubin CT (1999) Osteoclastogenesis is repressed by mechanical strain in an in vitro model. J Orthop Res 17:639–45.

88. Schock CC, Noyes FR, Villanueva AR (1972) Measurement of haversian bone remodeling by means of tetracycline labeling in rib of Rhesus monkeys. Henry Ford Hosp Med J 20:131–44.

89. Steiniche T, Christiansen P, Vesterby A, Hasling C, Ullerup R, Mosekilde L, et al. (1994) Marked changes in iliac crest bone structure in postmenopausal osteoporotic patients without any signs of disturbed bone remodeling or balance. Bone 15:73–9.

90. Steiniche T, Mosekilde L, Christensen MS, Melsen F (1989) Histomorphometric analysis of bone in idiopathic hypercalciuria before and after treatment with thiazide. Apmis 97:302–8.

91. Teitelbaum SL (2000) Bone resorption by osteoclasts. Science 289:1504–8.

92. Thomsen JS, Mosekilde L, Mosekilde E (1996) Quantification of remodeling parameter sensitivity – assessed by a computer simulation model. Bone 19:505–11.

93. Tran Van P, Vignery A, Baron R (1982) An electron-microscopic study of the bone-remodeling sequence in the rat. Cell Tissue Res 225:283–92.

94. Tran Van PT, Vignery A, Baron R (1982) Cellular kinetics of the bone remodeling sequence in the rat. Anat Rec 202:445–51.

95. Turner CH, Pavalko FM (1998) Mechanotransduction and functional response of the skeleton to physical stress: the mechanisms and mechanics of bone adaptation. J Orthop Sci 3:346–55.

96. Wehrli FW, Gomberg BR, Saha PK, Song HK, Hwang SN, Snyder PJ (2001) Digital topological analysis of in vivo magnetic resonance microimages of trabecular bone reveals structural implications of osteoporosis. J Bone Miner Res 16:1520–31.

97. Yeni YN, Brown CU, Wang Z, Norman TL (1997) The influence of bone morphology on fracture toughness of the human femur and tibia. Bone 21:453–9.

5.

Inflammatory Cytokines

Mark S. Nanes and Roberto Pacifici

Introduction

Inflammatory cytokines have a major role in bone disease. The estrogen deficiency of menopause results in an indolent inflammatory state with elevated production of cytokines, most notably tumor necrosis factor-α (TNF) and interleukin-1 (IL-1). A local effect of cytokines in inflammatory arthritis also contributes to periarticular bone destruction. Cytokines act as skeletal catabolic agents that stimulate osteoclastogenesis while simultaneously inhibiting osteoblast differentiation and function. The postmenopausal state is associated with infiltration of marrow by TNF-producing T cells, which percolate through bone and stimulate the production of an expanded local cytokine cascade. The skeletal catabolic state is achieved by cytokine regulation of genes in hematopoietic cells, marrow stromal cells, osteoblasts, and osteoclasts that tilt the balance of formation and resorption toward net bone loss. TNF and IL-1 engage initially distinct signaling pathways that converge with activation of the transcription factor, nuclear factor kappa B (NfκB), and stimulation of the mitogen-activated protein kinase (MAPK) system. The combined effect of these two cytokines provides a potent signal that stimulates differentiation and prolongs lifespan of osteoclasts, while inhibiting differentiation of osteoblasts and promoting their apoptosis. NfκB regulates an array of genes that include the receptor activator of NfκB ligand (RANKL) and its receptor, RANK, both necessary and sufficient for osteo-clastogenesis. NfκB suppresses the expression of osteoblast matrix protein genes, stimulates the production of matrix-degrading metalloproteinases, causes resistance to 1,25-dihydroxyvitamin D_3 (1,25-$(OH)_2D_3$) and inhibits the differentiation of osteoblast progenitors. Similarly, activation of MAPK by TNF and IL-1 leads to the phosphorylation of other transcription factors of the activator protein (AP-1) class that contribute to the catabolic direction of gene expression. This chapter will focus on the source of cytokines in bone during estrogen deficiency, cytokine intracellular signal pathways, and the molecular mechanism through which cytokines regulate the genes that result in bone loss. A large number of inflammatory cytokines contribute to skeletal pathology, but attention will be focused primarily on TNF and IL-1 as central players. Inflammatory cytokines and their signal pathways are important targets in the development of new therapies for osteoporosis.

Sources of Cytokines in Bone

Early Data that Estrogen Deficiency Stimulates Cytokine Production

A major focus of osteoporosis research has been to understand the reasons for accelerated bone resorption following menopause; thus, an obvious question has been how estrogen deficiency leads to increased osteoclast activity and ultimately osteoporosis. Early work by

McSheehy et al. and Thompson et al. showed that conditioned media derived from osteoblasts that were stimulated by a variety of factors increased osteoclastogenesis [142–144, 207, 208]. These results suggested that substances were produced by osteoblasts that mediated differentiation of osteoclast precursors. After several inflammatory cytokines were found capable of producing this response, research focused on discerning their relative contributions in estrogen deficiency bone loss. A lively debate ensued with proponents for IL-1, TNF, or IL-6 as the major players. The osteoclastogenic response to all three cytokines *in vitro* was based on sound data [138, 166]. However, the use of different experimental models may have yielded different results. Several reports suggested increased production of TNF by cultures of mononuclear cells derived from postmenopausal women, an effect reversed by estrogen replacement [167, 177, 180]. In this model, secretion of IL-1, but not always of IL-6, mirrored that of TNF [67, 180]. Experimental models in which estrogen did not seem to regulate TNF expression included cultured stromal cells, some osteoblastic cell lines, and bone biopsies [1, 37, 176, 178]. Although small amounts of TNF are produced by many of these cell types, the lack of regulation by estrogen in all but monocytes hinted at an uncertainty as to the genuine source. To add to the confusion, phytohemaglutinin stimulation was required to demonstrate increased TNF production from monocytes. Another level of complexity was evident in the study by Atkins et al., in which peripheral blood mononuclear cells were shown to secrete TNF, IL-1, and IL-6 after co-culture with the stromal-like cell line ST-2 [6]. Thus, cytokine production is also modulated by cell-cell contact and/or paracrine events in the bone microenvironment. More recent data revealed the presence of membrane anchored RANKL, part of a potent osteoclastogenic system that is, itself, dependent on TNF (discussed in detail below).

Weitzman et al. have suggested that IL-7 also contributes to bone loss following estrogen deficiency [226, 227]. Ovariectomy increases the level of IL-7 in mice and neutralization of IL-7 *in vivo* blocks ovariectomy-induced bone loss. Exactly where IL-7 is synthesized and where it fits into the scheme of skeletal regulation is unclear. At the physiologic level, IL-7 stimulates T-cell production of other cytokines, including TNF and RANKL. T-cell-deficient nude mice do not respond to IL-7 with bone loss, though they do so after adoptive T-cell transfer [211]. Whether the *in vivo* action of IL-7 requires production of TNF is, as yet, unknown. Surprisingly, IL-7 inhibits osteoclastogenesis in an ex vivo system of cultured marrow cells [125]. Marrow cells from IL-7-deficient mice exhibit an increased osteoclastogenic response to a variety of stimuli, including 1,25-dihydroxyvitamin D, PTH, and mCSF/RANKL. To make matters more confusing, marrow cells derived from IL-7-receptor-deficient mice had the opposite outcome [125]. Thus, the exact role of IL-7 in bone is yet to be established. Understanding IL-7 may require knowing both its systemic action on T-cell expansion and direct local actions on skeletal cells.

In premenopausal women the production of TNF, interleukin-1, -4, -6, and IFNγ by blood cells varies inversely with the estrogen level. Interestingly, the plasma levels of these cytokines also correlate inversely with bone density after menopause; this strengthens the hypothesis that cytokines play an important role in menopausal bone loss [186, 220, 242].

Central Role for TNF in Estrogen Deficiency Bone Loss

Substantial *in vitro* and *in vivo* evidence suggests that TNF is a central player in the pathophysiology of skeletal loss following menopause [82, 166]. As noted above, TNF and IL-1 are potent stimuli for the formation of osteoclasts *in vitro*. This is also true in animal models with reference to ectopic bone formation, estrogen-deficiency-induced bone loss, and to periarticular bone destruction in the inflamed joint. In these animal models, blockade of TNF or IL-1 action alleviates bone loss, thus confirming the role played by TNF and IL-1 in stimulating osteoclastogenesis [33, 35, 106–108, 110, 167]. The most definitive findings in support of the central role of TNF in mediating osteoporosis came from experiments that showed that TNF-deficient and TNF receptor knockout mice are resistant to ovariectomy-induced bone loss [106, 107, 183]. Comparable findings from IL-6 or IL-1 knockout mice were less definitive. In the wild-type mouse, the rise in TNF following ovariectomy is immediately followed by increases in IL-6 and IL-1, which, in turn, magnify the stimulus to osteoclastogenesis [17, 37, 77, 178, 182].

T-Cells as a TNF Source in Estrogen Deficiency Bone Loss

Substantial evidence is accumulating to suggest that T cells play a pivotal role in bone loss caused by estrogen deficiency [33]. T cells are a major source of TNF, and ovariectomy enhances the production of T-cell-derived TNF. The concept that the T cell is the source of TNF is consistent with other models of T-cell-dependent immunity [187]. TNF acts through the TNF receptor, TNFR1 (p55), to augment RANKL-induced osteoclastogenesis and osteoclast activity [58]. Athymic, T-cell-deficient nude mice are completely protected against the bone loss and the increase in bone turnover induced by ovariectomy [33, 183] (Figure 5.1). Reconstitution studies in nude mice have shown that the relevant T-cell subpopulation is made up of CD4+ cells, but not of CD+8 cells, because only CD4+ cells, when implanted in nude mice, restored ovariectomy-induced bone loss transfer of CD4+. It is thus apparent that CD4+ T cells are an essential mediator of the bone-wasting effect that is the result of estrogen deficiency *in vivo*. The ovariectomy induced increase in T-cell production raises the TNF level to a point where it can augment RANKL-induced osteoclastogenesis [33]. TNF may also be pivotal in disrupting the coupling between bone resorption and bone formation, not only by synergizing with RANKL to stimulate bone resorption, but also by repressing the compensatory increase in bone formation.

Evidence is accumulating to suggest that T cells also regulate bone resorption in humans. For example, RANKL-expression by T cells is up-regulated by estrogen deficiency and correlates with increases in bone resorption markers and inversely with serum 17β-estradiol [47].

Estrogen Effects on TNF Production and Action

Estrogen Regulation of T-Cell Clonal Expansion

As discussed above, estrogen regulates the increase in the mass of TNF-producing cells [33, 183]. Estrogen also causes the lymphocyte populations to shift toward clones that produce anti-inflammatory TH2 cytokines (IL-4, IL-10), thereby causing fewer clones that produce inflammatory TH1 cytokines (IL-2, IFNγ)). In postmenopausal women, production of cytokines representative of TH1 lymphocytes is increased, an effect reversed by supplemental estrogen [97].

The mechanism by which estrogen regulates T-cell clonal expansion is shown in Figure 5.2.

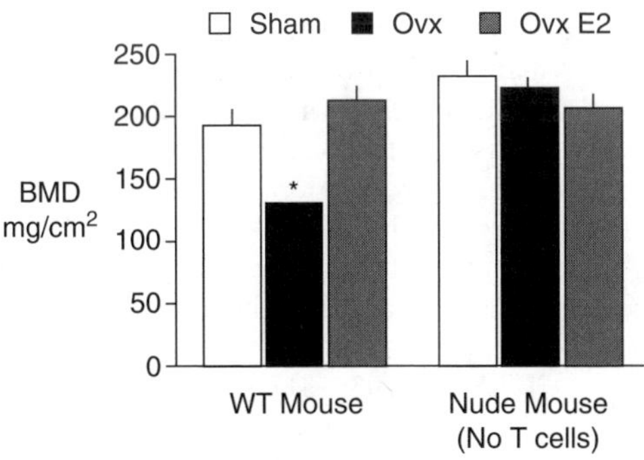

Figure 5.1 T-cell-deficient mice are protected against ovariectomy-induced bone loss. Reproduced with permission from Cenci S, Weitzmann MN, Roggia O, et al. Estrogen deficiency induces bone loss by enhancing T-cell production of TNF-alpha. J Clin Invest 2000 Nov;106(10):1203–4.

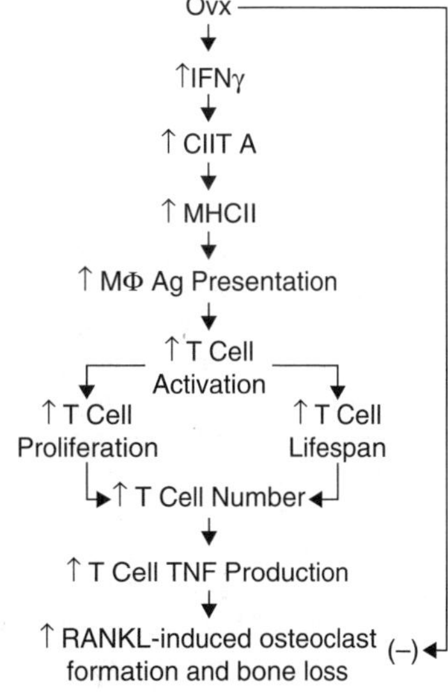

Figure 5.2 Schematic representation of the mechanism by which ovariectomy causes bone loss.

Ovariectomy increases T-cell activation. This in turn causes an expansion of the T-cell pool in bone marrow, spleen and in lymph nodes. T-cell activation occurs by enhancing antigen presentation by bone marrow macrophages. This in turn is due to the up-regulation of the expression of MHCII that occurs in estrogen deficiency. The mechanism of T-cell activation elicited by estrogen deficiency is similar to that triggered by infections, but the intensity of events that follow estrogen withdrawal is significantly less. With estrogen withdrawal, CD4+ clones of T cells double. Modulation of antigen presentation by estrogen is specific for macrophages, since no change occurs in B cells and dendritic cells, the other two antigen presenting-cell populations (APC) [32].

The relevance of this mechanism *in vivo* has been established by utilizing DO11.10 mice, a strain in which all T cells recognize a single peptide epitope of chicken albumin (ovalbumin), which is not expressed in mice. In the absence of ovalbumin, the APC of DO11.10 mice cannot induce T-cell activation. Therefore, if APC are targeted by estrogen, the DOLL.10 mice should be protected from increased T-cell proliferation and the bone loss that follows ovariectomy. Injection of ovalbumin leads to the generation of the appropriate MHC-peptide antigen for the DOLL.10 mouse T cells. This restores the series of events in which ovariectomy causes the T-cell pool to expand and to induce bone loss. It is therefore apparent that the generation of appropriate peptide-MHC complexes is critical to the process by which ovariectomy increases T-cell proliferation and lifespan and leads to bone loss. Furthermore, the finding that T cells from ovariectomized mice exhibit an increased response to ovalbumin demonstrates that ovariectomy increases the reactivity of APC to endogenous antigens rather than stimulating the production of a new antigen or modulating antigen levels.

The effects of ovariectomy on antigen presentation and the resulting changes in T-cell activation, proliferation, and lifespan come about because, as a result of ovariectomy, there is an increased expression of the gene that encodes Class II Transactivator (CIITA). The product of the CIITA gene is a non-DNA binding factor that functions as a transcriptional coactivator when recruited to the MHC II promoter by interaction with promoter-bound factors [18, 152, 153]. CIITA expression is, indeed, required and sufficient for the stimulation of antigen presentation in macrophages. CIITA expression is regulated by four distinct promoters that direct the transcription of four separate first exons spliced to a common second exon [149, 150]. Initially it was thought that IFNγ expression in murine macrophages is regulated exclusively by promoter IV [149, 150, 165]. However, it is now recognized that promoters I and IV together account for IFNγ induced CIITA *in vitro* and *in vivo* [168, 225].

CIITA is constitutively expressed in B and dendritic cells, but not in bone marrow macrophages. IFNγ induces CIITA in macrophages. Increased CIITA expression in bone marrow macrophages from ovariectomized mice is the result of ovariectomy leading to an increase in both T-cell production of IFNγ and the responsiveness of the CIITA gene to IFNγ [32].

That ovariectomy increases T-cell production of IFNγ was demonstrated by measuring the cytokine concentration in the media of purified T cells and by fluorescent-activated cell sorting (FACS) analysis of unfractionated bone marrow. IFNγ production by T cells is induced either by a cyclosporin-A sensitive T-cell receptor (TCR)-dependent mechanism, mediated by T-cell activation, or by the cytokines IL-12 and IL-18. The expression of the IL-12 and IL-18 genes in BMM is induced by Nf-κB and AP-1, nuclear proteins whose transcriptional activity is directly repressed by estrogen [4, 60, 194]. Unstimulated bone marrow macrophages, such as those from estrogen-replete mice, express low or undetectable levels of NFκB and AP-1 [148]. Ovariectomy potently increases secretion of IL-12 and IL-18, whereas treatment with 17β estradiol represses it. Thus, estrogen represses CIITA by decreasing IFNγ production via an inhibitory effect on the production of IL-12 and IL-18. Also, because CIITA expression in T cells increases IFNγ production, and because IFNγ stimulates its own inducers, IL-18 and IL-12 and IL-12 receptor expression, ovariectomy triggers an amplification loop that leads to a further increase in the level of IFNγ and to the induction of CIITA [68, 105, 151].

Regulation of IFNγ By Estrogen and Skeletal Effects of IFNγ

IFNγ is a key factor in a complex pathway by which ovariectomy leads to increased T-cell proliferation and T-cell TNF production.

Ovariectomy up-regulates IFNγ production *in vivo*, even though estrogen stimulates IFNγ gene expression *in vitro* [55]. The discordance between *in vitro* and *in vivo* data is further exemplified by the finding that IFNγ represses osteoclast formation *in vitro* [56]. *In vivo*, IFNγ stimulates osteoclast formation by increasing the T-cell production of TNF. IFNγ receptor knock-out mice are entirely protected against ovariectomy-induced bone loss. Furthermore, ovariectomy fails to increase CIITA expression in IFNγ receptor knock out mice [32]. Thus, the data strongly suggest that in estrogen deficiency the indirect pro-resorptive effects of IFNγ prevail over the direct repression of osteoclastogenesis. This is consistent with earlier reports that indicated bone resorption and/or bone loss increased in models of IFNγ overexpression [9, 136]. Other studies that have shown IFNγ decreases bone resorption *in vivo* have been carried out in T-cell deficient mice [188, 209]. This again demonstrates that the T-cell-mediated indirect effects are more potent than direct repression by IFNγ. IFNγ has been shown in one study to repress bone resorption in a T-cell replete model, but the only *in vivo* data presented were obtained on the calvaria of newborn mice [203]. Further work will be needed to sort out possible maturation stage dependent effects of IFNγ.

Estrogen Repression Of TNF Gene Expression and Action

Estrogen not only suppresses T-cell proliferation, but also inhibits monocyte TNF production and TNF action [197]. In a study using RAW 264.7 cells (a monocytic precursor that can be stimulated to acquire the osteoclast phenotype), estrogen decreased transcriptional activity of the TNF promoter. Mutation of an AP-1 binding site in the promoter abolished the inhibitory effect of estrogen. Furthermore, the expression of the AP-1 family proteins cJUN, JUND, and also the binding of AP-1 proteins to the promoter were selectively decreased after estrogen stimulation, as was the activity of JUN kinase (JNK), a kinase that would normally enhance the AP-1 transcriptional signal. Shevde et al. confirmed this in cultured monocytes and RAW 264.7 pre-osteoclastic cells, where the osteoclastogenic stimulus was RANKL, the membrane anchored protein that binds the TNF-family receptor RANK [194]. Estrogen also inhibits TNF-α-stimulated JNK activity in nonskeletal cells [26]. Thus, estrogen decreases the pool of TNF-producing T-cells, suppresses TNF transcription in monocytes, and decreases sensitivity to the TNF /RANKL stimulus.

Cytokine Signal Pathways in Skeletal Cells

Complex intracellular pathways transmit cytokine signals from cell surface receptors to gene activation. Here we will restrict the discussion to the signal pathways for TNF and IL-1 as they directly affect osteoblast and osteoclast function. Although these cytokines initiate their signals via unique membrane receptor families, the different signals converge in similar intracellular pathways. These include the activation of the transcription factor Nf-κB, activation of mitogen-activated protein kinase (MAPK), and the regulation of the apoptotic caspase cascade. Once activated, NFκB and MAPK elicit cell-specific responses in osteoblasts and osteoclasts that include a divergent response with regard to cell survival.

TNF Signaling

A trimeric form of TNF binds one of two cell surface receptors, TNFR1 (TNFRSF1A, p55) and TNFR2 (TNFRSF1B, p75), to initiate a signal cascade that causes inflammatory gene activation, selective gene repression, and for the TNFR1, an apoptotic response (Figure 5.3). Both of these receptors are expressed on osteoblasts and osteoclasts. From receptor to gene, numerous signal pathways provide an opportunity for divergence of the skeletal response. As will be discussed below, the TNF signal pathways include features linked specifically to stimulation of bone resorption, as well as inhibition of bone formation. Stimulation of bone resorption is due to protease production by osteoblasts and the escalation of osteoclastogenesis. Inhibition of bone formation is due to the inhibition of osteoblast differentiation, suppression of mature osteoblast function, and the induction of osteoblast resistance to 1,25-$(OH)_2D_3$. TNFR1 is the functional form of the receptor in both osteoblasts and osteoclasts. Both Abu-Amer et al. [2] and Roggia et al. [183] have reported that TNF fails to stimulate osteoclastogenesis in TNFR1 receptor knockout mice (R1$^{-/-}$).

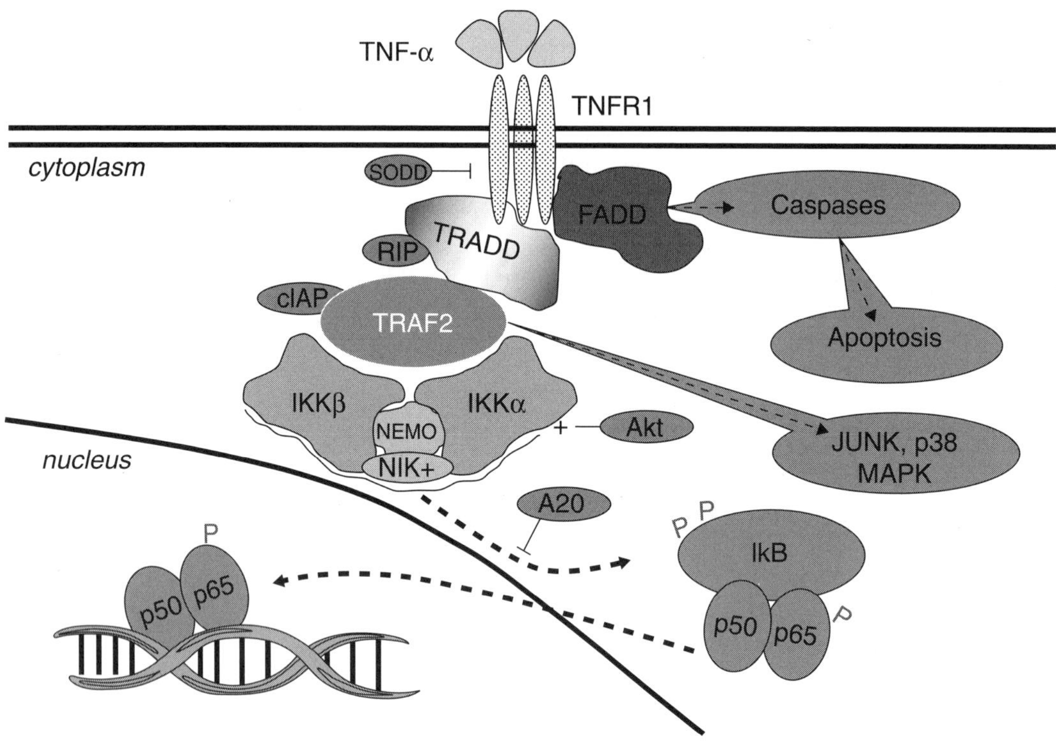

Figure 5.3   TNF signaling pathways. TNF binds as a trimer to its receptor to activate several intracellular pathways. Aggregation of a protein complex, including TRAF2, transduces the signal along the IkB pathway leading to phosphorylation of IkB with liberation of the transcription factor Nf-kB for nuclear entry and regulation of gene transcription. Additional pathways are activated via TRAF, including JNK and p38 MAPK. The apoptotic pathway is simultaneously activated by TNF through FADD and the caspase cascade. Modulator proteins include inhibitory SODD at the TNF receptor, cIAP, which attenuates the apoptotic response, RIP, and NEMO. Reprinted from Gene, vol. 321, Nanes MS. Tumor necrosis factor-alpha: molecular and cellular mechanisms in skeletal pathology, 1–15 (2003), with permission from Elsevier.

$R1^{+/+}R2^{-/-}$ knockout cells respond like the wild-type cells *in vitro*, whereas $R1^{-/-}/R2^{-/-}$ cells are resistant to TNF action, as expected. Similarly, TNF inhibition of osteoblastogenesis in bone marrow stromal cells requires the TNFR1. Although not required for action, TNFR2 may still contribute to the sensitivity toward TNF [62]. In addition, stimulation of TNFR2 could activate additional paracrine factors that affect the osteoblast; thus, a role for TNFR2 *in vivo* cannot be excluded. The skeletal phenotype of $R1^{-/-}$ mice is normal [219]. $R2^{-/-}$ mice are also grossly normal, although they have not been evaluated by histomorphometry. TNF therefore does not seems to be involved in the regulation of early skeletal differentiation, notwithstanding its role in the pathophysiology of osteoporosis and inflammatory joint disease.

Once the TNF trimer is bound, the receptor associates with cytosolic proteins that couple to downstream signals. One of the first associations is with the mediator "TNF receptor-associated death domain" (TRADD), a cytosolic protein that directs the flow of information along two well-known pathways: The first of these activates TRAFs 1 and 2. These regulate a large cytosolic complex that contains the I kappa B kinases (α and β), IκB (α, β, and ϵ), and the transcription factor NfκB. The specific TRAF family members activated by TNF stimulation provide selectivity through preferential activation by TNF family members. TNF-α signaling is mediated by TRAF 2 in many nonskeletal cells and possibly in osteoblasts [30]. TRAF 6, which is activated by the RANK and CD40 receptors, stimulates osteoclastogenesis [41, 59,

96]. The association of TRAF6 with the RANK receptor, rather than the TNFR1, is conferred by a unique TRAF6 sequence [41]. Interestingly, IL-1 stimulation of osteoclastogenesis also requires TRAF6 association with the IL1R-stimulated mediator IRAK [29]. More work will be needed to determine if the dissimilar effects of TNF as compared with RANKL are the result of selective selection of TRAFs. In addition to inducing NfκB activation, TRAFs signal via JNK, p38 kinase, and protein kinase C (PKC). p38 enhances the transcriptional potency of Nf-κB [16, 214]. Indeed, inhibitors of p38 MAPK reduce TNF stimulation of osteoclastogenesis [117].

On the basis of electrophoretic mobility shift assays (EMSA), TNF robustly and rapidly activates Nf-κB and AP-1 proteins in osteoblasts. The proteins that compose the Nf-κB and AP-1 complexes in osteoblasts can be shown by antibody supershift on EMSA to be predominantly p65/p50 (not c-Rel or Rel-B) and predominantly JunD/Fra-2, respectively (Nanes, unpublished). The second pathway that spirals off from TRADD is induced when the fas-activated death domain (FADD) is activated. FADD is a protein that triggers the pro-apoptotic caspases, leading to death in most cells, including osteoblasts. These pathways are not exclusive, inasmuch as TRAF-mediated activation of the anti-apoptotic protein, c-IAP, tempers the TNF apoptotic signal. Thus, gene regulation in osteoblasts by TNF via Nf-κB may in one view, be limited to apoptotic suicide, or in another, the apoptotic response may be tempered by Nf-κB activation. Activation of these two major pathways has made the study of TNF action difficult, because knockout or suppression of Nf-κB is often lethal *in vivo* and *in vitro*.

Unique and TNF-Redundant Signaling Pathways of IL-1

IL-1α and β bind receptors of the IL-1R/Toll-like receptor family to initiate a cascade that culminates in end points similar to that of TNF (Figure 5.4). IL-1 binding to its receptor preferentially activates interleukin receptor-associated kinase-1 (IRAK-1), a member of a family of intracellular proteins that possess active serine-threonine kinase activity. Surprisingly, IRAK-1 can activate Nf-κB independently of its kinase activity (for review, see [88]). In both osteoblasts and osteoclasts, IL-1-stimulated Nf-κB is translocated to the nucleus as described for TNF stimulation [93, 94]. Jeffries et al. investigated the interactions of intracellular proteins in the IL-1 signal cascade and showed that transfection of IRAK-1, TRAF-6, or MyD88 all caused Nf-κB translocation and transactivation of a p65-dependent transcriptional response [90]. Transfection of dominant negatives of any one of these proteins blocks IL-1 action, suggesting that all proteins may be needed for activation. This conclusion is also supported by the lack of an IL-1 response in MyD88- or IRAK-1-deficient cells. The small G protein Rac-1 may also function downstream of the IRAK-1/TRAF-6/MyD88 signal, as shown in experiments that utilize dominant negative or constitutively active mutants of Rac-1 in the presence of the three upstream proteins. Rac1 interacts directly with MyD88 and the IL-1 receptor accessory protein. MyD88 acts to facilitate inclusion of IRAK-4 in the complex. Unlike the other IRAKS, which have dispensable kinase activity, IRAK-4 has an essential kinase that phosphorylates IRAK-1. Exactly which IRAK functions in bone cells is unknown. Further investigation reveals that the cytosolic protein Tollip, which anchors the IL-1R to MyD88 and other adapters, is an active component of the complex [25]. Once IL-1 stimulates an active cytosolic complex, the signal is transduced inward. An IRAK-1-activated and mobile complex includes Tab1, Tab2, and Tak1, which associate with TRAF6. This is followed by the expected phosphorylation of the IκB kinases, IκB, and liberation of Nf-κB for nuclear entry [91, 175, 201]. Following activation, membrane-associated IRAK is degraded [235].

TRAF-6 interaction with IRAK-1 depends on a Pro-X-Glu-XX-(aromatic/acidic residue) sequence shared by RANK [238]. Thus, IκB is ultimately phosphorylated and Nf-κB enters the nucleus through this "double-barreled" IL-1 and TNF intracellular signal pathway. As with TNF stimulation, IL-1 may also signal via activation of p38 MAPK [117]. The TRAF6/Tab/Takk1 cytoplasmic complex directly phosphorylates MKK 3, 4, and 6. This leads to the downstream activation of JNK and p38. The IL-1 and TNF pathways may also cross-stimulate via IRAK-1, as shown in IRAK-1-deficient cells. In this model, TNF activity was lost but was restored through expression of IRAK-1 [206, 222].

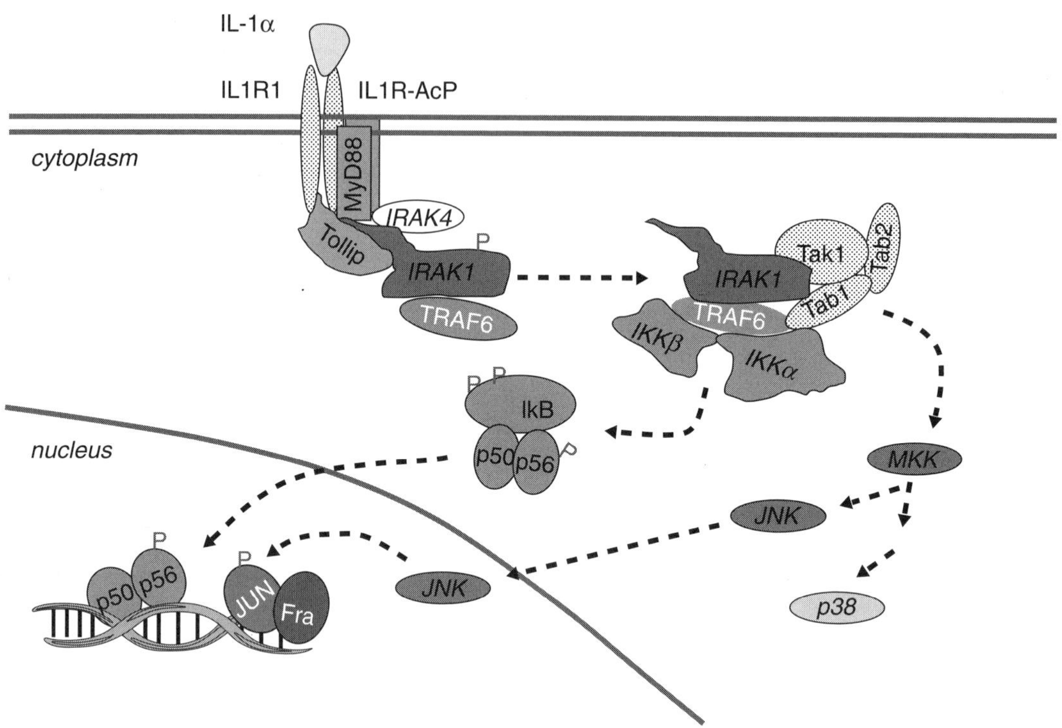

Figure 5.4   IL-1 signaling pathway. IL-1 binds its Toll-like receptor to activate IRAK-1. Successful activation of NFkB downstream requires a complex that includes TRAF-6 and MyD88. IRAK-4 has an essential kinase activity that phosphorylates IRAK-1. The protein, Tollip, serves to anchor the IL-1R to MyD88 and other members of the signal complex. An active complex becomes mobile, incorporates Tab1, Tab2, and Tak1, and transduces the signal inward. TRAF6 now associates with the IKKa and b to phosphorylate IkB and release NFkB similarly to TNF stimulation. The mobile TRAF6/Tak/Tab complex also phosphorylates MKK and activates JNK and p38 as described in the text. Reprinted from Gene, vol. 321, Nanes MS. Tumor necrosis factor-alpha: molecular and cellular mechanisms in skeletal pathology, 1–15 (2003), with permission from Elsevier.

Cytokine Effects on Osteoclast Differentiation and Survival

The Relationship Between TNF and RANKL in Osteoclastogenesis

Osteoclasts are derived from myeloid progenitors of the monocyte macrophage lineage, as shown in Figure 5.5. The role of TNF as a stimulator of osteoclastogenesis has been confirmed by numerous investigators [116, 138, 166]. As discussed above, the effect of TNF may be indirect via osteoblast signals, but it may also be direct [112, 116]. The expression of a number of transcription factors, including the prototypical p65/p50 Nf-κB, is critical to osteoclastogenesis (for detailed review see [7, 80, 82]). The work of Boyce et al. showed that Nf-κB was an essential stimulus to osteoclastogenesis [19]. Because p50/p65 knockout is lethal in midgestation, Boyce created a p50/p52 double knockout, depriving Nf-κB of its p50 subunit, and also of a potentially redundant p52 substitution. The double knockout animals develop osteopetrosis in the absence of osteoclasts. Interestingly, TNF-α and TNF-β knockout animals do not exhibit the osteopetrotic phenotype; this suggests that additional activators of Nf-κB must exist.

Later work defined the regulatory pathway for osteoclast differentiation in more detail, including very early steps required to launch the osteoclastic trajectory of differentiation from the myelomonocytic progenitors. Mouse knockout models confirm a role for Mi and PU.1 in the early stages of hematopoietic selection along this lineage [53, 134, 162, 210]. The early progenitors in the marrow then embark on a path toward pre-osteoclasts or monocytes/

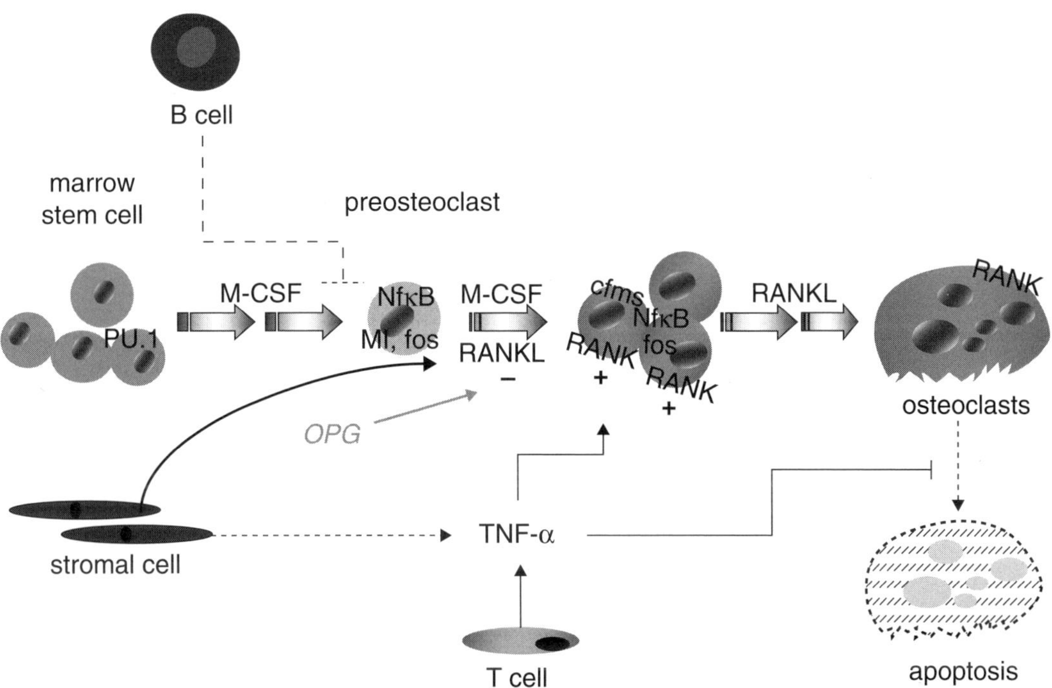

Figure 5.5 Role of TNF in osteoclast differentiation. Hematopoietic stem cells differentiate along the myelo-monocytic pathway with M-CSF stimulation. Differentiating cells continue along a trajectory toward the osteoclast phenotype under the influence of RANKL, which signals through the transcription factor NfkB. RANKL continues to support survival of the mature functional osteoclast. TNF induces the RANKL receptor, RANK, to increase responsiveness to RANKL. Additional factors in regulation include transcription factors PU.1, Mi, and fos; and the M-CSF receptor, cfms. Further details can be found in the text. Reprinted from Gene, vol. 321, Nanes MS. Tumor necrosis factor-alpha: molecular and cellular mechanisms in skeletal pathology, 1–15 (2003), with permission from Elsevier.

macrophages under the influence of M-CSF, while the soluble factors TNF, IL-1, and RANKL promote a downstream progression toward the functional osteoclast phenotype, signaling via the receptors, c-fms, TNFR1, IL1R, and RANK, respectively. Once the receptors are occupied, the transcription factors c-fos and Nf-κB enter the nucleus to regulate gene transcription [19, 57, 224, 228, 231, 232, 239] (also see detailed reviews [7, 20, 199]). In this way, genes that code for the mature osteoclast phenotype are activated. These include tartrate- resistant acid phosphatase, carbonic anhydrase II, and the receptors for calcitonin and vitronectin, to name a few.

RANKL, RANK (the RANKL receptor), and the soluble decoy, OPG, form a particularly potent system to regulate osteoclastogenesis, as confirmed by experiments using transgenic knockouts. Evidence confirmed a significant role for RANKL in skeletal ontogeny and in the ovariectomy-induced acute loss of skeletal mass. Additional studies quickly established that both OPG levels and the OPG/RANKL ratio were regulated by estrogen or androgen. In one interesting clinical trial, provision of OPG to patients with osteoporosis or rheumatoid arthritis reduced biochemical markers of bone resorption [11]. This confirmed a role for the RANKL system in postmenopausal osteoporosis [103, 129, 194, 196]. However, early work demonstrating an important role for TNF in osteoclastogenesis had to be reconciled with data that indicated the importance of the newly discovered RANKL system. In particular, what are the relative contributions of TNF and RANKL in osteoclastogenesis and do these two signals interact?

Recent work suggests that the RANK/RANKL system and TNF expression are interdependent in mice. TNF stimulates expression of the RANK receptor and of RANKL. This action in turn leads to reciprocal stimulation of TNF by means of feedback [81, 112, 241, 243], and may enhance the osteoclastogenic response after estrogen withdrawal, at least in mice. Indeed, even in mice, these experimental results may be strain-dependent. Zou et al. found that the RANKL requirement for TNF co-stimulation was observed in Balb/c, but not in C57BL/6 mice, strains that differ in the magnitude of their inflammatory response [243].

On the whole, RANKL only weakly stimulates osteoclastogenesis in murine marrow cells that have been derived from TNFR1 knockout mice. Similarly, TNF is only weakly osteoclastogenic in the absence of or at very low concentrations of RANKL [8, 111, 123, 241]. The weight of the evidence therefore suggests that synergy of RANKL and TNF is required for osteoclastogenesis to occur. Requiring both TNF and RANKL makes for more precise control of the number of osteoclasts because it involves selective signaling of the precursor cells via the two different receptors, and synergism in the stimulation of Nf-κB and JNK signaling. Interestingly, both TNF and IL-1 increase the expression of OPG, the soluble RANKL receptor. This could be the result of a feedback loop that tempers the potent RANKL stimulation of osteoclastogenesis [22, 221].

Cytokines Increase Osteoclast Survival

Several investigators have shown that TNF and IL-1 have potent anti-apoptotic effects in osteoclasts. Prolongation of osteoclast lifespan may be an important contribution toward accelerated bone resorption. The antiapoptotic action of IL-1 is associated with NfκB activation and blocked by inhibition of IκB degradation [94]. IL-1 inhibits apoptosis induced by caspase activation [164].

The exact signaling that leads from TNF or IL-1 to apoptosis is now known. Miyazaki et al. have shown that blockade of Nf-κB prevented bone-resorbing activity but did not prevent IL-1 induced apoptosis, for which ERK was required [148]. Lee et al. have confirmed that ERK is required for TNF- or IL-1-stimulated OC survival [124, 126]. These authors have also suggested that AKT is involved, because inhibition of the PI3kinase, an upstream activator of AKT,

prevented the prolongation of the osteoclast lifespan by TNF.

Effect of TNF on Osteoblasts

The maintenance of a healthy skeleton requires a balance of bone resorption and formation rates. To achieve this, bone formation by osteoblasts must increase in response to the resorptive stimulus of TNF; however, this does not occur. TNF assails bone by stimulating resorption while simultaneously inhibiting new bone formation. Even though the bone formation rate increases somewhat after ovariectomy, the increase is inadequate to compensate for the increase in bone resorption [107]. TNF blunts osteoblastic bone formation in four ways: (1) by suppressing mature osteoblast function, such as the production of a matrix competent for mineralization, (2) by blocking osteoblast differentiation from progenitor cells, (3) by promoting apoptosis of mature osteoblasts, and (4) by inducing osteoblast resistance to $1,25\text{-}(OH)_2D_3$.

Cytokine Regulation of Osteoblast Gene Expression

Table 5.1 lists some osteoblast genes subject to cytokine regulation. As can be seen, the genes that are stimulated by TNF are associated with increased bone resorption, while genes inhibited by TNF are associated with reduced bone formation. TNF and IL-1 inhibit the production of type I collagen from cultured calvaria and long bone explants from isolated fetal calvaria osteoblasts, and osteoblastic clonal cell lines [14, 15, 28, 34, 158, 195]. The inhibitory effect of TNF on collagen synthesis has been demonstrated by measuring ^{3}[H]-proline incorporation into TCA precipitable protein and by northern analysis of $\alpha1(I)$ collagen mRNA. Surprisingly, few transcriptional studies on TNF regulation of collagen gene transcription (COL1A1 or COL1A2) have been performed in osteoblasts. However, a detailed analysis TNF regulation of the collagen promoter has been reported, using transient transfection of dermal fibroblasts or hepatic stellate cells [73, 74]. These studies have identified putative regulatory regions of the COL1A1 and COL1A2 promoters that confer

Table 5.1.   Inhibitory and stimulatory effects of cytokines on genes in skeletal cells.
TNF-regulated genes

TNF-inhibited Inhibition of Bone Formation	mRNA:	TNF-stimulated Stimulation of Bone Resorption	mRNA:
αl collagen	[28, 34, 158, 169, 195]	Interleukin-6	[37, 77, 120, 130, 154, 172]
Osteocalcin	[70, 118, 119, 127, 159]	Inducible nitric oxide synthase	[83]
Alkaline phosphatase	[28, 34, 70, 114, 119, 155, 198, 240]	Tissue plasminogen activator/ uPA Plasminogen activator inhibitor-1, Gelatinases	[132, 169, 170]
Insulin-like growth factor-1	[63, 190, 236]	Matrix metalloproteinases Tissue inhibitor of matrix metalloproteinases	[23, 31, 215]
Vitamin D receptor	[140]	Receptor activator of NfκB	[112, 241, 243]
Parathyroid hormone receptor	[100, 192]	ICAM-1	[120]
PDGFR	[114]	Colony-stimulating factors: CSF-1, GM-CSF, G-CSF	[37, 52, 86, 98, 131, 237]
N-cadherin	[213]	Cyclooxygenase 2	[174, 223]
RUNX2	[64]	Interleukin-11	[184]
Osterix	[65]		

IL-1-regulated genes

IL-1-inhibited Inhibition of Bone Formation	mRNA:	IL-1-stimulated Stimulation of Bone Resorption	mRNA:
αl collagen	[73]	Interleukin-6	[21, 122]
Platelet derived growth factor receptor	[114, 230]	ICAM-1	[163]
		Matrix metalloproteinases 2,3,9,13	[121, 145]
		Cyclooxygenase 2	[174, 223]
		Phospholipase A2	[174]

TNF inhibitory action. For the COL1A1 promoter, Mori identified two TNF-responsive regions in the proximal promoter that bind nuclear proteins and inhibit transcription [147]. Additional studies have shown that the TNF-stimulated transcription factor cEBPβ is bound to the proximal promoter and that this effect is blocked by the naturally occurring dominant negatives cEBPδ and p20cEBPβ [75, 76]. TNF also reduces the binding of Sp-1 to the 5′-untranslated region of COL1A1 [75, 76, 85]. In the COL1A2 promoter, TNF similarly down-regulates Sp1 binding while stimulating AP-1 and Nf-κB (p65/p50) binding to a downstream region, that has been identified as a TGFβ responsive site [40, 84, 95, 115]. Mutational analysis of these promoters confirms the role of Nf-κB as a trans-acting regulator.

IL-1 also inhibits type 1 collagen synthesis and transcription of the Col1A1 promoter. Studies in mice bearing a collagen promoter-chloramphenicol acetyltransferase transgene suggest that IL-1 inhibition of transcription requires new protein synthesis, and may be partly mediated by prostaglandins [73].

Osteocalcin is another skeletal matrix protein, second in abundance to type 1 collagen. Osteocalcin is 1,25-$(OH)_2D_3$-responsive and is produced almost exclusively by osteoblasts. The skeletal specificity of osteocalcin and its use as a marker of the osteoblast phenotype has focused attention on the regulation of its promoter. TNF decreases the expression of osteocalcin mRNA in primary cultures of osteoblasts and in clonal osteoblastic cell lines, an action due to transcriptional repression by Nf-κB [70,

118, 127, 157, 159]. In contrast to TNF inhibition of type I collagen expression, TNF inhibition of osteocalcin does not involve Nf-κB binding to the osteocalcin promoter [157]. Here the inhibitory mechanism is indirect with TNF causing resistance to 1,25-(OH)$_2$D$_3$ stimulation of the promoter (discussed in detail below). This mechanism may explain why some investigators report that TNF only weakly inhibits osteocalcin secretion, whereas TNF inhibition of 1,25-(OH)$_2$D$_3$-stimulated secretion is relatively more potent [70, 119, 127, 159, 200]. IL-1 has been reported to inhibit constitutive and vitamin D-stimulated osteocalcin secretion by trabecular osteoblasts, but not of periosteal-derived osteoblasts [14, 119, 198].

Alkaline phosphatase, which is required for normal mineralization, is inhibited by TNF by a complex mechanism [28, 34, 70, 119, 155, 169, 198, 240]. TNF regulation of alkaline phosphatase occurs at several levels. Although TNF will decrease alkaline phosphatase mRNA and protein, TNF can also acutely stimulate alkaline phosphatase release. TNF-induced apoptosis of osteoblasts is associated with an immediate release of soluble alkaline phosphatase [49]. TNF may also stimulate retinoic acid-mediated increases in alkaline phosphatase gene transcription, but simultaneously causes an accumulation of mature mRNA in the cytoplasm, possibly with translational suppression [135]. Nevertheless, the net effect of TNF is inhibition of skeletal alkaline phosphatase activity. Similarly, IL-1, but not IL-6, inhibits alkaline phosphatase activity in human periosteal osteoblasts [119].

TNF also suppresses IGF-1 mRNA and secretion [190]. The effect of TNF on IGF-1 expression is post-transcriptional, since basal and PTH-stimulated activity of the IGF upstream promoter is not reduced by TNF. In addition, IGF-1 mRNA stability is not changed by TNF [236]. A role as a potential TNF target for the second downstream IGF-1 promoter has not been published.

Additional TNF-regulated skeletal genes, shown in Table 5.1, include nuclear receptors for vitamin D (VDR), which are post-transcriptionally decreased by TNF [140]; PDGFR-α, decreased by a pre-translational mechanism [114]; and PTHR, decreased by an unknown mechanism [71, 100, 192]. TNF decreases cell surface N-cadherins, which may compromise cell-cell communication among osteoblasts

[213]. The cytokine targets described above all contribute to osteoblast bone formation; thus, the function of the mature osteoblast is compromised in the TNF excess state.

An increase in the expression of genes that contribute to the activation of resorption occurs simultaneously with cytokine inhibition of bone-forming osteoblast genes. Both IL-1 and TNF stimulate the activation phase of the bone remodeling cycle by stimulating expression of proteolytic enzymes that degrade surface osteoid. The degradation of osteoid is quickly followed by attachment of bone-resorbing osteoclasts. These proteolytic enzymes include matrix metalloproteinases (MMP-1 through 9) and their inhibitors (TIMPs) [42, 45, 121, 132, 145, 169, 170, 179, 181, 193, 215]. Stimulation of metalloproteinase genes by TNF and IL-1 could increase the frequency of activation of bone remodeling units in the skeleton, thereby contributing to a net increase in resorption [216].

Synthesis of prostaglandin and of the key prostaglandin synthetic enzyme, cyclooxygenase 2 (COX2), is increased by IL-1 and TNF and may contribute to bone resorption in some species [44, 48, 74, 101, 104, 139, 146, 174, 202, 204, 205, 223, 233].

Many signals that promote the differentiation of osteoclasts are, in fact, osteoblast and marrow stromal cell products. These include the TNF-induced IL-6, MCSF (CSF-1), RANK, and RANKL [81, 112, 241]. TNF potently stimulates IL-6 expression by stromal cells and osteoblasts through a transcriptional Nf-κB-dependent mechanism [37, 66, 67, 77, 87, 99, 120, 130, 182, 218]. A TNF-stimulated pathway that includes Nf-κB activation via TRAF2 has been reported for dendritic cells [137]. Studies in bone and dendritic cells have provided additional evidence to support a role for p38 kinase and PKC in TNF stimulation of the IL-6 promoter [117, 154]. The way in which TNF stimulates MCSF is more controversial [52]. Kaplan et al. [98], have reported a transcriptional effect of TNF on MCSF expression. Furthermore, a putative Nf-κB binding site in the CSF-1 promoter can be shown to bind the p50 (but not the transactivational p65) subunit of Nf-κB [237]. However, inhibition of Nf-κB activation by N-acetyl cysteine fails to prevent TNF stimulation of both membrane and soluble forms of MCSF, and TNF does not regulate activity of a large MCSF promoter-reporter construct; this adds uncertainty to understanding the mechanism [86]. Deletion of the homologous Nf-κB consensus region in the MCSF promoter does not change transcriptional rate [185]. TNF also stimulates secretion of another member of the CSF factors, GM-CSF, which, in turn, increases secretion of TNF in an autocrine manner [37, 51, 69].

Effects of Cytokines on Osteoblast Differentiation

The steady-state number of osteoblasts results from a balance between their rate of differentiation and their rate of disappearance (Figure 5.6). Disappearance from the osteoblast pool may occur by apoptosis or progression to the osteocyte phenotype. TNF affects both the differentiation rate of osteoblasts from mesenchymal precursor cells and also their apoptosis. Osteoblasts are derived from pluripotent stem cells capable of differentiating to adipocytes, chondrocytes, fibroblasts, skeletal muscle cells, or tendon cells. Factors that stimulate differentiation in an osteoblastic direction, include the secreted proteins, insulin-like growth factor 1 (IGF-1), bone morphogenic proteins (BMPs), and the transcription factors RUNX2 (AML-3, Pepb2αA) and osterix (Osx). Gilbert et al. [63] have shown that TNF blocks osteoblast differentiation in three experimental models: fetal calvaria precursor cells, bone marrow stromal cells, and in the clonal MC3T3-E1 pre-osteoblast cell line. The critical period of sensitivity to TNF occurs when precursor cells commit to differentiate along an osteoblastic trajectory. The block to differentiation involves inhibition of IGF-1, RUNX2 (or Cbfa-1), and Osx, but not of BMPs-2, 4, or 6 [63, 65]. IGF-1 may act by expanding the pre-osteoblast pool through a mitogenic effect and by providing an anti-apoptotic stimulus. However, treatment with IGF-1 does not overcome the inhibitory effect of TNF. These results suggest that TNF acts downstream of the IGF-1 stimulus. TNF inhibits RUNX2 [64], a transcription factor that binds skeletal-specific enhancers in the osteocalcin promoter [10, 46, 113]. RUNX2 plays a critical role in skeletal development, because in the transgenic knockout there is no bone that mineralizes, only a cartilaginous skeletal pattern

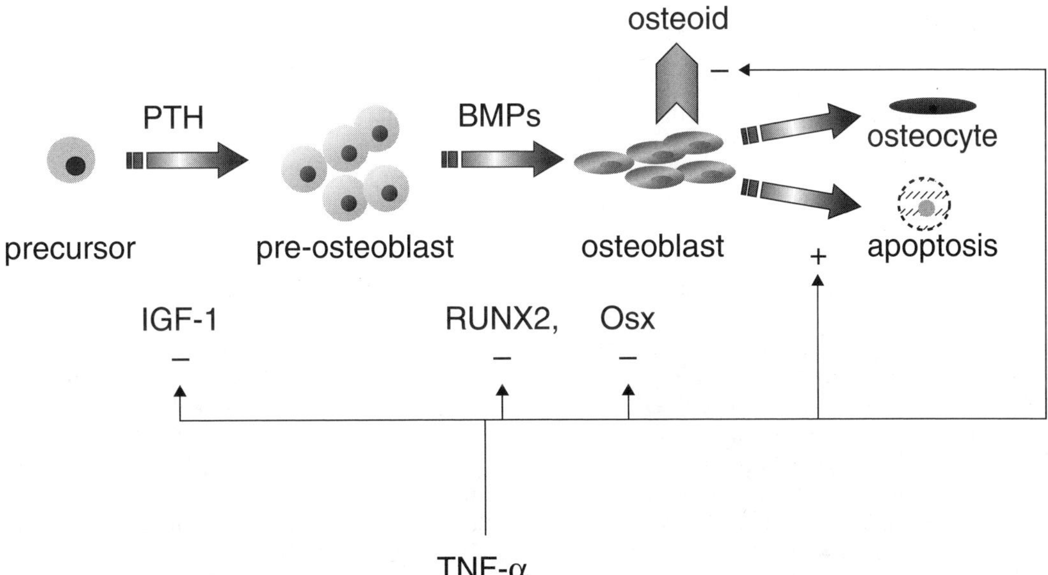

Figure 5.6　Role of TNF in osteoblast differentiation and survival. PTH and IGF-1 increase the pool of pluripotent precursor cells of mesenchymal origin. BMP signals the differentiation along an osteoblast/chondrocyte direction. The expression of the transcription factors RUNX2 and Osx is required for commitment to the osteoblast phenotype. TNF inhibits osteoblast differentiation by suppression of IGF-1, RUNX2, and Osx expression. Apoptosis of mature osteoblasts is stimulated. Functional consequences of TNF in mature osteoblasts include inhibition of bone-forming genes, increased expression of genes contributing to bone resorption, and vitamin D resistance. Reprinted from Gene, vol. 321, Nanes MS. Tumor necrosis factor-alpha: molecular and cellular mechanisms in skeletal pathology, 1–15 (2003), with permission from Elsevier.

devoid of marrow cavity. Many skeletal genes require RUNX2 for expression. These include alkaline phosphatase, osteopontin, bone sialoprotein, and COL1A1, and the transcription factor cEBPδ, all factors important for new bone formation [10, 13, 89, 102, 141, 189]. Interestingly, TNF inhibition of RUNX2 is isoform-specific. TNF almost completely inhibits mRNA and nuclear protein levels of the ubiquitous short form of RUNX2 (type 1), while inhibition of the longer osteoblastic-specific form (type 2, Til-1) is only 50% [64]. These results suggest that additional targets of TNF may exist that contribute to the blockade of differentiation. The TNF effect on RUNX2 includes both transcriptional suppression and mRNA destabilization [62, 64]. Although the RUNX2 distal promoter contains an Nf-κB homologous binding sequence, deletion of this sequence does not abolish TNF action. An area of the proximal promoter is required for the inhibition of RUNX2 transcription by TNF and also by Nf-κB [64]. Osx, an Sp-1 family protein that is up-regulated by BMP-2, is required downstream of RUNX2 for skeletal development, as knockout of Osx results in a phenotype similar to that of RUNX2 knockout despite RUNX2 expression [156, 234]. The mechanism of Osx inhibition by TNF has not been determined.

Although TNF inhibits osteoblast differentiation, the influence of this action on the bone formation rate in the postmenopausal skeleton has not been evaluated by histomorphometry. Gerstenfeld et al. found that fracture healing was delayed in TNF receptor-deficient mice [61]. In this model, the inflammatory action of TNF may be needed to replace fracture callus with new bone. Uy et al. did not find an effect of TNF on bone formation as measured by histomorphometry of nude mice bearing TNF-producing CHO cell tumors [216]. Neither of these models is representative of bone in the estrogen-deficient state, but the evidence suggests that the physiologic effect of TNF on bone formation may be complex. A lack of effect of TNF on basal bone formation rate would not preclude a possible inhibitory action in the postmenopausal skeleton in the estrogen-deficient state.

Effects of Cytokines on Osteoblast Survival

Most studies [78, 92, 109] (see also references in Hock et al. [79]) support the notion that TNF

and IL-1 induce apoptosis in osteoblasts. As noted above, a receptor death domain, as found in TNFR1, must signal through FADD to activate the caspase cascade. TNF (and IL-1) can also augment more powerful apoptotic stimuli that are induced by Fas ligand or cycloheximide [212]. Pascher et al. [171] did not find an effect of TNF alone on apoptosis of human osteoblasts; however, pretreatment of cells with 1,25-$(OH)_2D_3$ rendered the cells TNF-sensitive. In an interesting report by Bellido et al. [12], calbindin-D28k, a vitamin D-stimulated intracellular protein, was found to attenuate TNF-induced apoptosis by directly binding caspase-3. The experimental designs used by Pascher et al. and Bellido were quite different, with a very prolonged exposure to vitamin D in the former. Additional factors that block or attenuate TNF-induced apoptosis include dexamethasone, fluid shear stress, BMP-2 and BMP-4, and transforming growth factor β (TGFβ) [36, 38, 39, 173]. The relative contribution of apoptosis and rate of differentiation in regulating the pool of functioning osteoblasts remains controversial. Little is known about the effect of cytokines, or other factors, on further differentiation of osteoblasts to osteocytes.

TNF Induction of Vitamin D Resistance

The active metabolite of vitamin D_3, 1,25-$(OH)_2D_3$, contributes to skeletal health by stimulating intestinal calcium absorption and also by regulating gene transcription in bone cells. Aging and the postmenopausal state are associated with some resistance to 1,25-$(OH)_2D_3$ action. This can be attributed in part to a reduction in VDR number [5, 128, 229]. A rightward shift in the vitamin D dose-response has been reported in aged or osteoporotic patients with respect to calbindin-9_k expression, lymphocyte mitogenesis, and intestinal calcium absorption. This shift may not be entirely due to a decrease in VDR number [128, 160]. TNF has been shown to decrease vitamin D receptor number post-transcriptionally, and to decrease 1,25-$(OH)_2D_3$-stimulated receptor transactivation in osteoblastic cells [140, 159]. Interestingly, TNF treatment reduced the ligand-stimulated binding of the VDR/RXR (retinoid X receptor) heterodimer to the VDRE of the osteocalcin promoter. Deletion analysis of the osteocalcin promoter revealed that the vitamin D-responsive element (VDRE) conferred TNF suppression, even when the VDRE was cloned into a heterologous viral promoter [118, 157]. Transcriptional activation by a liganded VDR can therefore be suppressed by TNF-stimulated signals. Subsequently, Farmer et al. have shown that transcriptional suppression can be induced by forced expression of the p65 subunit of Nf-κB, but not by the p50 subunit [50]. A reciprocal suppression of Nf-κB transactivation of the IL-8 promoter by 1,25(OH)$_2$D$_3$ may involve a mechanism that inhibits Nf-κB binding to its cognate response element [72].

The regulation of VDR function by Nf-κB is not surprising, inasmuch as a similar transrepression of glucocorticoid receptors (GR) and retinoid X receptor (RXR) transactivation has been reported [3, 27, 54, 191]. The interaction between the GR and Nf-κB is reciprocal. Steroid receptors[1] that repress Nf-κB transactivation include the GR, progesterone receptor (PR), and the VDR [27, 72]. The mechanism of Nf-κB regulation of steroid receptor function is controversial. An Nf-κB response element in the target gene is not required for Nf-κB repression of either VDR or GR transactivation. The repression mechanism therefore may involve a protein-protein interaction. Further support for this concept is that GR repression of Nf-κB is limited to the α isoform of the GR and localizes to a region of the GR that encompasses the coactivator interface [24, 217]. Possible mechanisms for Nf-κB trans-repression include (1) direct binding of Nf-κB to steroid receptors; (2) Nf-κB competition or co-occupancy of general transcription proteins, including CBP or SRC-1; (3) competition for other nuclear proteins that bridge the steroid receptor-DNA complex to polymerase II; or (4) direct modification of polymerase II activity by TNF or Nf-κB. De Bosscher et al. have reported that GR repression of Nf-κB, or the reciprocal p65 repression of GR, occurs regardless of the level of CBP or SRC-1 in the cell, a finding that does not exclude potential competition for other nuclear coactivators [43]. Nissen et al. [161] have reported that the GR zinc finger domain (including the coactivator interface) can bind directly to the coactivator interface of p65. From the available data it seems that the transcriptional complex is co-

occupied by the steroid receptor and Nf-κB and as a result blunts transcriptional activation.

The p65 subunit of Nf-κB does not directly bind the VDR (Nanes, unpublished). Nf-κB repression of VDR has recently been shown to require the Rel homology domain of p65, which includes one of the CBP binding regions [133]. Thus, involvement of coactivator interface for both p65 and steroid receptors is required for transrepression. Lu et al. [133] have identified an additional midmolecular region of p65 that is also required for transrepression of VDR. This region includes a number of serine and tyrosine phosphorylation targets previously found to be required for p65 transcriptional activity. Deletion of this region or of individual serine or tyrosines reverses most of the p65 repression of VDR. These results add support to the concept that p65 interacts with nuclear proteins that are shared by the VDR transcriptional complex so as to reduce transactivational potency of the VDR. What coactivators are involved has not been determined.

Conclusion

Although many cytokines contribute to the pathophysiology of bone loss, TNF has an important and central role. A normally coupled resorption/formation system, important for the homeostasis of bone, is disturbed in the presence of elevated TNF. Such elevations may be acute, as in a flare of inflammatory arthritis, or insidious, as with estrogen loss and aging. Increased production of TNF damages bone by increasing bone resorption while simultaneously inhibiting bone-forming osteoblasts. This dual effect of TNF is a potent stimulus to skeletal loss that ultimately leads to microarchitectural deterioration and increased fracture risk. As discussed above, no single mechanism is responsible for TNF action on bone cells; rather, activation of a complex signal pathway drives gene transcription toward a skeletal catabolic state. TNF cooperates with other signal pathways activated by IL-1 and additional cytokines and the RANKL system, and also suppresses vitamin D action to impair bone at the cell, tissue, and physiologic levels. The accumulated evidence suggests that targeting of cytokine action by interfering with signal pathways from the TNFR1 or IL-1 receptors, through TRAFs, IRAKs, and finally Nf-κB, remains an important

---

[1] The term *steroid receptor* is used here to represent the nuclear receptors of the thyroid/retinoid/estrogen superfamily including the VDR.

goal for the treatment of osteoporosis. Many questions remain to be answered about cytokine action in bone. What are the key early genes that are activated (or suppressed) by TNF and IL-1? How can we capitalize on the mechanism of TNF stimulation of RANK/RANKL to block osteoclastogenesis? Can we circumvent TNF suppression of osteoblastogenesis to promote increased bone formation rates? Further investigation of cytokine action in bone is needed to answer these questions and provide interventions for bone loss in the aging skeleton.

References

1. Abrahamsen B, Shalhoub V, Larson EK, Eriksen EF, Beck-Nielsen H, Marks SC, Jr. (2000) Cytokine RNA levels in transiliac bone biopsies from healthy early postmenopausal women. Bone 26:137–45.
2. Abu-Amer Y, Erdmann J, Alexopoulou L, Kollias G, Ross FP, Teitelbaum SL (2000) Tumor necrosis factor receptors types 1 and 2 differentially regulate osteoclastogenesis. J Biol Chem 275:27307–10.
3. Adcock IM, Shirasaki H, Gelder CM, Peters MJ, Brown CR, Barnes PJ (1994) The effects of glucocorticoids on phorbol ester and cytokine stimulated transcription factor activation in human lung. Life Sci 55:1147–53.
4. An J, Ribeiro RC, Webb P, Gustafsson JA, Kushner PJ, Baxter JD, et al. (1999) Estradiol repression of tumor necrosis factor-α transcription requires estrogen receptor activation function-2 and is enhanced by coactivators. Proc Natl Acad Sci USA 96:15161–6.
5. Armbrecht HJ, Boltz MA, Christakos S, Bruns ME (1998) Capacity of 1,25-dihydroxyvitamin D to stimulate expression of calbindin D changes with age in the rat. Arch Biochem Biophys 352:159–64.
6. Atkins GJ, Haynes DR, Geary SM, Loric M, Crotti TN, Findlay DM (2000) Coordinated cytokine expression by stromal and hematopoietic cells during human osteoclast formation. Bone 26:653–61.
7. Aubin JE, Bonnelye E (2000) Osteoprotegerin and its ligand: a new paradigm for regulation of osteoclastogenesis and bone resorption. Osteoporos Int 11:905–13.
8. Azuma Y, Kaji K, Katogi R, Takeshita S, Kudo A (2000) Tumor necrosis factor-α induces differentiation of and bone resorption by osteoclasts. J Biol Chem 275:4858–64.
9. Baker PJ, Dixon M, Evans RT, Dufour L, Johnson E, Roopenian DC (1999) CD4(+) T cells and the proinflammatory cytokines gamma interferon and interleukin-6 contribute to alveolar bone loss in mice. Infect Immun 67:2804–9.
10. Banerjee C, McCabe LR, Choi JY, Hiebert SW, Stein JL, Stein GS, et al. (1997) Runt homology domain proteins in osteoblast differentiation: AML3/CBFA1 is a major component of a bone-specific complex. J Cell Biochem 66:1–8.
11. Bekker PJ, Holloway D, Nakanishi A, Arrighi M, Leese PT, Dunstan CR (2001) The effect of a single dose of osteoprotegerin in postmenopausal women. J Bone Miner Res 16:348–60.
12. Bellido T, Huening M, Raval-Pandya M, Manolagas SC, Christakos S (2000) Calbindin-D28k is expressed in osteoblastic cells and suppresses their apoptosis by inhibiting caspase-3 activity. J Biol Chem 275:26328–32.
13. Benson MD, Aubin JE, Xiao G, Thomas PE, Franceschi RT (1999) Cloning of a 2.5 kb murine bone sialoprotein promoter fragment and functional analysis of putative Osf2 binding sites. J Bone Min Res 14:396–405.
14. Beresford JN, Gallagher JA, Gowen M, Couch M, Poser J, Wood DD, et al. (1984) The effects of monocyte-conditioned medium and interleukin 1 on the synthesis of collagenous and non-collagenous proteins by mouse bone and human bone cells in vitro. Biochim Biophys Acta 801:58–65.
15. Bertolini DR, Nedwin GE, Bringman TS, Smith DD, Mundy GR (1986) Stimulation of bone resorption and inhibition of bone formation in vitro by human tumour necrosis factors. Nature 319:516–18.
16. Birkenkamp KU, Tuyt LM, Lummen C, Wierenga AT, Kruijer W, Vellenga E (2000) The p38 MAP kinase inhibitor SB203580 enhances nuclear factor-kappa B transcriptional activity by a non-specific effect upon the ERK pathway. Br J Pharmacol 131:99–107.
17. Bodine PV, Vernon SK, Komm BS (1996) Establishment and hormonal regulation of a conditionally transformed preosteocytic cell line from adult human bone. Endocrinology 137:4592–604.
18. Boss JM, Jensen PE (2003) Transcriptional regulation of the MHC class II antigen presentation pathway. Curr Opin Immunol 15:105–11.
19. Boyce BF, Xing L, Franzoso G, Siebenlist U (1999) Required and nonessential functions of nuclear factor-kappa B in bone cells. Bone 25:137–9.
20. Boyle WJ, Simonet WS, Lacey DL (2003) Osteoclast differentiation and activation. Nature 423:337–42.
21. Bradford PG, Maglich JM, Kirkwood KL (2000) IL-1 beta increases type 1 inositol trisphosphate receptor expression and IL-6 secretory capacity in osteoblastic cell cultures. Mol Cell Biol Res Commun 3:73–5.
22. Brandstrom H, Jonsson KB, Vidal O, Ljunghall S, Ohlsson C, Ljunggren O (1998) Tumor necrosis factor-α and -beta upregulate the levels of osteoprotegerin mRNA in human osteosarcoma MG-63 cells. Biochem Biophys Res Commun 248:454–7.
23. Brennan FM, Browne KA, Green PA, Jaspar JM, Maini RN, Feldmann M (1997) Reduction of serum matrix metalloproteinase 1 and matrix metalloproteinase 3 in rheumatoid arthritis patients following anti-tumour necrosis factor-α (cA2) therapy. Br J Rheumatol 36:643–50.
24. Brogan IJ, Murray IA, Cerillo G, Needham M, White A, Davis JR (1999) Interaction of glucocorticoid receptor isoforms with transcription factors AP-1 and Nf-κB: lack of effect of glucocorticoid receptor beta. Mol Cell Endocrinol 157:95–104.
25. Burns K, Clatworthy J, Martin L, Martinon F, Plumpton C, Maschera B, et al. (2000) Tollip, a new component of the IL-1RI pathway, links IRAK to the IL-1 receptor. Nat Cell Biol 2:346–51.
26. Burow ME, Weldon CB, Tang Y, McLachlan JA, Beckman BS (2001) Oestrogen-mediated suppression

of tumour necrosis factor α -induced apoptosis in MCF-7 cells: subversion of Bcl-2 by anti-oestrogens. J Steroid Biochem Mol Biol 78:409–18.

27. Caldenhoven E, Liden J, Wissink S, Van de Stolpe A, Raaijmakers J, Koenderman L, et al. (1995) Negative cross-talk between RelA and the glucocorticoid receptor: a possible mechanism for the antiinflammatory action of glucocorticoids. Mol Endocrinol 9: 401–12.

28. Canalis E (1987) Effects of tumor necrosis factor on bone formation in vitro. Endocrinology. 121:1596–604.

29. Cao Z, Xiong J, Takeuchi M, Kurama T, Goeddel DV (1996) TRAF6 is a signal transducer for interleukin-1. Nature 383:443–6.

30. Carpentier I, Beyaert R (1999) TRAF1 is a TNF inducible regulator of Nf-κB activation. FEBS Lett 460:246–50.

31. Catrina AI, Lampa J, Ernestam S, af Klint E, Bratt J, Klareskog L, et al. (2002) Anti-tumour necrosis factor (TNF)-_α therapy (etanercept) down-regulates serum matrix metalloproteinase (MMP)-3 and MMP-1 in rheumatoid arthritis. Rheumatology (Oxford) 41: 484–9.

32. Cenci S, Toraldo G, Weitzmann MN, Roggia C, Gao Y, Qian WP, et al. (2003) Estrogen deficiency induces bone loss by increasing T cell proliferation and lifespan through IFN-gamma-induced class II transactivator. Proc Natl Acad Sci USA 100:10405–10.

33. Cenci S, Weitzmann MN, Roggia C, Namba N, Novack D, Woodring J, et al. (2000) Estrogen deficiency induces bone loss by enhancing T-cell production of TNF-α. J Clin Invest 106:1229–37.

34. Centrella M, McCarthy TL, Canalis E (1988) Tumor necrosis factor-α inhibits collagen synthesis and alkaline phosphatase activity independently of its effect on deoxyribonucleic acid synthesis in osteoblast-enriched bone cell cultures. Endocrinology 123:1442–8.

35. Chabaud M, Miossec P (2001) The combination of tumor necrosis factor α blockade with interleukin-1 and interleukin-17 blockade is more effective for controlling synovial inflammation and bone resorption in an ex vivo model. Arthritis Rheum 44:1293–303.

36. Chae HJ, Chae SW, Kang JS, Bang BG, Cho SB, Park RK, et al. (2000) Dexamethasone suppresses tumor necrosis factor-α – induced apoptosis in osteoblasts: possible role for ceramide. Endocrinology 141:2904–13.

37. Chaudhary LR, Spelsberg TC, Riggs BL (1992) Production of various cytokines by normal human osteoblast-like cells in response to interleukin-1 beta and tumor necrosis factor-α: lack of regulation by 17 beta-estradiol. Endocrinology 130:2528–34.

38. Chen S, Guttridge DC, Tang E, Shi S, Guan K, Wang CY (2001) Suppression of tumor necrosis factor-mediated apoptosis by nuclear factor kappaB-independent bone morphogenetic protein/Smad signaling. J Biol Chem 276:39259–63.

39. Chua CC, Chua BH, Chen Z, Landy C, Hamdy RC (2002) TGF-beta1 inhibits multiple caspases induced by TNF-α in murine osteoblastic MC3T3-E1 cells. Biochim Biophys Acta 1593:1–8.

40. Chung KY, Agarwal A, Uitto J, Mauviel A (1996) An AP-1 binding sequence is essential for regulation of the human α2(I) collagen (COL1A2) promoter activity by transforming growth factor-beta. J Biol Chem 271: 3272–8.

41. Darnay BG, Ni J, Moore PA, Aggarwal BB (1999) Activation of Nf-κB by RANK requires tumor necrosis factor receptor-associated factor (TRAF) 6 and Nf-κB -inducing kinase. Identification of a novel TRAF6 interaction motif. J Biol Chem 274:7724–31.

42. de Bart AC, Quax PH, Lowik CW, Verheijen JH (1995) Regulation of plasminogen activation, matrix metalloproteinases and urokinase-type plasminogen activator-mediated extracellular matrix degradation in human osteosarcoma cell line MG63 by interleukin-1 α. J Bone Miner Res 10:1374–84.

43. De Bosscher K, Vanden Berghe W, Vermeulen L, Plaisance S, Boone E, Haegeman G (2000) Glucocorticoids repress Nf-κB -driven genes by disturbing the interaction of p65 with the basal transcription machinery, irrespective of coactivator levels in the cell. Proc Natl Acad Sci USA 97:3919–24.

44. de Brum-Fernandes AJ, Laporte S, Heroux M, Lora M, Patry C, Menard HA, et al. (1994) Expression of prostaglandin endoperoxide synthase-1 and prostaglandin endoperoxide synthase-2 in human osteoblasts. Biochem Biophys Res Commun 198:955–60.

45. Delaisse JM, Eeckhout Y, Vaes G (1988) Bone-resorbing agents affect the production and distribution of procollagenase as well as the activity of collagenase in bone tissue. Endocrinology 123:264–76.

46. Ducy P, Zhang R, Geoffroy V, Ridall AL, Karsenty G (1997) Osf2/Cbfa1: a transcriptional activator of osteoblast differentiation Cell 89:747–54.

47. Eghbali-Fatourechi G, Khosla S, Sanyal A, Boyle WJ, Lacey DL, Riggs BL (2003) Role of RANK ligand in mediating increased bone resorption in early postmenopausal women. J Clin Invest 111:1221–30.

48. Evans DB, Bunning RA, Russell RG (1990) The effects of recombinant human interleukin-1 beta on cellular proliferation and the production of prostaglandin E2, plasminogen activator, osteocalcin and alkaline phosphatase by osteoblast-like cells derived from human bone. Biochem Biophys Res Commun 166:208–16.

49. Farley JR, Stilt-Coffing B (2001) Apoptosis may determine the release of skeletal alkaline phosphatase activity from human osteoblast-line cells. Calcif Tissue Int 68:43–52.

50. Farmer PK, He X, Schmitz ML, Rubin J, Nanes MS (2000) Inhibitory effect of Nf-κB on 1,25-dihydroxyvitamin D(3) and retinoid X receptor function. Am J Physiol Endocrinol Metab 279:E213–20.

51. Felix R, Cecchini MG, Hofstetter W, Guenther HL, Fleisch H (1991) Production of granulocyte-macrophage (GM-CSF) and granulocyte colony-stimulating factor (G-CSF) by rat clonal osteoblastic cell population CRP 10/30 and the immortalized cell line IRC10/30-myc1 stimulated by tumor necrosis factor α. Endocrinology 128:661–7.

52. Felix R, Fleisch H, Elford PR (1989) Bone-resorbing cytokines enhance release of macrophage colony-stimulating activity by the osteoblastic cell MC3T3-E1. Calcif Tissue Int 44:356–60.

53. Feng X, Teitelbaum SL, Quiroz ME, Cheng SL, Lai CF, Avioli LV, et al. (2000) Sp1/Sp3 and PU.1 differentially regulate beta(5) integrin gene expression in macrophages and osteoblasts. J Biol Chem 275:8331–40.

54. Fernandez-Martin JL, Kurian S, Farmer P, Nanes MS (1998) Tumor necrosis factor activates a nuclear

inhibitor of vitamin D and retinoid-X receptors. Mol Cell Endocrinol 141:65–72.

55. Fox HS, Bond BL, Parslow TG (1991) Estrogen regulates the IFN-gamma promoter. J Immunol 146:4362–7.

56. Fox SW, Chambers TJ (2000) Interferon-gamma directly inhibits TRANCE-induced osteoclastogenesis. Biochem Biophys Res Commun 276:868–72.

57. Franzoso G, Carlson L, Xing L, Poljak L, Shores EW, Brown KD, et al. (1997) Requirement for Nf-κB in osteoclast and B-cell development. Genes Dev 11:3482–96.

58. Fuller K, Murphy C, Kirstein B, Fox SW, Chambers TJ (2002) TNF α potently activates osteoclasts, through a direct action independent of and strongly synergistic with RANKL. Endocrinology 143:1108–18.

59. Galibert L, Tometsko ME, Anderson DM, Cosman D, Dougall WC (1998) The involvement of multiple tumor necrosis factor receptor (TNFR)-associated factors in the signaling mechanisms of receptor activator of Nf-κB, a member of the TNFR superfamily. J Biol Chem. 273:34120–7.

60. Galien R, Garcia T (1997) Estrogen receptor impairs interleukin-6 expression by preventing protein binding on the Nf-κB site. Nucleic Acids Res 25:2424–9.

61. Gerstenfeld LC, Cho TJ, Kon T, Aizawa T, Cruceta J, Graves BD, et al. (2001) Impaired intramembranous bone formation during bone repair in the absence of tumor necrosis factor-α signaling. Cells Tissues Organs 169:285–94.

62. Gilbert L, Brantley A, Rubin J, Nanes MS (2002) The p55 TNF receptor mediates TNF inhibition of osteoblast differentiation. J Bone Miner Res 17:SU205.

63. Gilbert L, He X, Farmer P, Boden S, Kozlowski M, Rubin J, et al. (2000) Inhibition of osteoblast differentiation by tumor necrosis factor-α. Endocrinology 141:3956–64.

64. Gilbert L, He X, Farmer P, Rubin J, Drissi H, van WAJ, et al. (2002) Expression of the osteoblast differentiation factor RUNX2 (Cbfa1/AML3/Pebp2 αA) is inhibited by tumor necrosis factor-α. J Biol Chem 277:2695–701.

65. Gilbert LC, He, X., Kauppi, A., Rubin, J., Nanes, M.S. (2003) Inhibition of osteoblast differentiation by TNF-α is associated with suppression of osterix expression. J Bone Mineral Res 18:SU177.

66. Gimble JM, Hudson J, Henthorn J, Hua XX, Burstein SA (1991) Regulation of interleukin 6 expression in murine bone marrow stromal cells. Exp Hematol 19:1055–60.

67. Girasole G, Jilka RL, Passeri G, Boswell S, Boder G, Williams DC, et al. (1992) 17 beta-estradiol inhibits interleukin-6 production by bone marrow-derived stromal cells and osteoblasts in vitro: a potential mechanism for the antiosteoporotic effect of estrogens. J Clin Invest 89:883–91.

68. Gourley T, Roys S, Lukacs NW, Kunkel SL, Flavell RA, Chang CH (1999) A novel role for the major histocompatibility complex class II transactivator CIITA in the repression of IL-4 production. Immunity 10:377–86.

69. Gowen M, Chapman K, Littlewood A, Hughes D, Evans D, Russell G (1990) Production of tumor necrosis factor by human osteoblasts is modulated by other cytokines, but not by osteotropic hormones. Endocrinology 126:1250–5.

70. Gowen M, MacDonald BR, Russell RG (1988) Actions of recombinant human gamma-interferon and tumor necrosis factor α on the proliferation and osteoblastic characteristics of human trabecular bone cells in vitro. Arthritis Rheum 31:1500–7.

71. Hanevold CD, Yamaguchi DT, Jordan SC (1993) Tumor necrosis factor α modulates parathyroid hormone action in UMR-106-01 osteoblastic cells. J Bone Miner Res 8:1191–200.

72. Harant H, Andrew PJ, Reddy GS, Foglar E, Lindley IJ (1997) 1 α,25-dihydroxyvitamin D₃ and a variety of its natural metabolites transcriptionally repress nuclear-factor-kappaB-mediated interleukin-8 gene expression. Eur J Biochem 250:63–71.

73. Harrison JR, Kleinert LM, Kelly PL, Krebsbach PH, Woody C, Clark S, et al. (1998) Interleukin-1 represses COLIA1 promoter activity in calvarial bones of transgenic ColCAT mice in vitro and in vivo. J Bone Miner Res 13:1076–83.

74. Harrison JR, Lorenzo JA, Kawaguchi H, Raisz LG, Pilbeam C (1994) Stimulation of prostaglandin E2 production by interleukin-1α and transforming growth factor α in osteoblastic MC3T3-E1 cells. J Bone Miner Res 9:817–23.

75. Hatamochi A, Mori K, Ueki H (1994) Role of cytokines in controlling connective tissue gene expression. Arch Dermatol Res 287:115–21.

76. Hernandez I, de la Torre P, Rey-Campos J, Garcia I, Sanchez JA, Munoz R, et al. (2000) Collagen α1(I) gene contains an element responsive to tumor necrosis factor-α located in the 5′ untranslated region of its first exon. DNA Cell Biol 19:341–52.

77. Hierl T, Borcsok I, Sommer U, Ziegler R, Kasperk C (1998) Regulation of interleukin-6 expression in human osteoblastic cells in vitro. Exp Clin Endocrinol Diabetes 106:324–33.

78. Hill PA, Tumber A, Meikle MC (1997) Multiple extracellular signals promote osteoblast survival and apoptosis. Endocrinology 138:3849–58.

79. Hock JM, Krishnan V, Onyia JE, Bidwell JP, Milas J, Stanislaus D (2001) Osteoblast apoptosis and bone turnover. J Bone Miner Res 16:975–84.

80. Hofbauer LC, Heufelder AE (2001) Role of receptor activator of nuclear factor-kappaB ligand and osteoprotegerin in bone cell biology. J Mol Med 79:243–53.

81. Hofbauer LC, Lacey DL, Dunstan CR, Spelsberg TC, Riggs BL, Khosla S (1999) Interleukin-1beta and tumor necrosis factor-α, but not interleukin-6, stimulate osteoprotegerin ligand gene expression in human osteoblastic cells. Bone 25:255–9.

82. Horowitz MC, Xi Y, Wilson K, Kacena MA (2001) Control of osteoclastogenesis and bone resorption by members of the TNF family of receptors and ligands. Cytokine Growth Factor Rev 12:9–18.

83. Hukkanen M, Hughes FJ, Buttery LD, Gross SS, Evans TJ, Seddon S, et al. (1995) Cytokine-stimulated expression of inducible nitric oxide synthase by mouse, rat, and human osteoblast-like cells and its functional role in osteoblast metabolic activity. Endocrinology 136:5445–53.

84. Inagaki Y, Truter S, Tanaka S, Di Liberto M, Ramirez F (1995) Overlapping pathways mediate the opposing actions of tumor necrosis factor-α and transforming growth factor-beta on α2(I) collagen gene transcription. J Biol Chem 270:3353–8.

85. Iraburu MJ, Dominguez-Rosales JA, Fontana L, Auster A, Garcia-Trevijano ER, Covarrubias-Pinedo A, et al. (2000) Tumor necrosis factor α down-regulates expression of the α1(I) collagen gene in rat hepatic stellate cells through a p20C/EBPbeta- and C/EBPdelta-dependent mechanism. Hepatology 31:1086–93.

86. Isaacs SD, Fan X, Fan D, Gewant H, Murphy TC, Farmer P, et al. (1999) Role of NFkappaB in the regulation of macrophage colony stimulating factor by tumor necrosis factor-α in ST2 bone stromal cells. J Cell Physiol 179:193–200.

87. Ishimi Y, Miyaura C, Jin CH, Akatsu T, Abe E, Nakamura Y, et al. (1990) IL-6 is produced by osteoblasts and induces bone resorption. J Immunol 145:3297–303.

88. Janssens S, Beyaert R (2003) Functional diversity and regulation of different interleukin-1 receptor-associated kinase (IRAK) family members. Mol Cell 11:293–302.

89. Javed A, Barnes GL, Jasanya BO, Stein JL, Gerstenfeld L, Lian JB, et al. (2001) runt homology domain transcription factors (Runx, Cbfa, and AML) mediate repression of the bone sialoprotein promoter: evidence for promoter context-dependent activity of Cbfa proteins. Mol Cell Biol 21:2891–905.

90. Jefferies C, Bowie A, Brady G, Cooke EL, Li X, O'Neill LA (2001) Transactivation by the p65 subunit of Nf-κB in response to interleukin-1 (IL-1) involves MyD88, IL-1 receptor-associated kinase 1, TRAF-6, and Rac1. Mol Cell Biol 21:4544–52.

91. Jiang Z, Ninomiya-Tsuji J, Qian Y, Matsumoto K, Li X (2002) Interleukin-1 (IL-1) receptor-associated kinase-dependent IL-1-induced signaling complexes phosphorylate TAK1 and TAB2 at the plasma membrane and activate TAK1 in the cytosol. Mol Cell Biol 22:7158–67.

92. Jilka RL, Weinstein RS, Bellido T, Parfitt AM, Manolagas SC (1998) Osteoblast programmed cell death (apoptosis): modulation by growth factors and cytokines. J Bone Miner Res 13:793–802.

93. Jimi E, Ikebe T, Takahashi N, Hirata M, Suda T, Koga T (1996) Interleukin-1α activates all NF-kappa-b-like factor in osteoclast-like cells. Journal of Biological Chemistry 271:4605–4608.

94. Jimi E, Nakamura I, Ikebe T, Akiyama S, Takahashi N, Suda T (1998) Activation of Nf-κB is involved in the survival of osteoclasts promoted by interleukin-1. J Biol Chem 273:8799–805.

95. Kahari VM, Chen YQ, Su MW, Ramirez F, Uitto J (1990) Tumor necrosis factor-α and interferon-gamma suppress the activation of human type I collagen gene expression by transforming growth factor-beta 1. Evidence for two distinct mechanisms of inhibition at the transcriptional and posttranscriptional levels. J Clin Invest 86:1489–95.

96. Kaji K, Katogi R, Azuma Y, Naito A, Inoue JI, Kudo A (2001) Tumor necrosis factor α -induced osteoclastogenesis requires tumor necrosis factor receptor-associated factor 6. J Bone Miner Res 16:1593–9.

97. Kamada M, Irahara M, Maegawa M, Ohmoto Y, Murata K, Yasui T, et al. (2001) Transient increase in the levels of T-helper 1 cytokines in postmenopausal women and the effects of hormone replacement therapy. Gynecol Obstet Invest 52:82–8.

98. Kaplan DL, Eielson CM, Horowitz MC, Insogna KL, Weir EC (1996) Tumor necrosis factor-α induces transcription of the colony-stimulating factor-1 gene in murine osteoblasts. J Cell Physiol 168:199–208.

99. Kassem M, Harris SA, Spelsberg TC, Riggs BL (1996) Estrogen inhibits interleukin-6 production and gene expression in a human osteoblastic cell line with high levels of estrogen receptors. J Bone Miner Res 11:193–9.

100. Katz MS, Gutierrez GE, Mundy GR, Hymer TK, Caulfield MP, McKee RL (1992) Tumor necrosis factor and interleukin 1 inhibit parathyroid hormone-responsive adenylate cyclase in clonal osteoblast-like cells by down-regulating parathyroid hormone receptors. J Cell Physiol 153:206–13.

101. Kawaguchi H, Yavari R, Stover ML, Rowe DW, Raisz LG, Pilbeam CC (1994) Measurement of interleukin-1 stimulated constitutive prostaglandin G/H synthase (cyclooxygenase) mRNA levels in osteoblastic MC3T3-E1 cells using competitive reverse transcriptase polymerase chain reaction. Endocr Res 20:219–33.

102. Kern B, Shen J, Starbuck M, Karsenty G (2001) Cbfa1 contributes to the osteoblast-specific expression of type I collagen genes. J Biol Chem 276:7101–7.

103. Khosla S, Atkinson EJ, Dunstan CR, O'Fallon WM (2002) Effect of estrogen versus testosterone on circulating osteoprotegerin and other cytokine levels in normal elderly men. J Clin Endocrinol Metab 87:1550–4.

104. Kim CH, Kang BS, Lee TK, Park WH, Kim JK, Park YG, et al. (2002) IL-1beta regulates cellular proliferation, prostaglandin E2 synthesis, plasminogen activator activity, osteocalcin production, and bone resorptive activity of the mouse calvarial bone cells. Immunopharmacol Immunotoxicol 24:395–407.

105. Kim YM, Im JY, Han SH, Kang HS, Choi I (2000) IFN-gamma up-regulates IL-18 gene expression via IFN consensus sequence-binding protein and activator protein-1 elements in macrophages. J Immunol 165:3198–205.

106. Kimble RB, Bain S, Pacifici R (1997) The functional block of TNF but not of IL-6 prevents bone loss in ovariectomized mice. J Bone Miner Res 12:935–41.

107. Kimble RB, Matayoshi AB, Vannice JL, Kung VT, Williams C, Pacifici R (1995) Simultaneous block of interleukin-1 and tumor necrosis factor is required to completely prevent bone loss in the early postovariectomy period. Endocrinology 136:3054–61.

108. Kimble RB, Srivastava S, Ross FP, Matayoshi A, Pacifici R (1996) Estrogen deficiency increases the ability of stromal cells to support murine osteoclastogenesis via an interleukin-1and tumor necrosis factor-mediated stimulation of macrophage colony-stimulating factor production. J Biol Chem 271:28890–7.

109. Kitajima I, Soejima Y, Takasaki I, Beppu H, Tokioka T, Maruyama I (1996) Ceramide-induced nuclear translocation of NF-kappa B is a potential mediator of the apoptotic response to TNF-α in murine clonal osteoblasts. Bone 19:263–70.

110. Kitazawa R, Kimble RB, Vannice JL, Kung VT, Pacifici R (1994) Interleukin-1 receptor antagonist and tumor necrosis factor binding protein decrease osteoclast formation and bone resorption in ovariectomized mice. J Clin Invest 94:2397–406.

111. Kobayashi K, Takahashi N, Jimi E, Udagawa N, Takami M, Kotake S, et al. (2000) Tumor necrosis factor α stimulates osteoclast differentiation by a mechanism inde-

pendent of the ODF/RANKL-RANK interaction. J Exp Med 191:275–86.

112. Komine M, Kukita A, Kukita T, Ogata Y, Hotokebuchi T, Kohashi O (2001) Tumor necrosis factor-α cooperates with receptor activator of nuclear factor kappaB ligand in generation of osteoclasts in stromal cell-depleted rat bone marrow cell culture. Bone 28:474–83.

113. Komori T, Yagi H, Nomura S, Yamaguchi A, Sasaki K, Deguchi K, et al. (1997) Targeted disruption of Cbfa1 results in a complete lack of bone formation owing to maturational arrest of osteoblasts. Cell 89:755–64.

114. Kose KN, Xie JF, Carnes DL, Graves DT (1996) Pro-inflammatory cytokines downregulate platelet derived growth factor-α receptor gene expression in human osteoblastic cells. J Cell Physiol 166:188–97.

115. Kouba DJ, Chung KY, Nishiyama T, Vindevoghel L, Kon A, Klement JF, et al. (1999) Nuclear factor-kappa B mediates TNF-α inhibitory effect on α2(I) collagen (COL1A2) gene transcription in human dermal fibroblasts. J Immunol 162:4226–34.

116. Kudo O, Fujikawa Y, Itonaga I, Sabokbar A, Torisu T, Athanasou NA (2002) Proinflammatory cytokine (TNFα /IL-1α) induction of human osteoclast formation. J Pathol 198:220–7.

117. Kumar S, Votta BJ, Rieman DJ, Badger AM, Gowen M, Lee JC (2001) IL-1- and TNF-induced bone resorption is mediated by p38 mitogen activated protein kinase. J Cell Physiol 187:294–303.

118. Kuno H, Kurian SM, Hendy GN, White J, deLuca HF, Evans CO, et al. (1994) Inhibition of 1,25-dihydroxyvitamin D_3 stimulated osteocalcin gene transcription by tumor necrosis factor-α: structural determinants within the vitamin D response element. Endocrinology 134:2524–31.

119. Kuroki T, Shingu M, Koshihara Y, Nobunaga M (1994) Effects of cytokines on alkaline phosphatase and osteocalcin production, calcification and calcium release by human osteoblastic cells. Br J Rheumatol 33:224–30.

120. Kurokouchi K, Kambe F, Yasukawa K, Izumi R, Ishiguro N, Iwata H, et al. (1998) TNF-α increases expression of IL-6 and ICAM-1 genes through activation of Nf-κB in osteoblast-like ROS17/2.8 cells. J Bone Miner Res 13:1290–9.

121. Kusano K, Miyaura C, Inada M, Tamura T, Ito A, Nagase H, et al. (1998) Regulation of matrix metalloproteinases (MMP-2, -3, -9, and -13) by interleukin-1 and interleukin-6 in mouse calvaria: association of MMP induction with bone resorption. Endocrinology 139:1338–45.

122. Lacey DL, Grosso LE, Moser SA, Erdmann J, Tan HL, Pacifici R, et al. (1993) IL-1-induced murine osteoblast IL-6 production is mediated by the type 1 IL-1 receptor and is increased by 1,25 dihydroxyvitamin D_3. J Clin Invest 91:1731–42.

123. Lam J, Takeshita S, Barker JE, Kanagawa O, Ross FP, Teitelbaum SL (2000) TNF-α induces osteoclastogenesis by direct stimulation of macrophages exposed to permissive levels of RANK ligand. J Clin Invest 106:1481–8.

124. Lee SE, Chung WJ, Kwak HB, Chung CH, Kwack KB, Lee ZH, et al. (2001) Tumor necrosis factor-α supports the survival of osteoclasts through the activation of Akt and ERK. J Biol Chem 276:49343–9.

125. Lee SK, Kalinowski JF, Jastrzebski SL, Puddington L, Lorenzo JA (2003) Interleukin-7 is a direct inhibitor of in vitro osteoclastogenesis. Endocrinology 144:3524–31.

126. Lee ZH, Lee SE, Kim CW, Lee SH, Kim SW, Kwack K, et al. (2002) IL-1α stimulation of osteoclast survival through the PI 3-kinase/Akt and ERK pathways. J Biochem (Tokyo) 131:161–6.

127. Li YP, Stashenko P (1992) Proinflammatory cytokines tumor necrosis factor-α and IL-6, but not IL-1, downregulate the osteocalcin gene promoter. J Immunol 148:788–94.

128. Liel Y, Shany S, Smirnoff P, Schwartz B (1999) Estrogen increases 1,25-dihydroxyvitamin D receptors expression and bioresponse in the rat duodenal mucosa. Endocrinology 140:280–5.

129. Lindberg MK, Erlandsson M, Alatalo SL, Windahl S, Andersson G, Halleen JM, et al. (2001) Estrogen receptor alpha, but not estrogen receptor beta, is involved in the regulation of the OPG/RANKL (osteoprotegerin/receptor activator of NF-kappa B ligand) ratio and serum interleukin-6 in male mice. J Endocrinol 171:425–33.

130. Littlewood AJ, Russell J, Harvey GR, Hughes DE, Russell RG, Gowen M (1991) The modulation of the expression of IL-6 and its receptor in human osteoblasts in vitro. Endocrinology 129:1513–20.

131. Logan TF, Gooding W, Kirkwood JM, Shadduck RK (1996) Tumor necrosis factor administration is associated with increased endogenous production of M-CSF and G-CSF but not GM-CSF in human cancer patients. Exp Hematol 24:49–53.

132. Lorenzo JA, Pilbeam CC, Kalinowski JF, Hibbs MS (1992) Production of both 92- and 72-kDa gelatinases by bone cells. Matrix 12:282–90.

133. Lu X, Fiester, P., Rubin, J., Nanes M.S. (2003) NfkB suppression of VDR transactivaation requires the Rel Homology Domain of p65. J Bone Mineral Res 18:F459.

134. Luchin A, Suchting S, Merson T, Rosol TJ, Hume DA, Cassady AI, et al. (2001) Genetic and physical interactions between Microphthalmia transcription factor and PU.1 are necessary for osteoclast gene expression and differentiation. J Biol Chem 276:36703–10.

135. Manji SS, Zhou H, Findlay DM, Martin TJ, Ng KW (1995) Tumor necrosis factor-α facilitates nuclear actions of retinoic acid to regulate expression of the alkaline phosphatase gene in preosteoblasts. J Biol Chem 270:8958–62.

136. Mann GN, Jacobs TW, Buchinsky FJ, Armstrong EC, Li M, Ke HZ, et al. (1994) Interferon-gamma causes loss of bone volume *in vivo* and fails to ameliorate cyclosporin A-induced osteopenia. Endocrinology 135:1077–1083.

137. Mann J, Oakley F, Johnson PW, Mann DA (2002) CD40 induces interleukin-6 gene transcription in dendritic cells: regulation by TRAF2, AP-1, NF-kappa B, AND CBF1. J Biol Chem 277:17125–38.

138. Manolagas SC (1995) Role of cytokines in bone resorption. Bone 17:63S–67S.

139. Marusic A, Kalinowski JF, Harrison JR, Centrella M, Raisz LG, Lorenzo JA (1991) Effects of transforming growth factor-beta and IL-1α on prostaglandin synthesis in serum-deprived osteoblastic cells. J Immunol 146:2633–8.

140. Mayur N, Lewis S, Catherwood BD, Nanes MS (1993) Tumor necrosis factor-α decreases 1,25-dihydroxyvitamin D_3 receptors in osteoblastic ROS 17/2.8 cells. J Bone Miner Res 8:997–1003.

141. McCarthy TL, Ji C, Chen Y, Kim KK, Imagawa M, Ito Y, et al. (2000) Runt domain factor (Runx)-dependent effects on CCAAT/ enhancer-binding protein delta expression and activity in osteoblasts. J Biol Chem 275: 21746–53.

142. McSheehy PM, Chambers TJ (1986) Osteoblastic cells mediate osteoclastic responsiveness to parathyroid hormone. Endocrinology 118:824–8.

143. McSheehy PM, Chambers TJ (1986) Osteoblast-like cells in the presence of parathyroid hormone release soluble factor that stimulates osteoclastic bone resorption. Endocrinology 119:1654–9.

144. McSheehy PM, Chambers TJ (1987) 1,25-Dihydroxyvitamin D$_3$ stimulates rat osteoblastic cells to release a soluble factor that increases osteoclastic bone resorption. J Clin Invest 80:425–9.

145. Meikle MC, Bord S, Hembry RM, Reynolds JJ (1995) The synthesis of collagenase, gelatinase-A (72 kDa) and -B (95 kDa), and TIMP-1 and -2 by human osteoblasts from normal and arthritic bone. Bone 17: 255–60.

146. Min YK, Rao Y, Okada Y, Raisz LG, Pilbeam CC (1998) Regulation of prostaglandin G/H synthase-2 expression by interleukin-1 in human osteoblast-like cells. J Bone Miner Res 13:1066–75.

147. Mori K, Hatamochi A, Ueki H, Olsen A, Jimenez SA (1996) The transcription of human α1(I) procollagen gene (COL1A1) is suppressed by tumour necrosis factor-α through proximal short promoter elements: evidence for suppression mechanisms mediated by two nuclear-factorbinding sites. Biochem J 319 (Pt 3): 811–6.

148. Muegge K, Durum S (1990) Cytokines and Transcription Factors. [Review]. Cytokine 2:1–8.

149. Muhlethaler-Mottet A, Di Berardino W, Otten LA, Mach B (1998) Activation of the MHC class II transactivator CIITA by interferon-gamma requires cooperative interaction between Stat1 and USF-1. Immunity 8: 157–66.

150. Muhlethaler-Mottet A, Otten LA, Steimle V, Mach B (1997) Expression of MHC class II molecules in different cellular and functional compartments is controlled by differential usage of multiple promoters of the transactivator CIITA. Embo J 16:2851–60.

151. Murphy KM, Ouyang W, Farrar JD, Yang J, Ranganath S, Asnagli H, et al. (2000) Signaling and transcription in T helper development. Annu Rev Immunol 18: 451–94.

152. Nagarajan UM, Bushey A, Boss JM (2002) Modulation of gene expression by the MHC class II transactivator. J Immunol 169:5078–88.

153. Nagarajan UM, Lochamy J, Chen X, Beresford GW, Nilsen R, Jensen PE, et al. (2002) Class II transactivator is required for maximal expression of HLA-DOB in B cells. J Immunol 168:1780–6.

154. Nagy Z, Radeff J, Stern PH (2001) Stimulation of interleukin-6 promoter by parathyroid hormone, tumor necrosis factor -α, and interleukin-1beta in UMR-106 osteoblastic cells is inhibited by protein kinase C antagonists. J Bone Miner Res 16:1220–7.

155. Nakase T, Takaoka K, Masuhara K, Shimizu K, Yoshikawa H, Ochi T (1997) Interleukin-1 beta enhances and tumor necrosis factor-α inhibits bone morphogenetic protein-2-induced alkaline phosphatase activity in MC3T3-E1 osteoblastic cells. Bone 21:17–21.

156. Nakashima K, Zhou X, Kunkel G, Zhang Z, Deng JM, Behringer RR, et al. (2002) The novel zinc finger-containing transcription factor osterix is required for osteoblast differentiation and bone formation. Cell 108:17–29.

157. Nanes MS, Kuno H, Demay MB, Kurian M, Hendy GN, DeLuca HF, et al. (1994) A single up-stream element confers responsiveness to 1,25-dihydroxyvitamin D$_3$ and tumor necrosis factor-α in the rat osteocalcin gene. Endocrinology 134:1113–20.

158. Nanes MS, McKoy WM, Marx SJ (1989) Inhibitory effects of tumor necrosis factor-α and interferon-gamma on deoxyribonucleic acid and collagen synthesis by rat osteosarcoma cells (ROS 17/2.8). Endocrinology 124:339–45.

159. Nanes MS, Rubin J, Titus L, Hendy GN, Catherwood B (1991) Tumor necrosis factor-α inhibits 1,25-dihydroxyvitamin D$_3$-stimulated bone Gla protein synthesis in rat osteosarcoma cells (ROS 17/2.8) by a pretranslational mechanism. Endocrinology 128:2577–82.

160. Need AG, Morris HA, Horowitz M, Scopacasa E, Nordin BE (1998) Intestinal calcium absorption in men with spinal osteoporosis. Clin Endocrinol (Oxf) 48:163–8.

161. Nissen RM, Yamamoto KR (2000) The glucocorticoid receptor inhibits NFkappaB by interfering with serine-2 phosphorylation of the RNA polymerase II carboxy-terminal domain. Genes Dev 14:2314–29.

162. Nomura S, Sakuma T, Higashibata Y, Oboki K, Sato M (2001) Molecular cause of the severe functional deficiency in osteoclasts by an arginine deletion in the basic domain of Mi transcription factor. J Bone Miner Metab 19:183–7.

163. Okada Y, Morimoto I, Ura K, Watanabe K, Eto S, Kumegawa M, et al. (2002) Cell-to-Cell adhesion via intercellular adhesion molecule-1 and leukocyte function-associated antigen-1 pathway is involved in 1α,25(OH)$_2$D$_3$, PTH and IL-1α -induced osteoclast differentiation and bone resorption. Endocr J 49:483–95.

164. Okahashi N, Koide M, Jimi E, Suda T, Nishihara T (1998) Caspases (interleukin-1beta-converting enzyme family proteases) are involved in the regulation of the survival of osteoclasts. Bone 23:33–41.

165. O'Keefe GM, Nguyen VT, Ping Tang LL, Benveniste EN (2001) IFN-gamma regulation of class II transactivator promoter IV in macrophages and microglia: involvement of the suppressors of cytokine signaling-1 protein. J Immunol 166:2260–9.

166. Pacifici R (1996) Estrogen, cytokines, and pathogenesis of postmenopausal osteoporosis. J Bone Miner Res 11:1043–51.

167. Pacifici R, Brown C, Puscheck E, Friedrich E, Slatopolsky E, Maggio D, et al. (1991) Effect of surgical menopause and estrogen replacement on cytokine release from human blood mononuclear cells. Proc Natl Acad Sci USA 88:5134–8.

168. Pai RK, Askew D, Boom WH, Harding CV (2002) Regulation of class II MHC expression in APCs: roles of types I, III, and IV class II transactivator. J Immunol 169:1326–33.

169. Panagakos FS, Kumar S (1994) Modulation of proteases and their inhibitors in immortal human osteoblast-like cells by tumor necrosis factor-α in vitro. Inflammation 18:243–65.

170. Panagakos FS, Kumar S (1995) Differentiation of human osteoblastic cells in culture: modulation of pro-

teases by extracellular matrix and tumor necrosis factor-α. Inflammation 19:423–43.

171. Pascher E, Perniok A, Becker A, Feldkamp J (1999) Effect of 1α,25(OH)2-vitamin D$_3$ on TNF -α -mediated apoptosis of human primary osteoblast-like cells in vitro. Horm Metab Res 31:653–6.

172. Passeri G, Girasole G, Manolagas SC, Jilka RL (1994) Endogenous production of tumor necrosis factor by primary cultures of murine calvarial cells: influence on IL-6 production and osteoclast development. Bone Miner 24:109–26.

173. Pavalko FM, Gerard RL, Ponik SM, Gallagher PJ, Jin Y, Norvell SM (2003) Fluid shear stress inhibits TNF-α – induced apoptosis in osteoblasts: a role for fluid shear stress-induced activation of PI3-kinase and inhibition of caspase-3. J Cell Physiol 194:194–205.

174. Pruzanski W, Stefanski E, Vadas P, Kennedy BP, van den Bosch H (1998) Regulation of the cellular expression of secretory and cytosolic phospholipases A2, and cyclooxygenase-2 by peptide growth factors. Biochim Biophys Acta 1403:47–56.

175. Qian Y, Commane M, Ninomiya-Tsuji J, Matsumoto K, Li X (2001) IRAK-mediated translocation of TRAF6 and TAB2 in the interleukin-1-induced activation of NFkappa B. J Biol Chem 276:41661–7.

176. Ralston SH (1994) Analysis of gene expression in human bone biopsies by polymerase chain reaction: evidence for enhanced cytokine expression in post-menopausal osteoporosis. J Bone Miner Res 9:883–90.

177. Ralston SH, Russell RG, Gowen M (1990) Estrogen inhibits release of tumor necrosis factor from periph-eral blood mononuclear cells in postmenopausal women. J Bone Miner Res 5:983–8.

178. Ramalho AC, Jullienne A, Couttet P, Graulet AM, Morieux C, de Vernejoul MC, et al. (2001) Effect of oestradiol on cytokine production in immortalized human marrow stromal cell lines. Cytokine 16:126–30.

179. Rao VH, Singh RK, Delimont DC, Finnell RH, Bridge JA, Neff JR, et al. (1999) Transcriptional regulation of MMP-9 expression in stromal cells of human giant cell tumor of bone by tumor necrosis factor-α. Int J Oncol 14:291–300.

180. Rickard D, Russell G, Gowen M (1992) Oestradiol inhibits the release of tumour necrosis factor but not interleukin 6 from adult human osteoblasts in vitro. Osteoporos Int 2:94–102.

181. Rifas L, Halstead LR, Peck WA, Avioli LV, Welgus HG (1989) Human osteoblasts in vitro secrete tissue inhibitor of metalloproteinases and gelatinase but not interstitial collagenase as major cellular products. J Clin Invest 84:686–94.

182. Rifas L, Kenney JS, Marcelli M, Pacifici R, Cheng SL, Dawson LL, et al. (1995) Production of interleukin-6 in human osteoblasts and human bone marrow stromal cells: evidence that induction by interleukin-1 and tumor necrosis factor-α is not regulated by ovarian steroids. Endocrinology 136:4056–67.

183. Roggia C, Gao Y, Cenci S, Weitzmann MN, Toraldo G, Isaia G, et al. (2001) Up-regulation of TNF-producing T cells in the bone marrow: a key mechanism by which estrogen deficiency induces bone loss *in vivo*. Proc Natl Acad Sci USA 98:13960–5.

184. Romas E, Udagawa N, Zhou H, Tamura T, Saito M, Taga T, et al. (1996) The role of gp130-mediated signals in osteoclast development: regulation of interleukin 11 production by osteoblasts and distribution of its

185. Rubin J, Fan D, Wade A, Murphy TC, Gewant H, Nanes MS, et al. (2000) Transcriptional regulation of the expression of macrophage colony stimulating factor. Mol Cell Endocrinol 160:193–202.

186. Salamone LM, Whiteside T, Friberg D, Epstein RS, Kuller LH, Cauley JA (1998) Cytokine production and bone mineral density at the lumbar spine and femoral neck in premenopausal women. Calcif Tissue Int 63:466–70.

187. Salem ML, Hossain MS, Nomoto K (2000) Mediation of the immunomodulatory effect of beta-estradiol on inflammatory responses by inhibition of recruitment and activation of inflammatory cells and their gene expression of TNF-α and IFN-gamma. Int Arch Allergy Immunol 121:235–45.

188. Sato K, Satoh T, Shizume K, Yamakawa Y, Ono Y, Demura H, et al. (1992) Prolonged decrease of serum calcium concentration by murine gamma-interferon in hypercalcemic, human tumor (EC-GI)-bearing nude mice. Cancer Res 52:444–9.

189. Sato M, Morii E, Komori T, Kawahata H, Sugimoto M, Terai K, et al. (1998) Transcriptional regulation of osteopontin gene *in vivo* by PEBP2αA/CBFA1 and ETS1 in the skeletal tissues. Oncogene 17:1517–25.

190. Scharla SH, Strong DD, Mohan S, Chevalley T, Linkhart TA (1994) Effect of tumor necrosis factor-α on the expression of insulin-like growth factor I and insulin-like growth factor binding protein 4 in mouse osteo-blasts. Eur J Endocrinol 131:293–301.

191. Scheinman RI, Gualberto A, Jewell CM, Cidlowski JA, Baldwin AS, Jr. (1995) Characterization of mechanisms involved in transrepression of NF-kappa B by activated glucocorticoid receptors. Mol Cell Biol 15:943–53.

192. Schneider HG, Allan EH, Moseley JM, Martin TJ, Findlay DM (1991) Specific down-regulation of parathyroid hormone (PTH) receptors and responses to PTH by tumour necrosis factor -α and retinoic acid in UMR 106–06 osteoblast-like osteosarcoma cells. Biochem J 280 (Pt 2):451–7.

193. Shen V, Kohler G, Jeffrey JJ, Peck WA (1988) Bone-resorbing agents promote and interferon-gamma inhibits bone cell collagenase production. J Bone Miner Res 3:657–66.

194. Shevde NK, Bendixen AC, Dienger KM, Pike JW (2000) Estrogens suppress RANK ligand-induced osteoclast differentiation via a stromal cell independent mecha-nism involving c-Jun repression. Proc Natl Acad Sci USA 97:7829–34.

195. Smith DD, Gowen M, Mundy GR (1987) Effects of interferon-gamma and other cytokines on collagen synthesis in fetal rat bone cultures. Endocrinology 120:2494–9.

196. Srivastava S, Toraldo G, Weitzmann MN, Cenci S, Ross FP, Pacifici R (2001) Estrogen decreases osteoclast formation by down-regulating receptor activator of NF-kappa B ligand (RANKL)-induced JNK activation. J Biol Chem 276:8836–40.

197. Srivastava S, Weitzmann MN, Cenci S, Ross FP, Adler S, Pacifici R (1999) Estrogen decreases TNF gene expres-sion by blocking JNK activity and the resulting pro-duction of c-Jun and JunD. J Clin Invest 104:503–13.

198. Stashenko P, Obernesser MS, Dewhirst FE (1989) Effect of immune cytokines on bone. Immunol Invest 18:239–49.

199. Suda T, Kobayashi K, Jimi E, Udagawa N, Takahashi N (2001) The molecular basis of osteoclast differentiation and activation. Novartis Found Symp 232:235–47; discussion 247–50.

200. Taichman RS, Hauschka PV (1992) Effects of interleukin-1 beta and tumor necrosis factor-α on osteoblastic expression of osteocalcin and mineralized extracellular matrix in vitro. Inflammation 16:587–601.

201. Takaesu G, Ninomiya-Tsuji J, Kishida S, Li X, Stark GR, Matsumoto K (2001) Interleukin-1 (IL-1) receptor-associated kinase leads to activation of TAK1 by inducing TAB2 translocation in the IL-1 signaling pathway. Mol Cell Biol 21:2475–84.

202. Takaoka Y, Niwa S, Nagai H (1999) Interleukin-1beta induces interleukin-6 production through the production of prostaglandin E(2) in human osteoblasts, MG-63 cells. J Biochem (Tokyo) 126:553–8.

203. Takayanagi H, Ogasawara K, Hida S, Chiba T, Murata S, Sato K, et al. (2000) T-cell-mediated regulation of osteoclastogenesis by signalling cross-talk between RANKL and IFN-gamma. Nature 408:600–5.

204. Tatakis DN, Schneeberger G, Dziak R (1988) Recombinant interleukin-1 stimulates prostaglandin E2 production by osteoblastic cells: synergy with parathyroid hormone. Calcif Tissue Int 42:358–62.

205. Tatakis DN, Schneeberger G, Dziak R (1991) Recombinant interleukin-1 (IL-1) stimulates prostaglandin E2 production by osteoblastic cells: role of calcium, calmodulin, and cAMP. Lymphokine Cytokine Res 10:95–9.

206. Thomas JA, Allen JL, Tsen M, Dubnicoff T, Danao J, Liao XC, et al. (1999) Impaired cytokine signaling in mice lacking the IL-1 receptor-associated kinase. J Immunol 163:978–84.

207. Thomson BM, Mundy GR, Chambers TJ (1987) Tumor necrosis factors -α and β induce osteoblastic cells to stimulate osteoclastic bone resorption. J Immunol 138:775–9.

208. Thomson BM, Saklatvala J, Chambers TJ (1986) Osteoblasts mediate interleukin 1 stimulation of bone resorption by rat osteoclasts. J Exp Med. 164:104–12.

209. Tohkin M, Kakudo S, Kasai H, Arita H (1994) Comparative study of inhibitory effects by murine interferon gamma and a new bisphosphonate (alendronate) in hypercalcemic, nude mice bearing human tumor (LJC-1-JCK). Cancer Immunol Immunother 39:155–60.

210. Tondravi MM, McKercher SR, Anderson K, Erdmann JM, Quiroz M, Maki R, et al. (1997) Osteopetrosis in mice lacking haematopoietic transcription factor PU.1. Nature 386:81–4.

211. Toraldo G, Roggia C, Qian WP, Pacifici R, Weitzmann MN (2003) IL-7 induces bone loss in vivo by induction of receptor activator of nuclear factor kappa B ligand and tumor necrosis factor -α from T cells. Proc Natl Acad Sci USA 100:125–130.

212. Tsuboi M, Kawakami A, Nakashima T, Matsuoka N, Urayama S, Kawabe Y, et al. (1999) Tumor necrosis factor-α and interleukin-1beta increase the Fas-mediated apoptosis of human osteoblasts. J Lab Clin Med 134:222–31.

213. Tsutsumimoto T, Kawasaki S, Ebara S, Takaoka K (1999) TNF-α and IL-1beta suppress N-cadherin expression in MC3T3-E1 cells. J Bone Miner Res 14:1751–60.

214. Tuyt LM, Dokter WH, Birkenkamp K, Koopmans SB, Lummen C, Kruijer W, et al. (1999) Extracellular-regulated kinase 1/2, Jun N-terminal kinase, and c-Jun are involved in NF-kappa B-dependent IL-6 expression in human monocytes. J Immunol 162:4893–902.

215. Uchida M, Shima M, Shimoaka T, Fujieda A, Obara K, Suzuki H, et al. (2000) Regulation of matrix metalloproteinases (MMPs) and tissue inhibitors of metalloproteinases (TIMPs) by bone resorptive factors in osteoblastic cells. J Cell Physiol 185:207–14.

216. Uy HL, Mundy GR, Boyce BF, Story BM, Dunstan CR, Yin JJ, et al. (1997) Tumor necrosis factor enhances parathyroid hormone-related protein-induced hypercalcemia and bone resorption without inhibiting bone formation in vivo. Cancer Res 57:3194–9.

217. van der Saag PT, Caldenhoven E, van de Stolpe A (1996) Molecular mechanisms of steroid action: a novel type of cross-talk between glucocorticoids and NF-kappa B transcription factors. Eur Respir J Suppl 22:146s–153s.

218. Vargas SJ, Naprta A, Glaccum M, Lee SK, Kalinowski J, Lorenzo JA (1996) Interleukin-6 expression and histomorphometry of bones from mice deficient in receptors for interleukin-1 or tumor necrosis factor. J Bone Miner Res 11:1736–44.

219. Vargas SJ, Naprta A, Lee SK, Kalinowski J, Kawaguchi H, Pilbeam CC, et al. (1996) Lack of evidence for an increase in interleukin-6 expression in adult murine bone, bone marrow, and marrow stromal cell cultures after ovariectomy. J Bone Miner Res 11:1926–34.

220. Verthelyi D, Klinman DM (2000) Sex hormone levels correlate with the activity of cytokine-secreting cells in vivo. Immunology 100:384–90.

221. Vidal ON, Sjogren K, Eriksson BI, Ljunggren O, Ohlsson C (1998) Osteoprotegerin mRNA is increased by interleukin-1α in the human osteosarcoma cell line MG-63 and in human osteoblast-like cells. Biochem Biophys Res Commun 248:696–700.

222. Vig E, Green M, Liu Y, Donner DB, Mukaida N, Goebl MG, et al. (1999) Modulation of tumor necrosis factor and interleukin-1-dependent Nf-κB activity by mPLK/IRAK. J Biol Chem 274:13077–84.

223. Wadleigh DJ, Herschman HR (1999) Transcriptional regulation of the cyclooxygenase-2 gene by diverse ligands in murine osteoblasts. Biochem Biophys Res Commun 264:865–70.

224. Wagner EF (2002) Functions of AP1 (Fos/Jun) in bone development. Ann Rheum Dis 61 Suppl 2:1140–2.

225. Waldburger JM, Suter T, Fontana A, Acha-Orbea H, Reith W (2001) Selective abrogation of major histocompatibility complex class II expression on extrahematopoietic cells in mice lacking promoter IV of the class II transactivator gene. J Exp Med 194:393–406.

226. Weitzmann MN, Cenci S, Rifas L, Brown C, Pacifici R (2000) Interleukin-7 stimulates osteoclast formation by up-regulating the T-cell production of soluble osteoclastogenic cytokines. Blood 96:1873–8.

227. Weitzmann MN, Roggia C, Toraldo G, Weitzmann L, Pacifici R (2002) Increased production of IL-7 uncouples bone formation from bone resorption during estrogen deficiency. J Clin Invest 110:1643–50.

228. Wiktor-Jedrzejczak W, Urbanowska E, Aukerman SL, Pollard JW, Stanley ER, Ralph P, et al. (1991) Correction by CSF-1 of defects in the osteopetrotic op/op mouse suggests local, developmental, and humoral requirements for this growth factor. Exp Hematol 19:1049–54.

229. Wood RJ, Fleet JC, Cashman K, Bruns ME, Deluca HF (1998) Intestinal calcium absorption in the aged rat:

evidence of intestinal resistance to 1,25(OH)2 vitamin D. Endocrinology 139:3843–8.

230. Xie JF, Stroumza J, Graves DT (1994) IL-1 down-regulates platelet-derived growth factor-α receptor gene expression at the transcriptional level in human osteoblastic cells. J Immunol 153:378–83.

231. Xing L, Bushnell TP, Carlson L, Tai Z, Tondravi M, Siebenlist U, et al. (2002) Nf-κB p50 and p52 expression is not required for RANK-expressing osteoclast progenitor formation but is essential for RANK- and cytokine-mediated osteoclastogenesis. J Bone Miner Res 17:1200–10.

232. Xing L, Carlson L, Story B, Tai Z, Keng P, Siebenlist U, et al. (2003) Expression of either Nf-κB p50 or p52 in osteoclast precursors is required for IL-1-induced bone resorption. J Bone Miner Res 18:260–9.

233. Xu J, Cissel DS, Varghese S, Whipkey DL, Blaha JD, Graeber GM, et al. (1997) Cytokine regulation of adult human osteoblast-like cell prostaglandin biosynthesis. J Cell Biochem 64:618–31.

234. Yagi K, Tsuji K, Nifuji A, Shinomiya K, Nakashima K, DeCrombrugghe B, et al. (2003) Bone morphogenetic protein-2 enhances osterix gene expression in chondrocytes. J Cell Biochem 88:1077–83.

235. Yamin TT, Miller DK (1997) The interleukin-1 receptor-associated kinase is degraded by proteasomes following its phosphorylation. J Biol Chem 272:21540–7.

236. Yang C PC, Phillips LS, Rubin J, Nanes MS (1998) Paradoxical enhancement of PTH-stimulated IGF-1 gene transcription by TNF-α despite inhibition of IGF-1 mRNA. Bone 23:F041.

237. Yao GQ, Sun BH, Insogna KL, Weir EC (2000) Nuclear factor-kappaB p50 is required for tumor necrosis factor-α -induced colony-stimulating factor-1 gene expression in osteoblasts. Endocrinology 141:2914–22.

238. Ye H, Arron JR, Lamothe B, Cirilli M, Kobayashi T, Shevde NK, et al. (2002) Distinct molecular mechanism for initiating TRAF6 signalling. Nature 418:443–7.

239. Yoshida H, Hayashi S, Kunisada T, Ogawa M, Nishikawa S, Okamura H, et al. (1990) The murine mutation osteopetrosis is in the coding region of the macrophage colony stimulating factor gene. Nature 345:442–4.

240. Yoshihara R, Shiozawa S, Imai Y, Fujita T (1990) Tumor necrosis factor -α and interferon gamma inhibit proliferation and alkaline phosphatase activity of human osteoblastic SaOS-2 cell line. Lymphokine Res 9:59–66.

241. Zhang YH, Heulsmann A, Tondravi MM, Mukherjee A, Abu-Amer Y (2001) Tumor necrosis factor-α (TNF) stimulates RANKL-induced osteoclastogenesis via coupling of TNF type 1 receptor and RANK signaling pathways. J Biol Chem 276:563–8.

242. Zheng SX, Vrindts Y, Lopez M, De Groote D, Zangerle PF, Collette J, et al. (1997) Increase in cytokine production (IL-1 beta, IL-6, TNF-α but not IFN-gamma, GM-CSF or LIF) by stimulated whole blood cells in postmenopausal osteoporosis. Maturitas 26:63–71.

243. Zou W, Hakim I, Tschoep K, Endres S, Bar-Shavit Z (2001) Tumor necrosis factor-α mediates RANK ligand stimulation of osteoclast differentiation by an autocrine mechanism. J Cell Biochem 83:70–83.

6.

Genetics and Mutations Affecting Osteoclast Development and Function

Mark C. Horowitz, Melissa A. Kacena, and Joseph A. Lorenzo

Introduction

To understand the manner in which genetic background or DNA mutation affects osteoclast formation and function, it is necessary to possess a basic understanding of the cell biology of osteoclastogenesis. Osteoclasts are large, multinucleated, tartrate-resistant, acid phosphatase (TRAP)-positive cells that are responsible for bone resorption. They arise from hematopoietic stem cells and, like other hematopoietic cells, are thought to pass through a series of differentiation stages that culminate in large, multinucleated, bone-resorbing cells. Osteoclasts are the only true bone-resorbing cells. However, the specific stages and the regulation of their pathway development have not been completely elucidated. Osteoclasts arise from a bifurcation of the monocyte/macrophage lineage and thus evolve from the common myeloid progenitor. Using cells isolated from human bone marrow, Kurihara purified CD34$^+$ (a cell-surface marker found on myeloid progenitor cells, CFU-GMs) and treated them with granulocyte-macrophage colony-stimulating factor and 1,25-(OH)$_2$D$_3$. This resulted in the formation of osteoclasts, a result that suggests that the osteoclast precursor was the granulocyte-macrophage progenitor [95, 150]. However, Hattersley and Lee reported that a more primitive cell than the CFU-GM differentiated into osteoclasts [61, 101]. Udagawa showed that spleen or bone marrow cells are a

source of osteoclast precursors. It was possible to culture these cells with stromal cell lines or primary osteoblasts to induce the formation of multinucleated, TRAP$^+$ bone-resorbing osteoclast-like cells [177]. These authors also demonstrated that cell contact between the hematopoietic osteoclast precursor and the mesenchymal stromal/osteoblastic cell was required for osteoclast formation. These experiments formed the basis for the seminal work that demonstrated the requirement for interaction between the receptor activator of nuclear factor (NF)-κB (RANK)-receptor and the activator of NF-κB ligand (RANKL) for osteoclast precursors to differentiate terminally into functional osteoclast-like cells, a phenomenon that is aided by the presence of macrophage colony-stimulating factor (M-CSF) [5, 97, 200]. RANK is a member of the superfamily of TNF receptors; it is expressed on B and T cells, dendritic cells, osteoclast precursors, and mature osteoclasts [5]. RANKL is a type II transmembrane protein, expressed on stromal cells, osteoblasts, and T cells [97, 194, 200].

It has taken more than 30 years for bone biologists to understand how osteoclasts develop, become active and function. Modern molecular biology has made it possible to manipulate specific genes. The identification of spontaneous mutations and the ability to engineer overexpression or deletion of specific genes have brought valuable insights into how those genes affect the organism. This genetic approach has been used successfully in defining osteoclast biology.

In the Nucleus – Transcriptional Regulation

The molecular dissection of the differentiation pathway of hematopoietic cell lineages has been greatly facilitated by the identification of transcription factors required for successful maturation of a cell. An example of this occurs during B lymphopoiesis. In this process, numerous transcription factors, as well as specific protein–protein interactions that define their activities, are required for the progression of B cell differentiation to occur (Figure 6.1). Osteoclasts likely follow a similar, staged development. However, the transcription factors which control this progression have only been partially identified. This is particularly true for the early stages of development. Loss of these specific factors precludes cells from continued maturation, and causes cells at the latest stage of differentiation to accumulate prior to the arrest. PU.1 is one of the first in a series of transcription factors, which include E2A, Early B Cell Factor (EBF), and Pax5, that function in a specific maturation-dependent sequence that is required for B cell development. E2A appears to regulate transcription of the EBF gene and in turn EBF has been implicated in activating Pax5 [87, 135]. PU.1, a member of the ETS domain transcription factors, is required to regulate the proliferation and differentiation of B cell and macrophage lineage progenitors [6, 33]. PU.1–/– mice, in addition to having no B cells, fail to develop osteoclasts and macrophages [176]. PU.1 regulates these progenitors by controlling the expression of the IL-7 receptor and c-fms (the M-CSF receptor) [34, 33]. Low concentrations of PU.1 protein induce B cell differentiation, while high concentrations promote macrophage development and inhibit B cell progression [35]. In keeping with this hierarchical expression of PU.1 RNA, osteoclasts express higher levels of PU.1 mRNA than BM macrophage precursor cells [176]. PU.1 exerts additional control over osteoclast differentiation through its interaction with the microphthalmia transcription factor (MITF) [116]. This well-characterized locus has at least 16 different mutant alleles. Defects in the *mi, or* and *crc* alleles of MITF produce osteopetrosis [129, 167]. OC can be detected in mi/mi mice, however they fail to fuse and form multinucleated cells [54, 174]. These data indicate that defects in osteoclast formation in mi/mi mice occur later than in PU.1-deficient mice. In addition to the osteoclast defect, mi/mi mice are deficient in B cell precursors [169]. Co-culture of BM cells from mi/mi mice with stromal cells in the presence of IL-7 (the major growth and differentiation factor for B cells) resulted in B-cell differentiation. These results suggest that the defect in B-cell development in mi/mi mice was not in the precursors, but rather in the local microenvironment.

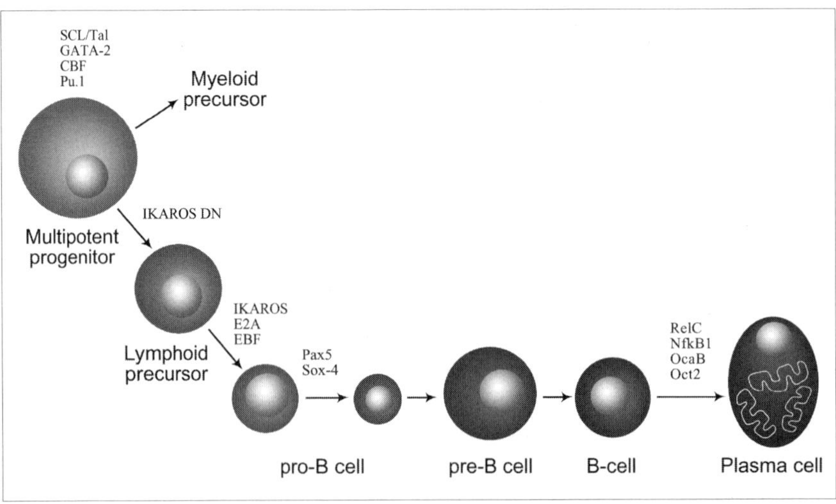

Figure 6.1 B-cell differentiation from hematopoietic stem cells is a multistep process requiring a program of transcription factors.

Two different, basic helix-loop-helix proteins encoded by the E2A and EBF genes play a critical role at the start of B cell differentiation. Absence of either of these proteins halts B cell development at the earliest stage, before the D_H-J_H rearrangement occurs [10, 108]. Although the skeletons of these mutant mice have not been extensively analyzed, EBF-deficient mice are runted (M. Horowitz, Hesslein, Lorenzo unpublished). This implies that their bones are pathologic.

Pax5 is a member of the multigene family that encodes the paired box transcription factors. The Pax5 gene encodes for the B cell lineage specific activation factor (BSAP). Pax5 is expressed exclusively in the B-lymphocyte lineage that leads from $B220^+$ pro-B cells to mature B cells. However, Pax5 is not present in terminally differentiated plasma cells [179]. When the Pax5 gene is deleted in mice, the most striking result, in addition to early postnatal lethality, is the loss of all B cell development beyond the early pro-B cell stage [134]. This developmental arrest of the B cell lineage leaves normal numbers of $B220^+$ pro-B cells in the BM. Pro-B cells isolated from Pax5–/– BM can be grown *in vitro* on stromal/osteoblast feeder cells in the presence of IL-7, a condition that maintains their undifferentiated phenotype [8]. With removal of IL-7 and stimulation with the appropriate cytokines, these cells can differentiate into multiple hematopoietic lineages [134]. Similarly, in normal BM, an early osteoclast progenitor ($Mac-1^+$ $c-fms^-$) can be induced to express a B-cell-like phenotype ($B220^+$) when cultured with a stromal/osteoblast cell line and treated with IL-7 [8]. Treatment of the Pax5–/– pro-B cells with M-CSF and RANKL induced the formation of osteoclast-like cells; this raises the possibility that Pax5 is involved in the regulation of osteoclast development [134]. Because cloned pro-B-cell lines can be used, these findings are the clearest indication that pro-B cells can be induced to form osteoclasts in the absence of Pax5. These observations and the severe runting of the homozygous mutant mice prompted us to examine Pax5–/– mice to determine whether they had a bone phenotype. Pax5–/– mice are severely osteopenic, missing more than 60% of their bone mass [67]. This condition is the result of a 3–5-fold increase in the number of osteoclasts in bone, even though the number of osteoblasts in Pax5–/– mice is the same as in control mice. *In vitro*, spleen cells from Pax5–/–

mice are enriched in osteoclast precursors. These data identify Pax5 as a transcription factor that is required for the normal regulation of osteoclast development. In addition, Pax5–/– mice represent a novel system in which to study the relationship of osteoclasts and B cell differentiation.

Recently, it was shown that loss or overexpression of certain transcription factors reprograms the fate of progenitor/precursor cells [196]. As an example, enforced expression in B cells of C/EBPα and C/EBPβ, a bZip family transcription factor, reprograms the cells into macrophages [196]. Conversely, macrophages from mice deficient in C/EBPβ exhibit functional defects [161]. At present it is unclear how changes in the expression of these transcription factors relates specifically to osteoclasts. However, it is not unreasonable to predict that these alterations may affect osteoclast differentiation. These findings are consistent with the idea that there exist networks of transcription factors, which together function as both positive and negative regulators of differentiation [139].

It is now known that NF-κB is a critical mediator of RANK signaling in most responsive cells, including osteoclasts and osteoclast precursors [5, 17, 195]. RANKL-RANK interaction signals TRAF-6, which activates NF-κB. NF-κB is also required for osteoclastic responses to IL-1 and TNF [197]. NF-κB transcription factors are dimers composed of various combinations of the structurally related proteins p50 (NFKB1), p52 (NFKB2), p65 (RelA), c-Rel (Rel), and RelB [49, 75]. Unlike the single knockout of either p50 or p52, which have no skeletal phenotype, p50/p52 double knockout mice fail to generate mature osteoclasts or B cells and have severe osteopetrosis. These mice are runted and their incisor teeth fail to erupt, both of which are additional signs of an osteoclast defect. The p50/p52 double-knockout mice also have markedly impaired thymic and splenic architectures and macrophage activity. Co-culture experiments show that the defect in these animals is in osteoclast precursors rather than in osteoclast induction. Hence, in this regard they resemble RANK- or RANKL-deficient mice.

c-fos is a proto-oncogene that is a component of the AP-1 transcription factor complex [7]. Overexpression of c-fos transforms chondroblasts and osteoblasts, but not osteoclasts/hematopoietic cells [58, 155, 186, 187]. Therefore, the fact that c-fos –/– mice develop osteopetrosis as a result of impaired osteoclast differentiation is unexpected [59]. In addition to having osteopetrosis, c-fos –/– mice are smaller, and have reduced body weight, presumably because lack of tooth eruption causes diminished food intake. These mice have a shorter snout and shorter limbs [188]. Interestingly, these mice also have a marked reduction (75%) in B220[+] B cells in their spleen. This is another example of a defect in osteoclast development that is paralleled by defects in B-cell development. Further investigation into the mechanism associated with the osteopetrotic phenotype of c-fos–/– mice has shown that there are no TRAP[+] cells in the long bones [59]. Osteoclast progenitors, but no differentiated multinucleated osteoclasts, were seen [59]. Interestingly, c-fos was found to cause a lineage shift between osteoclasts and macrophages, which resulted in an increase in the number of tissue macrophages. These studies clarified the role of c-fos as a transcriptional regulator of osteoclast and macrophage differentiation [59].

Nuclear factor of activated T cells-c1 (NFATc1) has recently been shown to be a critical signaling molecule in osteoclastogenic responses [76, 170]. NFATs are a family of transcription factors that shuttle between the cytoplasm and the nucleus. Activation, which allows entry to the nucleus [27], occurs when calcium activates the phosphatase calcineurin. This in turn, dephosphorylates cytoplasmic NFAT, and exposes a nuclear localization sequence in the molecule. This allows NFAT to be transported to the nucleus, where it binds DNA and activates transcription. Using embryonic stem cells to generate osteoclasts, Takayanagi et al. [170] demonstrated that ES cells from NFATc1-deficient mice, which have an embryonic lethal mutation, did not form osteoclasts when treated with M-CSF and RANKL. In contrast, M-CSF and RANKL stimulated abundant osteoclast formation in cultures of wild-type ES cells. Retroviral overexpression of NFATc1 in bone marrow cells induced osteoclastogenesis in the absence of RANKL stimulation [170]. This finding confirms the critical role of NFATc1 induction in RANKL responses. It also appears that NFAT is a downstream target of c-fos in RANK-mediated osteoclastogenesis [124]. Interestingly, in the absence of RANKL, stimulation of c-fos-deficient osteoclast precursor cells were insensitive to NFATc1-induced osteoclastogenesis. Hence, it appears that independent actions of both NFATc1 and c-fos are critical elements of normal osteoclast formation.

At the Cell Surface and Beyond – Cytokines, Receptors and Signaling

M-CSF, also known as colony-stimulating factor-1 (CSF-1), was originally found to be a regulator of macrophage formation [153]. However, a spontaneous mouse mutant with a phenotype of absent osteoclasts and defective macrophage-monocyte formation (the op/op mouse) was discovered to have a point mutation in the coding region of the M-CSF gene [46, 193, 202]. This mutation introduced a stop codon and prevented normal expression of a functional M-CSF protein. Injection of M-CSF into op/op mice corrected the defect in osteoclast formation and bone resorption [47], a result that confirmed the importance of this protein for osteoclast development. Recently, a mouse that lacked the receptor for M-CSF (c-fms a receptor tyrosine kinase) was generated and found to have a phenotype, that is similar to that of the op/op mouse [31].

Stimulators of bone resorption increase production of M-CSF in bone [45, 156, 191], with multiple transcripts of M-CSF produced by alternate splicing [29, 28]. The membrane-bound or cell-surface form of M-CSF differs from the soluble form because it lacks a cleavage site. Only forms with a cleavage site are subject to rapid proteolytic release of the ectodomain as a soluble protein. The membrane-bound form of M-CSF is regulated by stimulators of resorption and facilitates the differentiation of osteoclasts from precursor cells [156, 198].

The effect of M-CSF on the function of mature osteoclasts is controversial. Osteoclasts express c-fms [65] and initial reports concluded that M-CSF inhibited bone resorption in mature osteoclasts [62]. Subsequent studies have found that it increased cytoplasmic spreading, fusion of mononuclear osteoclast precursors into osteoclasts, and led to osteoclastic resorption [3, 102, 159]. M-CSF also induces proliferation of osteoclast precursors. While these precursor cells are proliferating in response to M-CSF, they do not differentiate into multinucleated bone-resorbing cells. This is one reason that osteoclastic bone resorption is inhibited by M-CSF. The ability of M-CSF to stimulate cytoplasmic spreading in osteoclasts appears to involve c-src because src kinase activity increased threefold after M-CSF treatment. Moreover, osteoclastic cytoplasmic spreading did not occur in c-src-deficient mice [72, 73]. M-CSF also appears to down-regulate the expression of c-fms.

The role of M-CSF in regulating osteoclast apoptosis has recently been examined. Addition of M-CSF to mature osteoclast cultures prolongs their survival [50, 80]. This response may be important for the development of the osteopetrotic phenotype in op/op mice because transgenic expression of bcl-2, which blocks apoptosis in myeloid cells, partially reversed the defects in osteoclast and macrophage development [99].

The role of osteoprotegerin (OPG) in bone was first established in studies with transgenic animals [164]. It was demonstrated that global overexpression of the protein in mice produced animals with markedly decreased bone resorption, increased bone mass, and few osteoclasts. OPG is a member of the tumor necrosis factor receptor superfamily (TNFRSF11b). It is a decoy receptor for RANKL [98, 201]. OPG inhibits OC formation and bone resorption by binding RANKL and preventing its interaction with RANK, its cognate receptor, on the surface of osteoclast precursor cells. Mice lacking OPG have severe osteoporosis, an increase in the number of osteoclasts, and, importantly, exhibit arterial calcification [24, 127]. Studies with OPG-deficient mice have shown that the active resorption of bone by osteoclasts is an ongoing process, which must be overtly held in check to maintain bone mass. One role of M-CSF in facilitating osteoclastogenesis is its ability to stimulate RANK expression on osteoclast precursor cells [8]. Once activated, RANK initiates a series of intracellular second messengers, including TNF-receptor associated factors (TRAF) family members, NF-κB, mitogen-activated protein kinases (MAPK), activator protein-1 (AP-1), NFATc1, and the src-AKT-phosphatidylinositol-3-OH kinase (PI(3)K) system [17].

Perhaps the most convincing evidence that RANKL and RANK are critical regulators of osteoclastogenesis comes from mice lacking these proteins. RANKL-deficient mice have significant osteopetrosis, no osteoclasts, a normal number of monocyte-macrophages, and extramedullary hematopoiesis [93]. They also have significant defects in B-cell lymphopoiesis, with markedly reduced numbers of pre-B-lymphocytes in their marrow. Remarkably, RANKL knockout mice lack lymph nodes and their T cells secrete less cytokines. These findings demonstrate that, in addition to its effects on osteoclastogenesis, RANKL is an important regulator of lymphocyte development.

RANK-deficient mice also have no osteoclasts and develop osteopetrosis and extramedullary hematopoiesis [38, 103]. In addition, like RANKL-deficient mice, they lack mature B-lymphocytes and have defects in lymph node development. Overexpression of a soluble form of RANK in transgenic mice produced a phenotype that was similar to that of OPG-overexpressing transgenic mice [68] and was characterized by osteopetrosis and a decreased number of osteoclasts in bone.

Our understanding of the <u>signaling</u> pathways utilized by RANK in the activation of osteoclasts has been greatly enhanced by the development of knockout mouse models that lack specific components of this signaling pathway. TRAFs 2, 5, and 6 all bind RANK, but only TRAF6 deficiency has been associated with osteopetrosis in mice [111, 133]. TRAF proteins

Table 6.1. Transgenic or Spontaneous Mutations in Mice with Alterations in Osteoclast Number/Physiology

Cathepsin k	Ion channels	Prostaglandin receptors
c-fos	IRAK	Pu.1
Cyclooxygenase	LIF receptor	RANKL
DAP-12	M-CSF	RANK
FcRγ	Micropthalmia transcription factors	SHP-1
gp130	NFAT	Src
IL-1 receptors	NF$_k$B	TNF receptors
Intergins ($\alpha_v\beta_3$)	OPG	TRAF5 and 6
Interferons	Pax 5	

are believed to be involved in mediating responses of TNF superfamily receptors like RANK. Two murine models of TRAF6 deficiency have now been produced [111, 133]. Curiously, in one mouse model, there was an almost complete absence of osteoclasts in bone [133], while in the other, osteoclasts were abundant in bone but appeared to function poorly and lacked contact with the bone surface [111]. Mice lacking TRAF6 also have impaired CD40 and lipopolysaccharide (LPS)-induced proliferation in their B cells, impaired nitric oxide induction in macrophages and impaired interleukin-1 (IL-1)-, CD40-, and LPS-induced activation of NF-κB and JNK. In addition, *in vitro* osteoclastogenesis from spleen cell precursors obtained from these mice was impaired [111, 133]. TRAF5-deficient mice demonstrate normal bone mass but delayed osteoclastogenic responses to RANKL and TNF *in vitro* and a delayed hypercalcemic response to PTH *in vivo* [84]. This finding demonstrates that TRAF5, while not critical for osteoclastogenic responses, is part of the signaling pathway in osteoclast precursor cells.

IL-1 is encoded by two separate gene products, α and β, which have identical activities [36]. IL-1 was the first polypeptide mediator of immune cell function that was found to regulate bone resorption [112]. It also increased prostaglandin synthesis in bone [112], an action that may account for some of its resorptive activity. IL-1 is the most potent known peptide stimulator of *in vitro* bone resorption [112]; it also has potent *in vivo* effects [18].

Two known receptors for IL-1, type I and type II, have been identified [37]. All known biologic responses to IL-1 appear to be mediated exclusively through the type I receptor [165]. Signaling through type I receptors involves activation of NF-κB and specific TRAFs [121, 41]. IL-1 receptor type I requires interaction with a second protein, interleukin-1 receptor accessory protein (IRAcP), to generate post-receptor signals [69, 94, 192]. IRAcP induces activation of interleukin-1 receptor-associated kinase (IRAK) [192]. Phosphorylated IRAK binds TRAF6 with subsequent downstream signaling. IRAKM, unlike other members of the family, lacks kinase activity and is a negative regulator of IL-1R signaling. IRAKM-deficient mice develop lower total bone mineral density than do wild-type controls; a 60% reduction in trabecular bone, as measured by micro-CT, along

with an almost fourfold increase in osteoclast number, has been reported [104]. IRAKM appears to down-regulate osteoclast differentiation and activation through NF-κB and MAPK signaling pathways. IL-1 receptor type II does not appear to have agonist activity. Rather, there is convincing evidence that it is a decoy receptor, which prevents activation of IL-1 type I receptors [30]. IL-1 receptor type II can also synergize with IL-1ra to inhibit activation of the IL-1 receptor type I [25]. IL-1 may play a role in estrogen-mediated bone loss, because the IL-1 antagonist IL-1ra blocks ovariectomy-induced bone loss [140]. This has been confirmed by studies demonstrating that mice lacking the IL-1 receptor type I (IL-1R1 −/−) did not lose bone mass following ovariectomy [113].

Like IL-1, tumor necrosis factor (TNF) consists of two related polypeptides (α and β) that are separate gene products [13, 138, 164]. TNF α and β have similar biologic activities, and both are potent stimulators of bone resorption [12, 36]. TNF is similar to IL-1 in its potency to induce bone resorption. Like IL-1, TNF also enhances the formation of osteoclast-like cells in bone marrow culture [143], and thus appears to regulate osteoclast precursor cell differentiation. TNFα is produced by human osteoblast-like cell cultures [55] and its production can be stimulated by IL-1, GM-CSF, and LPS, but not by PTH, 1,25-(OH)$_2$ vitamin D, or calcitonin. Recently, TNF was shown to stimulate osteoclast formation directly in an *in vitro* culture system. This effect was independent of the actions of RANK, because it occurred in cells from RANK-deficient mice [9, 90]. However, the functional significance of this finding is questionable because *in vivo* administration of TNF to RANK-deficient mice caused only an occasional osteoclast to form [81].

Like IL-1, TNF binds to two cell surface receptors, the TNF receptor 1 or p55 and the TNF receptor 2 or p75 [48]. In contrast to IL-1, both receptors transmit biologic responses. Mice deficient in either or both TNF receptors have been engineered [142, 154]. All of these animals appear healthy and breed normally, but lack selective immune responses. Bones from mice that lack either IL-1 receptor type I or TNF receptor 1 are similar to those of wild-type mice, except for a 36% increase in the total bone area of calvaria from IL-1 receptor type I-deficient mice [182]. Mice deficient in TNF receptors (TNF −/−) fail to lose bone mass after ovariectomy [149]. This finding appears significant because production of TNF by T lymphocytes appears responsible for some of the bone loss that occurs in mice after ovariectomy [149].

IL-6, like IL-1 and TNF, modulates immune cell function in many ways. It also affects the replication and differentiation of other cell types [2, 63]. The receptor for IL-6 is composed of two parts: a specific IL-6-binding protein (IL-6 receptor), which can be either membrane bound or soluble, and gp-130, an activator protein that is common to a number of cytokine receptors [88]. Production of the specific IL-6 receptor may be regulated, because bone cells do not always express it [171].

The ability of IL-6 to stimulate bone resorption *in vitro* is variable and depends on the assay system [1, 77, 109, 115]. The reasons for this variability are not known. A major function of IL-6 is to regulate the differentiation of osteoclast progenitor cells into mature osteoclasts [118, 151]. In an *in vitro* model of osteoclast differentiation from human bone marrow, IL-6 was found to be a potent stimulus of new osteoclast-like cell development by a mechanism that also was dependent on IL-1 [96]. In contrast, in a murine *in vitro* system, IL-6 was only effective when soluble IL-6 receptor was added to the cultures [171]. Implantation of Chinese hamster ovary (CHO) cells, which were genetically engineered to express murine IL-6, into nude mice produced a syndrome of hypercalcemia, cachexia, leukocytosis, and thrombocytosis [14]. The effects of IL-6 on resorption in this model were weak, but were potentiated significantly when the animals also were treated with PTHrP [32]. A major effect of IL-6 in these *in vivo* models was to increase the number of early osteoclast precursors (CFU-GM) in the bone marrow. IL-6 action may contribute to some of the increased bone resorption and bone pathology that are associated with the clinical syndromes of Paget's disease [152], hypercalcemia of malignancy [60], fibrous dysplasia [199], giant cell tumors of bone [147], and Gorham–Stout disease [55].

Ovariectomy-induced bone loss in mice has been associated with increased IL-6 production [79] and mice deficient in IL-6 failed to lose bone after ovariectomy [44].

IL-6 is a member of a group of cytokines that share the gp-130 activator protein in their receptor complex [119]. Each family member utilizes unique ligand receptors to generate specific binding. Besides IL-6, the cytokines of this family include interleukin 11 (IL-11), leukemia inhibitory factor (LIF), oncostatin M (OSM), ciliary neurotrophic factor (CNTF), and cardiotrophin-1 (CT-1). Except for CT-1, receptors for all other IL-6 family members have been detected in bone marrow stromal or osteoblastic cells [11]. In addition, IL-11-specific receptors are present in OC-like cells that are generated *in vitro*. Signal transduction through these receptors utilizes the JAK/STAT pathway [88].

Leukemia inhibitory factor (LIF) is produced by bone cells in response to a number of resorption stimuli [57, 78, 122]. However, production can be variable and depends on the model system that is being studied. The effects of LIF on bone resorption also are variable. In a number of *in vitro* model systems LIF stimulates resorption by a mechanism that is prostaglandin dependent [148], while in other *in vitro* assays, it has shown inhibitory effects [114, 180]. Up-regulation of RANKL production seems to be the mechanism by which LIF stimulates bone resorption in organ cultures, but the role of prostaglandins in this model remains unknown [141]. Mice that lack the specific LIF receptor and hence, cannot respond to LIF, exhibit reduced bone volume and a sixfold increase in osteoclast number [190].

The role of IL-6 family members in osteoclast formation recently has been reexamined in light of findings that demonstrated that, compared to wild-type animals, mice lacking the gp-130 activator protein have an increased number of osteoclasts [85]. Because gp-130 is an activator of signal transduction for all members of the IL-6 family, this result implies that one or more IL-6 family members inhibit osteoclast formation and bone resorption.

Prostaglandins are potent stimulators of bone resorption [145]. Curiously, they directly inhibit the resorbing activity of mature osteoclasts [26, 51]. However, they stimulate RANKL and inhibit OPG production by osteoblasts [20, 64, 184, 201]. This leads to increases in the number of osteoclasts and to a net increase in bone resorption.

Prostaglandins synergize with RANK-L and M-CSF to stimulate both the formation of osteoclasts from hematopoietic progenitors and the bone-resorbing activity of mature osteoclasts [189]. In mice that lack PGHS2, the inducible enzyme, which produces prostaglandins from arachidonic acid, there was a 60–70% decrease in the ability of PTH or 1,25-(OH)$_2$D$_3$ to stimulate an increase in osteoclast-like cell formation in bone marrow cultures [136]. Hence, prostaglandins appear to be involved in the resorptive responses of a number of agents.

Prostaglandin receptors are present on bone cells and of these the EP2 and EP4 receptors, which stimulate cyclic AMP, appear to mediate resorptive responses [168]. Interestingly, the enhancement of RANKL-mediated effects on osteoclast numbers exclusively involves interactions with EP2, because these effects did not occur in cells from EP2-deficient mice [105]. Prostaglandins are anabolic when given intermittently *in vivo* [86]. Significantly, the *in vivo* bone anabolic effects of prostaglandins appear to be mediated by the EP4 receptor, because these responses are absent in EP4-deficient mice [203].

Similar to other osteopetrotic mice such as the op/op mice [46, 91, 193], DAP12 –/– mice and DAP12 –/–FcRγ –/– double-knockout mice had osteopetrosis or severe osteopetrosis, respectively, as a result of impaired osteoclast differentiation [70, 83, 92, 128]. DAP12 and FcRγ (Fc receptor γ-chain) are both transmembrane proteins that contain an immunoreceptor tyrosine-based activation motif (ITAM).

DAP12 –/– mice exhibited mild osteopetrosis as evidenced by micro-CT and histomorphometric analysis, but were normal in terms of growth and fertility [70, 83, 92, 128]. *In vivo* osteoclast number was normal as was osteoclast morphology; however, *in vitro* the osteoclast number was significantly reduced when bone marrow cells were cultured in the presence of RANKL and M-CSF. The osteoclast morphology also was different, and the ability to resorb bone was severely reduced [70, 83, 92, 128]. Osteoclast formation can be rescued with retroviral expression of DAP12. In addition, when bone marrow cells were co-cultured with osteoblasts, osteoclastogenesis was partially restored. This suggests that osteoblasts can compensate, at least in part, for the loss of DAP12-mediated signaling.

A shorter stature and a more rounded face characterized the more severe osteopetrosis seen in DAP12 –/–FcRγ –/– mice. Interestingly, unlike what occurs is src –/– or RANKL –/– mice, teeth erupted normally in DAP12 –/– FcRγ –/– mice [93, 128, 166]. The osteoclast number was significantly reduced *in vivo*, indicating a

defect in osteoclast differentiation as opposed to a defect in activity. *In vitro*, few osteoclasts formed when precursors were stimulated with RANKL and M-CSF. Further, unlike in DAP12 –/– mice, co-culturing precursors with osteoblasts did not significantly elevate the number of osteoclasts formed *in vitro* [92, 128].

Two signaling pathways have been implicated as responsible for the severe inhibition of osteoclastogenesis in these mice. Mocsai et al. [128] demonstrated that during osteoclastogenesis, ITAM-signaling was dependent on Syk kinase. Further, Cbl and Pyk2 (signals downstream of Syk) previously had been implicated in osteoclast formation and/or function [43, 100, 158, 172]. In other studies, Koga et al. [92] confirmed that NFATc1 is a downstream target of FcRγ- and DAP12- ITAM-mediated signaling and that the induction of NFATc1 is required for RANK-induced osteoclast differentiation. These findings suggest that other ITAM-containing signaling adapters, or their downstream targets, also can play a role in regulating osteoclastogenesis (Figure 6.2).

As described earlier, deficiencies in osteoclast differentiation are responsible for the osteopetrosis seen in the op/op mice [46, 91, 193], PU.1 [14], NFκB [49, 197], and c-fos [59, 188] null mice. However, like the cathepsin K deficient mice [56, 157], c-src –/– mice have osteopetrosis that has resulted from impaired osteoclast function [4, 19, 66, 74, 166, 175]. The c-src proto-oncogene is a tyrosine kinase [23] that is highly expressed in osteoclasts and is used as a marker for the osteoclast phenotype [66]. Initially, c-src –/– mice died within the first few weeks after birth because of the failure of their incisors to erupt. Feeding mice ground-up chow and baby formula allowed them to survive and made possible long-term follow-up [19]. Osteopetrosis (up to a fourfold increase in unremodeled osteocartilaginous matrix in the vertebrae) resulted from the failure of osteoclasts to form ruffled borders [19, 175]. Similarly, studies show that c-src –/– osteoclasts did not exhibit a well-defined attachment ring [74]. Other studies demonstrated that pp60$^{c\text{-}src}$ (the gene product) was expressed in osteoclasts and even though other src family members (c-fyn, c-yes, and c-lyn) were similarly expressed in osteoclasts, this did not compensate for the absence of pp60$^{c\text{-}src}$ [66].

In other studies, investigators developed c-src –/– mice that expressed either wild-type or

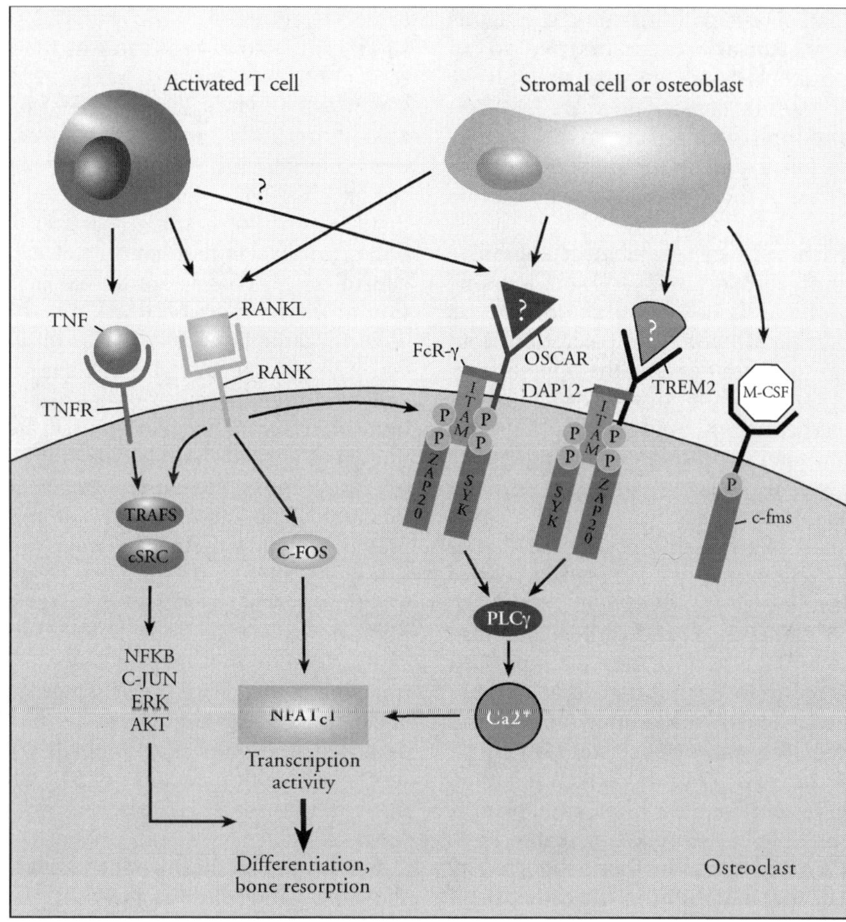

Figure 6.2   Immunoreceptor tyrosine-based activation motifs (ITAMs) are part of the signaling pathway leading to osteoclast formation.

mutant versions of src. Expression of the wild-type transgene rescued the osteopetrotic phenotype; osteoclasts from these mice exhibited ruffled borders and produced normal bone histology. Expression of a src allele that reduced activation of the kinase several fold also fully restored the normal bone phenotype in src–/– mice. However, expression of an src allele that severely impaired kinase activity only partially restored the bone phenotype. Osteoclast ruffled borders were formed in these mice, but fewer osteoclasts displayed them. These results suggest that *in vivo* c-src has important kinase-independent functions [160]. In mice that lack c-src, src inhibitors inhibit bone resorption *in vitro* and *in vivo* [126]. On the other hand, c-src –/– mice also display enhanced indices of bone

formation, which likely also contribute to the osteopetrotic phenotype [177]. In addition to the *in vivo* increase in osteoblast number described in c-src –/– mice, *in vitro* results have shown that incubation of osteoblasts with src-antisense oligodeoxynucleotides (~60% reduction in src levels) reduced cell proliferation [123]. Overall, these data suggest that c-src plays a dual role, regulating both bone formation and resorption.

Mice expressing the autosomal recessive motheaten (me/me) mutation are deficient in SHP-1 protein tyrosine phosphatase [163]. These mice have markedly reduced bone mineral density. Their trabecular and cortical thicknesses are decreased as a result of a 14% increase in osteoclast number [178]. Co-culture of normal osteoblasts with me/me BM cells (as a source of osteoclast precursors) led to an increase in osteoclasts as compared to controls. Notably, B cells from me/me mice are hyperresponsive and polyclonaly activated. Whether these B cells participate in the increased osteoclast formation in these animals remains to be shown.

To resorb bone, osteoclasts must solubilize both the inorganic mineral and the organic proteins of bone [15]. Inorganic mineral is efficiently removed with acid secretion, and lysosomal proteinases degrade the bone matrix proteins [131]. One of the lysosomal proteinases, cathepsin K, efficiently degrades several bone matrix proteins including type I collagen, type II collagen, osteopontin, and osteonectin [16, 22, 52, 82].

Cathepsin K is a cysteine proteinase that is highly and predominantly expressed in cells of the osteoclast lineage [21, 39, 106, 110, 162, 173]. Cathepsin B, cathepsin L, and cathepsin O also are cysteine proteinases, but they are expressed at low levels or are absent in osteoclasts. Cathepsin K has been cloned from rabbit, human, and murine osteoclasts and osteoclastomas [21, 40, 71, 106, 107, 146, 162, 173, 183]. Taken together, these observations suggest that cathepsin K plays a major role in osteoclast-mediated bone resorption. This idea was further supported by the discovery that mutations in the cathepsin K gene were responsible for the skeletal disorder, pycnodysostosis. The clinical presentation of that disease includes osteopetrosis, bone fragility, short stature, and multiple cranial facial and dental abnormalities [42, 53, 81, 120].

The role of cathepsin K was further elucidated by studies that examined cathepsin K knockout mice [56, 137, 157] and mice overexpressing cathepsin K [89]. Overexpression of cathepsin K resulted in a 36% reduction in trabecular bone volume. In these mice, osteoclast number and osteoclast surface were unchanged, but their functionality was not assessed either *in vivo* or *in vitro* [89]. Therefore, enhanced osteoclast function could provide an explanation for the reduction in bone volume that was observed. Conversely, cathepsin K null (−/−) mice developed osteopetrosis [56, 157]. Both cathepsin K −/− mouse models had a similar phenotype with a significant increase in trabecular (~3.5-fold increase) and cortical bone volume, and no alteration in osteoclast number. However, both articles report alterations in

osteoclast function. Saftig et al. [157] reported a significant, sixfold reduction in the number of resorption pits formed by cathepsin K −/− osteoclasts *in vitro*. The perimeter of these pits was significantly greater than in controls, but the volume and depth were significantly reduced. Gowen et al. [56] reported visualizing distinct zones of demineralization (osteoclast-bone interface) that were not apparent in control mice. This suggests that demineralization of the bone was normal, but that removal of the organic bone matrix was impaired. Conversely, Okaji et al. [137] visualized indistinct zones of demineralization at the osteoclast-bone interface on alveolar bone surfaces, and on that basis argued that alveolar bone resorption of both inorganic and organic bone was unaltered. The latter authors also reported that matrix metalloproteinase-9 levels were significantly elevated in the absence of cathepsin K, and thus may act as a compensatory proteinase. Further, osteoclast morphology was significantly different in cathepsin K −/− mice. In these mice the ruffled border was irregular, adhesion sites in the sealing zone were open and detached, and fine collagen fibrils were present in the resorption lacunae [157]; all of these observations are consistent with altered functionality.

Finally, the studies of Motyckova et al. [130] show that cathepsin K is a transcriptional target of MITF. As described above, mi/mi MITF mice are osteopetrotic. Osteoclasts from mi/mi mice are mononuclear, do not form ruffled-borders, exhibit impaired bone resorption, and contain decreased levels of TRAP [117, 132, 174, 185]. The latter observation is consistent with the report that Mif regulates osteoclast TRAP expression. Interestingly, these mice also have a significant reduction in cathepsin K mRNA and protein expression. On the other hand, overexpression of MITF up-regulated expression of cathepsin K in osteoclasts that formed *in vitro* [130]. These findings indicate that cathepsin K is a transcriptional target of MITF. In cathepsin K −/− mice, only bones formed by endochondral ossification were affected; in c-fos −/− mice, on the other hand, osteopetrosis was observed in all bones examined, including the skull [188].

Integrins are heterodimeric, transmembrane, adhesion receptors that mediate cell–matrix and cell–cell interactions [181]. The $\alpha_v\beta_3$ integrin is expressed in osteoclasts and plays an important role in bone resorption [125]. Mice deficient in the β_3 subunit (β_3 −/− mice) developed osteosclerosis and were hypocalcemic. Interestingly, the osteoclasts in these mice were normal in appearance, but their numbers had increased 3.5-fold. Despite their normal appearance, these osteoclasts were dysfunctional *in vitro* and *ex vivo* by a number of criteria. For example, they displayed a significant reduction in resorption potential, they failed to spread normally, and they showed a general inability to form normal ruffled borders or actin rings. Osteoclast number also was decreased *in vitro*, suggesting arrested differentiation [125]. Importantly, *in vitro* studies showed that addition of high-doses of M-CSF rescued the dysfunctions of osteoclasts generated from β_3 −/− mice [44]. *In vivo*, these mice produce elevated levels of M-CSF. This may account for the elevated osteoclast number seen *in vivo* versus the diminished osteoclast number seen *in vitro* [44]. It also was shown that bone marrow macrophages derived from β_3 −/− mice expressed decreased levels of c-fos, which may, in turn, account for the arrested differentiation of osteoclasts *in vitro* and possibly *in vivo* [44]. While overexpression of c-fos in osteoclasts generated from β_3 −/− mice also was able to normalize osteoclast number, these cells were unable to resorb bone. This showed that the $\alpha_v\beta_3$ integrin is required for bone resorption to take place [44].

Conclusion

It is clear from the work presented here that formation of bone-resorbing osteoclasts from progenitors is a highly ordered multi-step process. The identification of spontaneous genetic mutations and our ability to engineer gene expression has resulted in a quantum leap forward in our understanding of this process. Regulation of osteoclast formation can occur at many steps along the pathway leading to functional osteoclasts. This high degree of regulation suggests that osteoclast formation, and thereby the function that osteoclasts carry out, is important to the survival of the animal. Although much is now known about osteoclast formation and function, the ability to use genetic tools will, without question, allow identification of new regulatory molecules. Such discoveries will result in a detailed understanding of osteoclast biology, the consequence of which will be the development of new therapeutics that regulate the skeleton.

Acknowledgments

This work was supported by grants from the National Institutes of Health to J.A.L (AR38933, AR48714, AR49190) and to M.C.H (AR49109, AR47342) and the Yale Core Center for Musculoskeletal Disorders (AR46032).

References

1. Al-Humidan A, Ralston SH, Hughes DE, et al. (1991) Interleukin-6 does not stimulate bone resorption in neonatal mouse calvariae. J Bone Miner Res 6:3–8.
2. Akira S, Hirano T, Taga T, Kishimoto T (1990) Biology of multifunctional cytokines: IL-6 and related molecules (IL-1 and TNF). FASEB J 4:2860–7.
3. Amano H, Yamada S, Felix R (1998) Colony-stimulating factor-1 stimulates the fusion process in osteoclasts. J Bone Miner Res 13:846–53.
4. Amling M, Neff L, Priemel M, Schilling AF, Rueger JM, Baron R (2000) Progressive increase in bone mass and development of odontomas in aging osteopetrotic c-src-deficient mice. Bone 27:603–10.
5. Anderson DM, Maraskovsky E, Billingsley, et al. (1997) A homologue of the TNF receptor and its ligand enhance T-cell growth and dendritic-cell function. Nature 390:175–9.
6. Anderson KL, Smith KA, Pio F, et al. (1998) Neutrophils deficient in PU.1 do not terminally differentiate or become functionally competent. Blood 92:1576–85.
7. Angel P, Karin M (1991) The role of Jun, Fos and the AP-1 complex in cell-proliferation and transformation. Biochem Biophys Acta 1072, 129–57.
8. Arai F, Miyamoto T, Ohneda O, et al. (1999) Commitment and differentiation of osteoclast precursor cells by the sequential expression of c-Fms and receptor activator of nuclear factor $_\kappa$B (RANK) receptors. J Exp Med 12:1741–54.
9. Azuma Y, Kaji K, Katogi R, Takeshita S, Kudo A (2000) Tumor necrosis factor-alpha induces differentiation of and bone resorption by osteoclasts. J Biol Chem 275:4858–64.
10. Bain G, Robanus Maandag EC, Izon DJ, et al. (1994) E2A proteins are required for proper B cell development and initiation of immunoglobulin gene rearrangements. Cell 79:885–92.
11. Bellido T, Stahl N, Farruggella TJ, Borba V, Yancopoulos GD, Manolagas SC (1996) Detection of receptors for interleukin-6, interleukin-11, leukemia inhibitory factor, oncostatin M, and ciliary neurotrophic factor in bone marrow stromal osteoblastic cells. J Clin Invest 97:431–7.
12. Bertolini DR, Nedwin GE, Bringman TS, Smith DD, Mundy GR (1986) Stimulation of bone resorption and

inhibition of bone formation in vitro by human tumour necrosis factors. Nature 319:516–18.

13. Beutler B, Cerami A (1987) Cachectin: More than a tumor necrosis factor. N Eng J Med 316:379–85.

14. Black K, Garrett IR, Mundy GR (1991) Chinese hamster ovary cells transfected with the murine interleukin-6 gene cause hypercalcemia as well as cachexia, leukocytosis and thrombocytosis in tumor bearing nude mice. Endocrinology 128:2657–9.

15. Blair HC, Khan AJ, Crouch EC, Jeffrey JJ, Teitelbaum SL (1986) Isolated osteoclasts resorb the organic and inorganic components of bone. J Cell Biol 102:1164–72.

16. Bossard MJ, Tomaszek TA, Thompson SK, et al. (1996) Proteolytic activity of human osteoclast cathepsin I: Expression, purification, activation, and substrate identification. J Biol Chem 271:12517–24.

17. Boyle WJ, Simonet WS, Lacey DL (2003) Osteoclast differentiation and activation. Nature 423:337–42.

18. Boyce BF, Aufdemorte TB, Garrett R, Yates AJP, Mundy GR (1989) Effects of interleukin-1 on bone turnover in normal mice. Endocrinology 125:1142.

19. Boyce BF, Chen H, Soriano P, Mundy GR (1993) Histomorphometric and immunocytochemical studies of src-related osteopetrosis. Bone 14:335–40.

20. Brändström H, Jonsson KB, Vidal O, Ljunghall S, Ohlsson C, Ljunggren Ö (1998) Tumor necrosis factor-α and -β upregulate the levels of osteoprotegerin mRNA in human osteosarcoma MG-63 cells. Biochem Biophys Res Commun 248:454–7.

21. Bromme D, Okamoto K (1995) The baculovirus cysteine protease has a cathepsin B-like S2-subsite specificity. Biol Chem 376:611–15.

22. Bromme D, Okamoto K, Wang W, Biroc S (1996) Human cathepsin 02, a matrix protein-degrading cysteine protease expressed in osteoclasts: Functional expression of human cathepsin 02 in spodoptera frugiperda and characterization of the enzyme. J Biol Chem 271:2126–32.

23. Brown MT, Cooper JA (1996) Regulation, substrates, and functions of Src. BBA Rev. Cancer 1287:121–49.

24. Bucay N, Sarosi I, Dunstan CR, et al. (1998) Osteoprotegerin-deficient mice develop early onset osteoporosis and arterial calcification. Genes Dev 12:1260–8.

25. Burger D, Chicheportiche R, Giri JG, Dayer J-M (1995) The inhibitory activity of human interleukin-1 receptor antagonist is enhanced by type II interleukin-1 soluble receptor and hindered by type 1 interleukin-1 soluble receptor. J Clin Invest 96:38–41.

26. Chambers TJ, Fox S, Jagger CJ, Lean JM, Chow JWM (1999) The role of prostaglandins and nitric oxide in the response of bone to mechanical forces. Osteoarthritis Cartilage 7:422–3.

27. Crabtree GR, Olson EN (2002) NFAT signaling: Choreographing the social lives of cells. Cell 109 Suppl:S67–79.

28. Cerretti DP, Wignall J, Anderson D, Tushinski RJ, Gallis B, Cosman D (1990) Membrane bound forms of human macrophage colony stimulating factor (M-CSF, CSF-1). Prog Clin Biol Res 352:63–70.

29. Cerretti DP, Wignall J, Anderson D, et al. (1988) Human macrophage-colony stimulating factor: alternative RNA and protein processing from a single gene. Mol Immunol 25:761–70.

30. Colotta F, Re F, Muzio M, et al. (1993) Interleukin-1 type II receptor: A decoy target for IL-1 that is regulated by IL-4. Science 261:472–5.

31. Dai XM, Ryan GR, Hapel AJ, et al. (2002) Targeted disruption of the mouse colony-stimulating factor 1 receptor gene results in osteopetrosis, mononuclear phagocyte deficiency, increased primitive progenitor cell frequencies, and reproductive defects. Blood 99: 111–20

32. De La Mata J, Uy HL, Guise TA, et al. (1995) Interleukin-6 enhances hypercalcemia and bone resorption mediated by parathyroid hormone-related protein in vivo. J Clin Invest 95:2846–52.

33. DeKoter RP, Walsh JC, Singh H (1998) PU.1 regulates both cytokine-dependent proliferation and differentiation of granulocyte/macrophage progenitors. EMBO J 17:4456–68.

34. DeKoter RP, Lee H-J, Singh H (2002) PU.1 regulates expression of the interleukin-7 receptor in lymphoid progenitors. Immunity 16:297–309.

35. DeKoter RP, Singh H (2000) Regulation of B lymphocyte and macrophage development by graded expression of PU.1. Science 288:1439–41.

36. Dinarello CA (1991) Interleukin-1 and interleukin-1 antagonism. Blood 77:1627–52.

37. Dinarello CA (1993) Blocking interleukin-1 in disease. Blood Purif 11:118–27.

38. Dougall WC, Glaccum M, Charrier K, et al. (1999) RANK is essential for osteoclast and lymph node development. Genes Dev 13:2412–24.

39. Drake FH, Dodds RA, James IR, et al. (1996) Cathepsin K, but not cathepsins B, L, or S, is abundantly expressed in human osteoclasts. J Biol Chem 271:12511–16.

40. Drake FH, James IE, Connor JR, et al. (1994) Identification of a novel osteoclast-selective human cysteine proteinase. J Bone Miner Res 9:S177.

41. Eder J (1997) Tumour necrosis factor alpha and interleukin 1 signalling: do MAPKK kinases connect it all? Trends Pharmacol Sci 18:319–22.

42. Edelson JG, Obad S, Geiger R, On A, Artul HJ (1992) Pycnodysostosis. Orthopedic aspects with a description of 14 new cases. Clin Orthop Relat Res 280:264–76.

43. Faccio R, Novack DV, Zallone A, Ross FP, Teitelbaum SL (2003) Dynamic changes in the osteoclast cytoskeleton in response to growth factors and cell attachment are controlled by β_3 integrin. J Cell Biol 162:499–509.

44. Faccio R, Takeshita S, Zallone A, Ross FP, Teitelbaum SL (2003) C-Fms and the α_v-β_3 integrin collaborate during osteoclast differentiation. J Clin Invest 111: 749–58.

45. Felix R, Fleisch H, Elford PR (1989) Bone-resorbing cytokines enhance release of macrophage colony-stimulating activity by the osteoblastic cell MC3T3-E1. Calcif Tissue Int 44:356–60.

46. Felix R, Cecchini MG, Hofstetter W, Elford PR, Stutzer A, Fleisch H (1990) Impairment of macrophage colony-stimulating factor production and lack of resident bone marrow macrophages in the osteopetrotic op/op mouse. J Bone Miner Res 5:781–9.

47. Felix R, Cecchini MG, Fleisch H (1990) Macrophage colony stimulating factor restores in vivo bone resorption in the op/op osteopetrotic mouse. Endocrinology 127:2592–4.

48. Fiers W (1993) Tumor Necrosis Factor. In: Sim E (ed) The Natural Immune System: Humoral Factors. IRL Press at Oxford University Press, Oxford, pp 65–119.

49. Franzoso G, Carlson L, Xing L, et al. (1997) Requirement for NF-kappaB in osteoclast and B-cell development. Genes Dev 11:3482–96.

50. Fuller K, Owens JM, Jagger CJ, Wilson A, Moss R, Chambers TJ (1993) Macrophage colony-stimulating factor stimulates survival and chemotactic behavior in isolated osteoclasts. J Exp Med 178:1733–44.

51. Fuller K, Chambers TJ (1989) Effect of arachidonic acid metabolites on bone resorption by isolated rat osteoclasts. J Bone Miner Res 4:209–15.

52. Garnero PO, Borel IB, Ferreras M, et al. (1998) The collagenolytic activity of cathepsin K is unique among mammalian proteinases. J Biol Chem 273:32347–52.

53. Gelb BD, Shi G-P, Chapman HA, Desnick RJ (1996) Pycnodysostosis, a lysosomal disease caused by cathepsin K deficiency. Science 273:1236–8.

54. Glowacki J, Cox KA, Wilcon S (1989) Impaired osteoclast differentiation in subcutaneous implants of bone particles in osteopetrotic mutants. J Bone Miner Res 5:271–8.

55. Gowen M, Chapman K, Littlewood A, Hughes D, Evans D, Russell RGG (1990) Production of tumor necrosis factor by human osteoblasts is modulated by other cytokines, but not by osteotropic hormones. Endocrinology 126:1250–5.

56. Gowen M, Lazner F, Dodds R, et al. (1999) Cathepsin K knockout mice develop osteopetrosis due to a deficit in matrix degradation but not demineralization. J Bone Miner Res 14:1654–63.

57. Greenfield EM, Horowitz MC, Lavish SA (1996) Stimulation by parathyroid hormone of interleukin-6 and leukemia inhibitory factor expression in osteoblasts is an immediate-early gene response induced by cAMP signal transduction. J Biol Chem 271:10984–9.

58. Grigoriadis AE, Schellander K, Wang Z-Q, Wagner EF (1993) Osteoblasts are target cells for transformation in C-fos transgenic mice. J Cell Biol 122:685–701.

59. Grigoriadis AE, Wang Z-Q, Cecchini MG, et al. (1994) c-FOS: a key regulator of osteoclast-macrophage lineage determination and bone remodeling. Science 266:443–6.

60. Guise TA, Mundy GR (1998) Cancer and bone. Endocrine Reviews 19:18–54.

61. Hattersley G, Kerby JA, Chambers TJ (1991) Generation of osteoclast precursors in multilineage hematopoietic colonies. Endocrinology 128:259–62.

62. Hattersley G, Dorey E, Horton MA, Chambers TJ (1988) Human macrophage colony-stimulating factor inhibits bone resorption by osteoclasts disaggregated from rat bone. J Cell Physiol 137:199–203.

63. Hirano T, Akira S, Taga T, Kishimoto T (1990) Biological and clinical aspects of interleukin 6. Immunol Today 11:443–9.

64. Hofbauer LC, Dunstan CR, Spelsberg TC, Riggs BL, Khosla S (1998) Osteoprotegerin production by human osteoblast lineage cells is stimulated by vitamin D, bone morphogenetic protein-2, and cytokines. Biochem Biophys Res Commun 250:776–81.

65. Hofstetter W, Wetterwald A, Cecchini MC, Felix R, Fleisch H, Mueller C (1992) Detection of transcripts for the receptor for macrophage colony-stimulating factor, c-*fms*, in murine osteoclasts. Proc Natl Acad Sci USA 89:9637–41.

66. Horne WC, Neff L, Chatterjee D, Lomri A, Levy JB, Baron R (1992) Osteoclasts express high levels of pp60^{c-src} in association with intracellular membranes. J Cell Biology 119:1003–13.

67. Horowitz MC, Xi Y, Pflugh DL, et al. (2002) Severe osteopenia with increased osteoclast progenitors in Pax5 deficient mice. JBMR #1098:S148 (abst).

68. Hsu H, Lacey DL, Dunstan CR, et al. (1999) Tumor necrosis factor receptor family member RANK mediates osteoclast differentiation and activation induced by osteoprotegerin ligand. Proc Natl Acad Sci USA 96:3540–5.

69. Huang J, Gao X, Li S, Cao Z (1997) Recruitment of IRAK to the interleukin 1 receptor complex requires interleukin 1 receptor accessory protein. Proc Natl Acad Sci USA 94:12829–32.

70. Humphrey MB, Ogasawara K, Yao W, et al. (2004) The signaling adapter protein DAP12 regulates multinucleation during osteoclast development. J Bone Miner Res 19:224–34.

71. Inaoka T, Bilbe G, Ishibashi O, Tezuka K, Kumegawa M, Kokubo T (1995) Molecular cloning of human cDNA for cathepsin K: Novel cysteine proteinase predominately expressed in bone. Biochem Biophys Res Commun 206:89–96.

72. Insogna K, Tanaka S, Neff L, Horne W, Levy J, Baron R (1997) Role of c-Src in cellular events associated with colony-stimulating factor-1-induced spreading in osteoclasts. Mol Reprod Dev 46:104–8.

73. Insogna KL, Sahni M, Grey AB, et al. (1997) Colony-stimulating factor-1 induces cytoskeletal reorganization and c-src-dependent tyrosine phosphorylation of selected cellular proteins in rodent osteoclasts. J Clin Invest 100:2476–85.

74. Insogna K, Tanaka S, Neff L, Horne W, Levy J, Baron R (1997) Role of c-Src in cellular events associated with colony-stimulating factor-1-induced spreading in osteoclasts. Molecular Reproduction & Development 46:104–8.

75. Iotsova V, Caamano J, Loy J, Yang Y, Lewin A, Bravo R (1997) Osteopetrosis in mice lacking NF-kappaB1 and NF-kappaB2. Nat Med 3:1285–9.

76. Ishida N, Hayashi K, Hoshijima M, et al. (2002) Large scale gene expression analysis of osteoclastogenesis in vitro and elucidation of NFAT2 as a key regulator. J Biol Chem 277:41147–56.

77. Ishimi Y, Miyaura C, Jin CH, et al. (1990) IL-6 is produced by osteoblasts and induces bone resorption. J Immunol 145:3297–303.

78. Ishimi Y, Abe E, Jin CH, et al. (1992) Leukemia inhibitory factor/differentiation-stimulating factor (LIF/D-factor): Regulation of its production and possible roles in bone metabolism. J Cell Physiol 152:71–8.

79. Jilka RL, Hangoc G, Girasole G, et al. (1992) Increased osteoclast development after estrogen loss: mediation by interleukin-6. Science 257:88–91.

80. Jimi E, Shuto T, Koga T (1995) Macrophage colony-stimulating factor and interleukin-1α maintain the survival of osteoclast-like cells. Endocrinology 136:808–11.

81. Johnson MR, Polymeropoulos MH, Vos HL, Ortiz de Luna RI, Francomano CA (1996) A nonsense mutation in the cathepsin K gene observed in a family with pycnodysostosis. Genome Res 6:1050–5.

82. Kafienah W, Brömme D, Buttle DJ, Croucher LJ, Hollander AJ (1998) Human cathepsin K cleaves native type I and II collagens at the N-terminal end of the triple helix. Biochem 331:727–32.

83. Kaifu T, Nakahara J, Inui M, et al. (2003) Osteopetrosis and thalamic hypomyelinosis with synaptic degenera-

tion in DAP12-deficient mice. J Clin Invest 111:323–32.

84. Kanazawa K, Azuma Y, Nakano H, Kudo A (2003) TRAF5 functions in both RANKL- and TNFalpha-induced osteoclastogenesis. J Bone Miner Res 18: 443–50.

85. Kawasaki K, Gao YH, Yokose S, et al. (1997) Osteoclasts are present in gp130-deficient mice. Endocrinology 138:4959–65.

86. Kawaguchi H, Pilbeam CC, Harrison JR, Raisz LG (1995) The role of prostaglandins in the regulation of bone metabolism. Clin Orthop 313:36–46.

87. Kee BL, Murre C (1998) Induction of early B cell factor (EBF) and multiple B lineage genes by the basic helix-loop-helix transcription factor E12. J Exp Medicine 188:699–713.

88. Kishimoto T, Taga T, Akira S (1994) Cytokine signal transduction. Cell 76:253–62.

89. Kiviranta R, Morko J, Uusitalo H, Aro HT, Vuorio E, Rantakokko J (2001) Accelerated turnover of meta-physeal trabecular bone in mice overexpressing cathepsin K. J Bone Miner Res 16:1444–52.

90. Kobayashi K, Takahashi N, Jimi E, et al. (2000) Tumor Necrosis Factor alpha Stimulates Osteoclast Differentiation by a Mechanism Independent of the ODF/RANKL-RANK Interaction. J Exp Med 191:275–86.

91. Kodama H, Yamasaki A, Nose M, et al. (1991) Congen-ital osteoclast deficiency in osteopetrotic (op/op) mice is cured by injections of macrophage colony stimulat-ing factor. J Exp Med 173:269–72.

92. Koga T, Inul M, Inoue K, et al. (2004) Costimulatory signals mediated by the ITAM motif cooperate with RANKL for bone homeostasis. Nature 428:758–63.

93. Kong YY, Yoshida H, Sarosi I, et al. (1999) OPGL is a key regulator of osteoclastogenesis, lymphocyte develop-ment and lymph-node organogenesis. Nature 397:315–23.

94. Korherr C, Hofmeister R, Wesche H, Falk W (1997) A critical role for interleukin-1 receptor accessory protein in interleukin-1 signaling. Eur J Immunol 27:262–7.

95. Kurihara N, Chenu C, Civin CI, Roodman GD (1990) Identification of committed mononuclear precursors for osteoclast-like cells formed in long-term marrow cultures. Endocrinology 126:2733–41.

96. Kurihara N, Bertolini D, Suda T, Akiyama Y, Roodman GD (1990) IL-6 stimulates osteoclast-like multi-nucleated cell formation in long term human marrow cultures by inducing IL-1 release. J Immunol 144: 4226–30.

97. Lacey DL, Timms E, Tan H-L, et al. (1998) Osteoprote-gerin (OPG) ligand is a cytokine that regulates osteo-clast differentiation and activation. Cell 93:165–76.

98. Lacey DL, Tan HL, Lu J, et al. (2000) Osteoprotegerin ligand modulates murine osteoclast survival in vitro and in vivo. Am J Pathol 157:435–48.

99. Lagasse E, Weissman IL (1997) Enforced expression of Bcl-2 in monocytes rescues macrophages and partially reverses osteopetrosis in op/op mice. Cell 89:1021–31.

100. Lakkakorpi PT, Brett A, Lipfert L, Rodan GA, Duong Le T (2003) PYK2 atuophosphorylation, but not kinase activity, is necessary for adhesion-induced association with c-Src, osteoclast spreading, and bone resorption. J Biol Chem 278:11502–12.

101. Lee MY, Eyre DR, Osborne WR (1991) Isolation of murine osteoclast colony-stimulating factor. Proc Natl Acad Sci USA 88:8500–4.

102. Lees RL, Heersche JNM (1999) Macrophage colony stimulating factor increases bone resorption in dis-persed osteoclast cultures by increasing osteoclast size. J Bone Miner Res 14:937–45.

103. Li J, Sarosi I, Yan XQ, et al. (2000) RANK is the intrin-sic hematopoietic cell surface receptor that controls osteoclastogenesis and regulation of bone mass and calcium metabolism. Proc Natl Acad Sci USA 97: 1566–71.

104. Li H, Cuartas E, Cui W, et al. (2004) Irak-m is a nega-tive regulator of osteoclast. In: Proceedings: Advances in Skeletal Anabolic Agents for the Treatment of Osteo-porosis, ASBMR 35, 23 (Abstract).

105. Li X, Okada Y, Pilbeam CC, Lorenzo, et al. (2000) Knockout of the murine prostaglandin EP2 receptor impairs osteoclastogenesis in vitro. Endocinology 141:2054–61.

106. Li YP, Alexander M, Wucherpfennig AL, Yelick P, Chen W, Stashenko P (1995) Cloning and complete coding sequence of a novel human cathepsin expressed in giant cells of osteoclastomas. J Bone Miner Res 10:1197–2202.

107. Li YP, Chen W (1999) Characterization of mouse cathepsin K gene, the gene promoter, and the gene expression. J Bone Miner Res 14:487–99.

108. Lin H, Grosschedl R (1995) Failure of B-cell differenti-ation in mice lacking the transcription factor EBF. Nature 376:263–7.

109. Linkhart TA, Linkhart SG, MacCharles DC, Long DL, Strong DD (1991) Interleukin-6 messenger RNA expression and interleukin-6 protein secretion in cells isolated from normal human bone: regulation by inter-leukin-1. J Bone Miner Res 6:1285–94.

110. Littlewood EA, Kokubo T, Ishibashi O, et al. (1997) Localization of cathepsin K in human osteoclasts by in situ hybridization and immunohistochemistry. Bone 20:81–6.

111. Lomaga MA, Yeh WC, Sarosi I, et al. (1999) TRAF6 deficiency results in osteopetrosis and defective interleukin-1, CD40, and LPS signaling. Genes Dev 13:1015–24.

112. Lorenzo JA, Sousa S, Alander C, Raisz LG, Dinarello CA (1987) Comparison of the bone-resorbing activity in the supernatants from phytohemagglutinin-stimu-lated human peripheral blood mononuclear cells with that of cytokines through the use of an antiserum to interleukin 1. Endocrinology 121:1164–70.

113. Lorenzo JA, Naprta A, Rao Y, et al. (1998) Mice lacking the type I interleukin-1 receptor do not lose bone mass after ovariectomy. Endocrinology 139:3022–5.

114. Lorenzo JA, Sousa SL, Leahy CL (1990) Leukemia inhibitory factor (LIF) inhibits basal bone resorption in fetal rat long bone cultures. Cytokine 2:266–71.

115. Lowik CW, Van der PG, Bloys H, et al. (1989) Parathy-roid hormone (PTH) and PTH-like protein (PLP) stim-ulate interleukin-6 production by osteogenic cells: a possible role of interleukin-6 in osteoclastogeneis. Biochem Biophys Res Commun 162:1546–52.

116. Luchin A, Suchting S, Merson T, et al. (2001) Genetic and physical interactions between Microphthalmia transcription factor and PU.1 are necessary for osteo-clast gene expression and differentiation. J Biol Chem 276:36703–10.

117. Luchin A, Purdom G, Murphy K, et al. (2000) The microphthalmia transcription factor regulates expression of the tartrate-resistant acid phosphatase gene during terminal differentiation of osteoclasts. J Bone Miner Res 15:451–60.

118. Manolagas SC, Jilka RL (1995) Mechanisms of disease: Bone marrow, cytokines, and bone remodeling – Emerging insights into the pathophysiology of osteoporosis. N Engl J Med 332:305–11.

119. Manolagas SC, Bellido T, Jilka RL (1995) New insights into the cellular, biochemical, and molecular basis of postmenopausal and senile osteoporosis: Roles of IL-6 and gp130. Int'l J Immunopharm 17:109–16.

120. Maroteaux P, Lamy M (1962) Pyknodysostosis. Presse Med 70:999–1002.

121. Martin MU, Falk W (1997) The interleukin-1 receptor complex and interleukin-1 signal transduction. Eur Cytokine Netw 8:5–17.

122. Marusic A, Kalinowski JF, Jastrzebski S, Lorenzo JA (1993) Production of leukemia inhibitory factor mRNA and protein by malignant and immortalized bone cells. J Bone Miner Res 8:617–24.

123. Marzia M, Sims NA, Voit S, et al. (2000) Decreased c-Src expression enhances osteoblast differentiation and bone formation. J Cell Biology 151:311–20.

124. Matsuo K, Galson DL, Zhao C, et al. (2004) Nuclear Factor of Activated T-cells (NFAT) rescues osteoclastogenesis in precursors lacking c-Fos. J Biol Chem 279:26475–80.

125. McHugh KP, Hodivala-Dilke K, Zheng M-II, et al. (2000) Mice lacking [beta]3 integrins are osteosclerotic because of dysfunctional osteoclasts. J Clin Invest 105:433–44.

126. Missbach M, Jeschke M, Feyen J, et al. (1999) A novel inhibitor of the tyrosine kinase Src suppresses phosphorylation of its major cellular substrates and reduces bone resorption in vitro and in rodent models in vivo. Bone 24:437–49.

127. Mizuno A, Amizuka N, Irie K, et al. (1998) Severe osteoporosis in mice lacking osteoclastogenesis inhibitory factor/osteoprotegerin. Biochem Biophys Res Commun 247:610–15.

128. Mócsai A, Humphrey MB, Van Ziffle JAG, et al. (2004) The immunomodulatory adapter proteins DAP12 and Fc receptor γ-chain (FcRγ) regulate development of functional osteoclasts through the Syk tyrosine kinase. Proc Natl Acad Sci USA 101:6158–63.

129. Moore KJ (1995) Insight into the microphthalmia gene. Trends Genet 11:442–8.

130. Motyckova G, Weilbaecher KN, Horstmann M, Rieman DJ, Fisher DZ, Fisher DE (2001) Linking osteopetrosis and pycnodysostosis: regulation of cathepsin K expression by the microphthalmia transcription factor family. Proc Natl Acad Sci USA 98:5798–803.

131. Mundy GR (1989) Local factors in bone remodeling. Recent Prog Horm Res 45:507–27.

132. Murphy HM (1973) The osteopetrotic syndrome in the microphthalmic mutant mouse. Calcif Tissue Res 13:19–26.

133. Naito A, Azuma S, Tanaka S, et al. (1999) Severe osteopetrosis, defective interleukin-1 signaling and lymph node organogenesis in TRAF6-deficient mice. Genes Cells 4:353–62.

134. Nutt SL, Heavey B, Rolink AG, Busslinger M (1999) Commitment to the B-lymphoid lineage depends on the transcription factor Pax5. Nature 401:556–62.

135. O'Riordan M, Grosschedl R (1999) Coordinate regulation of B cell differentiation by the transcription factors EBF and E2A. Immunity 11:21–31.

136. Okada Y, Lorenzo JA, Freeman AM, et al. (2000) Prostaglandin G/H synthase-2 is required for maximal formation of osteoclast-like cells in culture. J Clin Invest 105:823–32.

137. Okaji M, Sakai H, Sakai E, et al. (2003) The regulation of bone resorption in tooth formation and eruption processes in mouse alveolar crest devoid of cathepsin K. J Pharmacol Sci 91:285–294.

138. Oliff A (1988) The role of tumor necrosis factor (cachectin) in cachexia. Cell 54:141–2.

139. Orkin SH (2000) Diversification of hematopoietic stem cells to specific lineages. Nat Rev Genet 1:57–64.

140. Pacifici R, Rifas L, McCracken R, Avioli LV (1990) The role of interleukin-1 in postmenopausal bone loss. Exp Gerontol 25:309–16.

141. Palmqvist P, Persson E, Conaway HH, Lerner UH (2002) IL-6, Leukemia Inhibitory Factor, and Oncostatin M Stimulate Bone Resorption and Regulate the Expression of Receptor Activator of NF-kappaB Ligand, Osteoprotegerin, and Receptor Activator of NF-kappaB in Mouse Calvariae. J Immunol 169:3353–62.

142. Pfeffer K, Matsuyama T, Kündig TM, et al. (1993) Mice deficient for the 55 kd tumor necrosis factor receptor are resistant to endotoxic shock, yet succumb to L. monocytogenes infection. Cell 73:457–67.

143. Pfeilschifter J, Chenu C, Bird A, Mundy GR, Roodman GD (1989) Interleukin-1 and tumor necrosis factor stimulate the formation of human osteoclast-like cells in vitro. J Bone Min Res 4:113–18.

144. Poli V, Balena R, Fattori E, et al. (1994) Interleukin-6 deficient mice are protected from bone loss caused by estrogen depletion. EMBO Journal 13:1189–96.

145. Raisz LG (1999) Prostaglandins and bone: physiology and pathophysiology. Osteoarthritis Cartilage 7:419–21

146. Rantakokko J, Aro HT, Savontaus M, Vuorio E (1996) Mouse cathepsin K: cDNA cloning and predominant expression of the gene in osteoclasts, and in some hypertrophying chondrocytes during mouse development. FEBS Lett 393:307–13.

147. Reddy SV, Takahashi S, Dallas M, Williams RE, Neckers L, Roodman GD (1994) Interleukin-6 antisense deoxyoligonucleotides inhibit bone resorption by giant cells from human giant cell tumors of bone. J Bone Miner Res 9:753–7.

148. Reid IR, Lowe C, Cornish J, et al. (1990) Leukemia inhibitory factor: a novel bone-active cytokine. Endocinology 126:1416–20.

149. Roggia C, Gao Y, Cenci S, et al. (2001) Up-regulation of TNF-producing T cells in the bone marrow: A key mechanism by which estrogen deficiency induces bone loss in vivo. Proc Natl Acad Sci USA 98:13960–5.

150. Roodman GD (1996) Advances in Bone Biology: The osteoclast. Endocrine Reviews 17:308–32.

151. Roodman GD (1992) Interleukin-6: an osteotropic factor? J Bone Miner Res 7:475–8.

152. Roodman GD, Kurihara N, Ohsaki Y, et al. (1992) A potential autocrine/paracrine factor in Paget's disease of bone. J Clin Invest 89:46–52.

153. Roth P, Stanley ER (1992) The biology of CSF-1 and its receptor. Curr Top Microbiol Immunol 181:141–67.

154. Rothe J, Lesslauer W, Lotscher H, et al. (1993) Mice lacking the tumour necrosis factor receptor 1 are resistant to TNF-mediated toxicity but highly susceptible to infection by Listeria monocytogenes. Nature 364: 798–802.

155. Röther U, Komitowski D, Schubert FR, Wagner EF (1989) c-fos expression induces bone tumors in transgenic mice. Oncogene 4:861–5.

156. Rubin J, Fan X, Thornton D, Bryant R, Biskobing D (1996) Regulation of murine osteoblast macrophage colony-stimulating factor production by 1,25(OH)2D3. Calcif Tissue Int 59:291–6.

157. Saftig P, Hunziker E, Wehmeyer O, et al. (1998) Impaired osteoclastic bone resorption leads to osteopetrosis in cathepsin-K-deficient mice. Proc Natl Acad Sci USA 95:13453–8.

158. Sanjay A, Houghton A, Neff L, et al. (2001) Cbl Associates with Pyk2 and Src to regulate Src kinase activity, $\alpha_v\beta_3$ integrin-mediated signaling, cell adhesion, and osteoclast motility. J Cell Biol 152:181–96.

159. Sarma U, Flanagan AM (1996) Macrophage colony-stimulating factor induces substantial osteoclast generation and bone resorption in human bone marrow cultures. Blood 88:2531–40.

160. Schwartzberg PL, Xing L, Hoffman O, et al. (1997) Rescue of osteoclast function by transgenic expression of kinase-deficient Src in src–/– mutant mice. Genes & Development 11:2835–44.

161. Screpanti I, Romani L, Musiani P, et al. (1995) Lymphoproliferative disorder and imbalance T-helper response in C-EBP beta-deficient mice. EMBO 14: 1932–41.

162. Shi GP, Chapman HA, Bhairi SM, DeLeeuw C, Reddy VY, Weiss SJ (1995) Molecular cloning of human cathepsin O, a novel endoproteinase and homologue of rabbit OC2. FEBS Lett 357:129–34.

163. Shultz LD, Schweitzer PA, Rajan TV, et al. (1993) Mutations at the murine motheaten locus are within the hematopoietic cell protein-tyrosine phosphates (Hcph) gene. Cell 73:1445–54.

164. Simonet WS, Lacey DL, Dunstan CR, et al. (1997) Osteoprotegerin: a novel secreted protein involved in the regulation of bone density. Cell 89:309–19.

165. Sims JE, Gayle MA, Slack JL, et al. (1993) Interleukin 1 signaling occurs exclusively via the type I receptor. Proc Natl Acad Sci USA 90:6155–9.

166. Soriano P, Montgomery C, Geske R, Bradley A (1991) Targeted disruption of the c-srd proto-oncogene leads to osteopetrosis in mice. Cell 64:693–702.

167. Steingrimsson E, Moore KJ, Lamoreux ML, et al. (1994) Molecular basis of mouse microphthalmia mi mutations helps explain their developmental and phenotypic consequences. Nat Genet. 8:256–63.

168. Suzawa T, Miyaura C, Inada M, et al. (2000) The role of prostaglandin E receptor subtypes (EP1, EP2, EP3, and EP4) in bone resorption: an analysis using specific agonists for the respective EPs. Endocrinology 141:1554–9.

169. Tagaya H, Kunisada T, Yamazaki H, et al. (2000) Intramedullary and extramedullary B lymphopoiesis in osteopetrotic mice. Blood 95:3363–70.

170. Takayanagi H, Kim S, Koga T, et al. (2002) Induction and Activation of the Transcription Factor NFATc1 (NFAT2) Integrate RANKL Signaling in Terminal Differentiation of Osteoclasts. Dev Cell 3:889–901.

171. Tamura T, Udagawa N, Takahashi N, et al. (1993) Soluble interleukin-6 receptor triggers osteoclast formation by interleukin 6. Proc Natl Acad Sci USA 90:11924–8.

172. Tanaka S, Amling M, Neff L, et al. (1996) c-Cbl is downstream of c-Src in a signaling pathway necessary for bone resorption. Nature 383:528–31.

173. Tezuka K, Tezuka Y, Maijima A, et al. (1994) Molecular cloning of a possible cytokine proteins predominantly expressed in osteoclasts. J Biol Chem 269:1106–9.

174. Thesingh CW, Scherft JP (1985) Fusion disability of embryonic osteoclast precursor cells and macrophages in the microphthalmic osteopetrotic mouse. Bone 6: 43–52.

175. Tiffee JC, Xing L, Nilsson S, Boyce BF (1999) Dental abnormalities associated with failure of tooth eruption in src knockout and op/op mice. Calcif Tissue Int 65:53–8.

176. Tondravi MM, McKercher, Anderson K, et al. (1997) Osteopetrosis in mice lacking haematopoietic transcription factor PU.1. Nature 386:81–4.

177. Udagawa N, Takahashi N, Akatsu, T, et al. (1989) The bone marrow-derived stromal cell lines MC3T3-G2/PA6 and ST2 support osteoclast-like cell differentiation in cocultures with mouse spleen cells. Endocrinology 125:1805–13.

178. Umeda S, Beamer WG, Takagi K, et al. (1999) Deficiency of SHP-1 protein-tyrosine phosphatase activity results in heightened osteoclast function and decreased bone density. Am J Pathol 155:223–33.

179. Urbanek P, Wang Z, Fetka I, et al. (1994) Complete block of early B cell differentiation and altered patterning of the posterior midbrain in mice lacking Pax5/BSAP. Cell 79:901–12.

180. Van Beek E, Van der Wee-Pals L, et al. (1993) Leukemia inhibitory factor inhibits osteoclastic resorption, growth, mineralization, and alkaline phosphatase activity in fetal mouse metacarpal bones in culture. J Bone Miner Res 8:191–8.

181. van der Flier A, Sonnenberg A (2001) Function and interactions of integrins. Cell Tissue Res 305:285–98.

182. Vargas SJ, Naprta A, Glaccum M, Lee SK, Kalinowski J, Lorenzo JA (1996) Interleukin-6 expression and histomorphometry of bones from mice deficient for receptors for interleukin-1 or tumor necrosis factor. J Bone Miner Res 11:1736–44.

183. Velasco G, Ferrando AA, Puente XS, Sanchez LM, Lopez-Otin CJ (1994) Human cathepsin O. Molecular cloning from a breast carcinoma, production of the active enzyme in Escherichia coli, and expression analysis in human tissues. J Biol Chem 269:27136–42.

184. Vidal ON, Sjögren K, Eriksson BI, Ljunggren Ö, Ohlsson C (1998) Osteoprotegerin mRNA is increased by interleukin-1α in the human osteosarcoma cell line MG-63 and in human osteoblast-like cells. Biochem Biophys Res Commun 248:696–700.

185. Walker DG (1975) Bone resorption restored in osteopetrotic mice by transplants of normal bone marrow and spleen cells. Science 190:784–5.

186. Wang Z-Q, Grigoriadis AE, Möhle-Steinlein U, Wagner EF (1991) A novel target cell for c-fos-induced oncogenesis: development of chondrogenic tumours in embryonic stem cell chimeras. EMBO 10:2437–50.

187. Wang Z-Q, Grigoriadis AE, Wagner EF (1993) Stable murine chondrogenic cell lines derived from c-fos-induced cartilage tumors. J Bone Miner Res 8:839–47.

188. Wang Z-Q, Ovitt C, Grigoriadis AE, et al. (1992) Bone and haematopoietic defects in mice lacking c-fos. Nature 360:741–5.
189. Wani MR, Fuller K, Kim NS, Choi YW, Chambers T (1999) Prostaglandin E₂ cooperates with TRANCE in osteoclast induction from hemopoietic precursors: Synergistic activation of differentiation, cell spreading, and fusion. Endocrinology 140:1927–35.
190. Ware CB, Horowitz MC, Renshaw BR, et al. (1995) Targeted disruption of the low-affinity leukemia inhibitory factor receptor gene causes placental, skeletal, neural and metabolic defects and results in perinatal death. Development 121:1283–99.
191. Weir EC, Horowitz MC, Baron R, Centrella M, Kacinski BM, Insogna KL (1993) Macrophage colony-stimulating factor release and receptor expression in bone cells. J Bone Miner Res 8:1507–18.
192. Wesche H, Korherr C, Kracht M, Falk W, Resch K, Martin MU (1997) The interleukin-1 receptor accessory protein (IL-1RAcP) is essential for IL-1-induced activation of interleukin-1 receptor-associated kinase (IRAK) and stress-activated protein kinases (SAP kinases). J Biol Chem 272:7727–31.
193. Wiktor Jedrzejczak W, Bartocci A, Ferrante AJr, et al. (1990) Total absence of colony-stimulating factor 1 in the macrophage-deficient osteopetrotic (op/op) mouse. Proc Natl Acad Sci USA 87:4828–32.
194. Wong BR, Rho J, Arron J, et al. (1997) TRANCE is a novel ligand of the tumor necrosis factor receptor family that activates c-jun N-terminal kinase in T cells. J Biol Chem 272:25190–4.
195. Wong BR, Josien R, Lee SY, Vologodskaia M, Steinman RM, Choi Y (1998) The TRAF family of signal transducers mediates NF-kappaB activation by the TRANCE receptor. J Biol Chem 273:28355–9.
196. Xie H, Ye M, Feng R, Graf T (2004) Stepwise reprogramming of B cells into macrophages. Cell 117:663–76.
197. Xing L, Bushnell TP, Carlson L, et al. (2002) NF-kappaB p50 and p52 expression is not required for RANK-expressing osteoclast progenitor formation but is essential for RANK- and Cytokine-Mediated Osteoclastogenesis. J Bone Miner Res 17:1200–10.
198. Yao GQ, Sun BH, Hammond EE, et al. (1998) The cell-surface form of colony-stimulating factor-1 is regulated by osteotropic agents and supports formation of multinucleated osteoclast-like cells. J Biol Chem 273: 4119–28.
199. Yamamoto T, Ozono K, Kasayama S, et al. (1996) Increased IL-6-production by cells isolated from the fibrous bone dysplasia tissues in patients with McCune-Albright syndrome. J Clin Invest 98: 30–5.
200. Yasuda H, Shima N, Nakagawa N, et al. (1998) Osteoclast differentiation factor is a ligand for osteoprotegerin/osteoclastogenesis-inhibitory factor and is identical to TRANCE/RANKL. Proc Natl Acad Sci USA 95:3597–602.
201. Yoshida H, Hayashi S, Kunisada T, et al. (1990) The murine mutation osteopetrosis is in the coding region of the macrophage colony stimulating factor gene. Nature 345:442–4.
202. Yoshida K, Oida H, Kobayashi T, et al. (2002) Stimulation of bone formation and prevention of bone loss by prostaglandin E EP4 receptor activation. Proc Natl Acad Sci USA 99:4580–5.

7.
Clinical Disorders Associated with Alterations in Bone Resorption

Janet Rubin and Mark S. Nanes

This chapter is dedicated to Dr. Gideon Rodan, whose sustained and significant contributions to the field of clinical bone disease are much admired by the authors.

Introduction

The osteoclast's specialized function is irreplaceable by other cells. It is the only cell that resorbs bone, dentine, and mineralized cartilage; therefore defects in osteoclast function lead to a wide array of disorders. In this chapter we will discuss diseases of unchecked osteoclast activity, which lead to excessive bone resorption and thus result in bone fragility. We will also discuss diseases that result from too little osteoclast activity, which cause bone mineral content to increase and lead to disordered bone structure (Figure 7.1). The altered material properties associated with either decreased bone density (osteoporosis) or increased bone density (osteopetrosis or osteosclerosis) can lead to skeletal failure and fracture. Some of these disorders result from causes extraneous to the osteoclast itself, such as hormonal changes, and some reflect inherited defects in osteoclast formation or function. Many genetic disorders resulting in osteoclast dysfunction have been duplicated in transgenic mice where alterations to a specific gene have led to abnormalities in bone remodeling (see Horowitz, Chapter 6).

We shall first consider diseases where the osteoclast is too active, resulting in decreased bone mineral density and increased fragility. These include epigenetic diseases, such as postmenopausal osteoporosis or hyperparathyroidism, and diseases with a genetic basis or predisposition such as Paget's disease. Table 7.1 lists genetic disorders of osteoclast overfunction.

In the second part of the chapter we will consider the largely genetic diseases where osteoclast function is decreased (Table 7.2). These vary in their phenotypic spectrum from positive effects on bone as in the fracture-resistant LRP5 families, to lethal effects that result from the absence of the marrow compartment necessary for hematopoiesis.

Further and continually updated clinical and genetic information regarding those inherited disorders covered in this chapter are referred to in "Online Mendelian Inheritance in Man" (OMIM) and are shown as numbers in the text and tables. The OMIM website can be accessed at: www.ncbi.nlm.nih.gov.

Increased Osteoclast Activity Resulting in Decreased Bone Mass or Disordered Skeletal Architecture

The clinical term *osteoporosis* refers to conditions in which a decrease in bone mineral density leads to decreased skeletal strength and

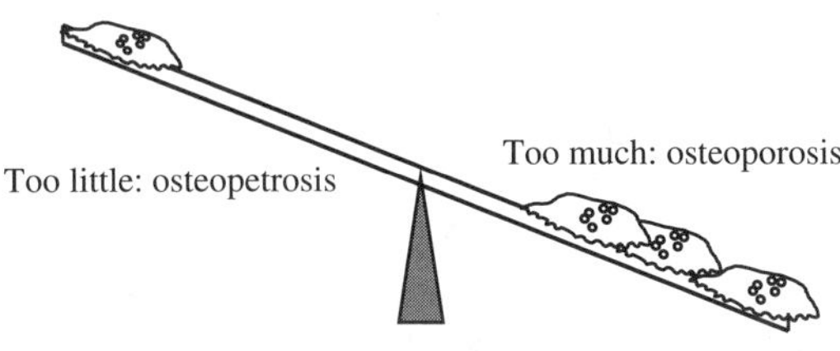

Figure 7.1 Bone remodeling.

increased risk of skeletal failure. The etiology of osteoporosis includes a large number of factors that result in either (a) an increase in osteoclast activity that leads to increased bone resorption, (b) decreased bone formation resulting from insufficient osteoblast activity, or (c) alterations in the tight coupling between the activities of osteoclast and osteoblast that normally permits the continual remodeling necessary to allow skeletons to respond to functional demands. Alterations in coupling can lead not only to reduced bone mineral density, but also to altered skeletal structure, as occurs in Paget's disease. Even though it is not possible operationally to separate the effects of osteoclast and osteoblast dysfunction when analyzing the

Table 7.1. Overactive Osteoclast Phenotype: Inherited

Disease	Gene	Protein affected	Osteoclast phenotype	OMIM#
Paget's disease	SQSTM1	p62 sequestosome	Increased numbers, hypernucleated	602080
Paget's disease, early onset	TNFRSF11A	RANK	As in PD	602080
Juvenile Paget's disease (hyperostosis corticalis deformans juvenalis)		Osteoprotegerin	Increased numbers, hyperactive	239000
Familial expansile osteolysis	TNFRSF11A	RANK	Hyperactive, enlarged	174810
Expansile skeletal hyperphosphatasia	TNFRSF11A	RANK	Increased numbers, enlarged	[118]
Polycystic lipomembranous osteodysplasia with sclerosing leukoencephalopathy (Nasu-Hakola disease)	DAP12 or TREM2	DAP12/TREM2	Impaired	221770
Rett syndrome	MECP2	Methyl-CpG-binding protein-2	Unknown	312750

Table 7.2. Underactive Osteoclast Phenotype Inherited

Disease	Gene	Protein affected	Osteoclast phenotype	OMIM#
Osteopetrosis, malignant	TC1RG1	Vacuolar proton pump	Number nl/↑	259700
Osteopetrosis, malignant	CLCN7	ClC-7 chloride channel	Number nl/↑	259700
Osteopetrosis, malignant	GL	Gray-lethal	Not known	259700
Osteopetrosis, autosomal dominant, type I	LRP5	Lipoprotein receptor protein 5	Reduced in number and size	607634
Osteopetrosis, autosomal dominant, type II (Albers-Schönberg disease)	CLCN7	ClC-7 chloride channel	Increase number and size	166600
Pycnodysostosis	CTSK	Cathepsin K	Normal	265800
Osteopetrosis w RTA	CA2	Carbonic anhydrase II	Normal	259730
Camurati–Engelmann	TGFB1	TGFβ1	Increased numbers *in vitro*	131300

ensuing bone phenotype (e.g., hyperparathyroidism), we have here selected to review those conditions in which the initial defect can be best ascribed directly to the osteoclast.

Endocrine Disorders

Sex Hormone Deficiency Leading to Increased Osteoclast Formation

Adult bone remodeling occurs continuously, permitting repair and allowing the skeleton to meet changing functional needs, whether in response to changes in load or to assure calcium homeostasis. Modeling begins on the quiescent bone surface at the time when osteoclasts are recruited locally. The osteoclastic resorption process forms a cutting cone in cortical bone, or a trench in cancellous bone. In the wake of this osteoclast activity, osteoblasts are recruited; they induce bone matrix synthesis followed by mineralization. This forms a "packet" of remodeled bone. The time for a packet to form from start to finish is nearly eight months; most of this time is spent forming new bone. The osteoclast's resorptive job is completed within the first two weeks. If the osteoblast response to osteoclastic bone destruction is not tightly coupled, i.e., if the activation frequency – initiation of osteoclast activity – is not followed by a sufficient osteoblastic response, bone resorption outpaces bone formation and bone mineral is lost [95]. This is, in fact, the situation that predominates in post-menopausal osteoporosis, and probably also occurs as a result of acute testosterone loss in men. When in post-menopausal osteoporosis resorption and formation is evaluated by biochemical markers, resorption is shown to increase by 90%, whereas formation markers increase by only 45% [32]. It is the resulting deterioration in bone microarchitecture and material properties that leads to an increased fracture risk (Figure 7.2: osteoporotic spine).

In the postmenopausal woman, bone loss is rapid within the first five years of estrogen deficiency. In the later menopause, the rate of bone loss approximates the slower, continuous decline associated with senile osteoporosis [53]. Acute estrogen deficiency increases the activation frequency so that more bone surface is covered by active osteoclasts. The many mechanisms by which estrogen deficiency increases osteoclastic activity are a topic of continued

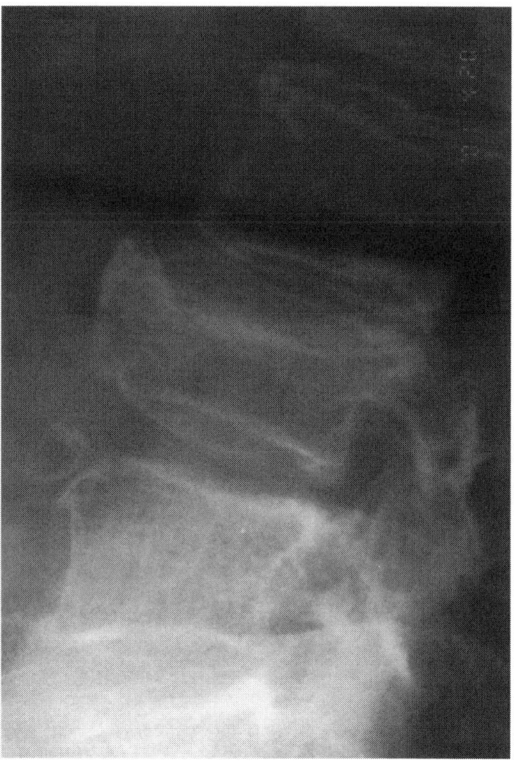

Figure 7.2 Post-menopausal osteoporosis resulting in osteopenia with vertebral compression fracture.

controversy [73, 85]. There are clear data that show estrogen promotes osteoclast apoptosis [48]. There are also data that show estrogen limits osteoclast formation *in vitro* by inhibiting osteoclast recruitment [39, 55]. Estrogen in addition regulates the expression of osteoactive factors such as osteoprotegerin or nitric oxide [91, 107]. Estrogen *in vivo* most probably modulates the RANKL:RANK:OPG axis. Estrogen deficiency is associated with increased RANKL expression by both stromal cells and circulating T cells [26]. Estrogen deficiency furthermore contributes to increased RANKL signaling by increasing cytokine production [18] (see also Chapter 5). Estrogen has effects within the target cell of RANKL: after RANKL activates RANK signaling (receptor activator of nuclear factor-$\kappa\beta$, or RANK, is the receptor for RANKL) in the osteoclast precursor, estrogen is able to mute the downstream signaling amplification, suggesting that estrogen deficiency will enhance response to RANKL [100, 106]. Estrogen appears to increase osteoprotegerin levels, thus providing an anti-resorptive factor [46]; interestingly, in the ovariectomized rat, osteoprotegerin levels have been shown to rise along with RANKL [49]; this may represent the skeleton's attempt to restrain rampant osteoclastogenesis.

Estrogen deficiency also seems to contribute to an impaired mechanical response of bone cells to signals generated during normal daily physical loading. This loss of a remodeling response to a load appears to be largely processed by osteocytes and osteoblasts [27]. For example, the estrogen receptor alpha knockout mouse is unable to mount an anabolic response to loading in terms of periosteal apposition or osteoblast proliferation [66]. There are also many reports that show that estrogen-deficient women, rats and pigs have reduced anabolic responses to exercise measured in the skeleton [5, 63, 123]. Androgen deficiency may also lead to alterations in the mechanostat response to loading [62]. In summary, estrogen modulates osteoclast activity indirectly through modulation of osteoclastogenic factors, and through regulation of the anabolic response to exercise.

Hyperparathyroidism

Hyperparathyroidism is a frequently diagnosed (1/25,000) endocrine disease, which presents in most patients as hypercalcemia. The hypercalcemia arises because of parathyroid hormone (PTH)-induced osteoclastic bone resorption (Figure 7.3) and changes in calcium absorption and excretion. Elevations in serum calcium that are less than 1.5 mg per deciliter above normal are not usually associated with skeletal disease [9]. Higher elevations of calcium, either due to a parathyroid secreting adenoma or parathyroid hyperplasia, generate a spectrum of disease from renal stones due to an increase in the filtered calcium in the renal collecting duct system, to gastrointestinal complaints, to neurological symptoms that can progress to stupor and coma. PTH synthesis and release is largely controlled by the parathyroid gland calcium receptor sensing decreased serum calcium levels [13]. When serum calcium rises, the calcium receptor generates intracellular calcium signals, which inhibit PTH release. Alternatively, when serum calcium drops, intracellular calcium also drops, causing the release of PTH. To increase extracellular calcium, released PTH raises calcium resorption in the kidney,

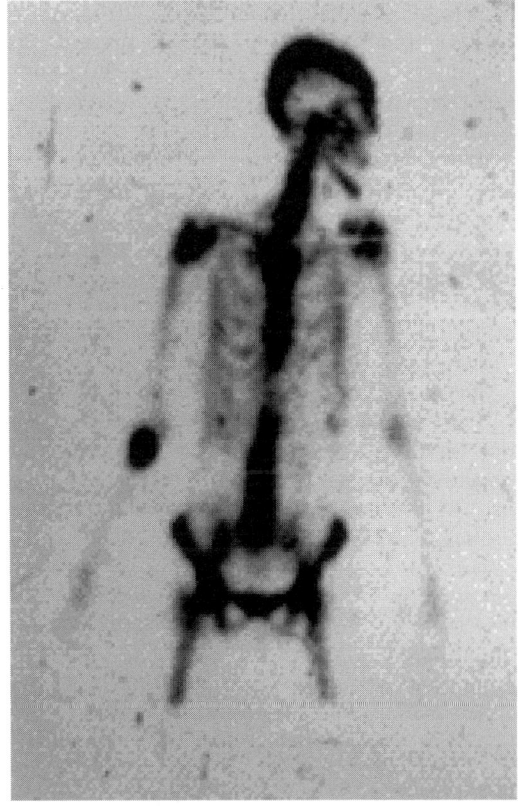

Figure 7.3 Hyperparathyroidism: Scintigraphy with technetium 99m shows increased bone activity throughout the skeleton of a hyperparathyroid patient.

increases 1,25-$(OH)_2D_3$ synthesis, which in turn increases intestinal calcium absorption, and finally affects release of calcium from skeletal stores. The target of PTH in bone is the stromal/osteoblast cell, which responds by increasing expression of RANKL [68], with an increase in the osteoclast recruitment from the hematopoietic pool.

The skeletal lesion of hyperparathyroidism is distinguished by osteitis fibrosa cystica. This condition is seen today most commonly in the hyperparathyroidism accompanying renal failure. Histopathological examination shows intense osteoclastic resorption resulting in bone destruction that leaves a picture of peritrabecular fibrosis within an enlarged marrow space.

The etiology of primary hyperparathyroidism is unknown. In two familial syndromes parathyroid hyperplasia is associated with other endocrine abnormalities. One is the syndrome of multiple endocrine neoplasia I (MEN1) (OMIM 131100), which presents as parathyroid, enteropancreatic neuroendocrine, anterior pituitary, or foregut carcinoid tumors. MEN1 is caused by a mutation in the menin gene [20] and germline MEN1 mutations have been identified in many MEN families [75]. Most germline and somatic mutations in MEN1 mutations lead to inactivating mutations of menin, suggesting that MEN1 may be a tumor suppressor gene such that stepwise inactivation of both menin alleles will lead to cell cycle entry. Indeed, menin interacts with the junD transcription factor during cell division [75]. MEN2 (OMIM 171400) also is associated with hyperparathyroidism, and stems from a mutation in the ret proto-oncogene, a tyrosine kinase [31]. The ret proto-oncogene mutation, besides inducing parathyroid hyperplasia, also causes pheochromocytoma and medullary cancer of the thyroid. The skeletal lesions and hypercalcemia in both MEN syndromes are indistinguishable from those of primary hyperparathyroidism.

Hyperthyroidism

Hyperthyroidism triggers increased bone remodeling, producing a skeletal syndrome in which the osteoclastic lesion predominates [40]. Practicing endocrinologists know that hyperthyroidism can cause hypercalcemia in as many as 20% of cases; indeed, von Recklinghausen recognized hyperthyroidism as a risk fracture for osteoporosis a century ago [50]. Bone mineral density is significantly decreased in patients with untreated hyperthyroidism and returns to normal upon treatment [111]. Thyroid hormone has direct effects on bone cells, and indeed thyroid hormone can induce the expression of RANKL in bone cells [78]. However, thyroid-stimulating hormone (TSH) may play the primary role in osteoclast recruitment here. Osteoclasts and their precursors have been found to express the TSH receptor. A 50% reduction in expression produced a profound osteoporosis in heterozygote TSH-receptor knockout mice [1]. Indeed, TSH itself inhibited osteoclast formation *in vitro*. TSH also appears to promote osteoblast differentiation, presumably directed via TSH receptors also demonstrated on these cells. Thus, in the hyperthyroid state, where TSH is severely suppressed, failure to stimulate the pre-osteoclast TSH-receptor may enhance osteoclast formation. The physiology of TSH control of bone cell function will be of great interest to endocrinologists in the coming years.

Glucocorticoid Excess

In 1932 Harvey Cushing described a connection between osteoporosis and the overproduction of cortisol by the adrenal glands [24]. Corticosteroid therapy for inflammatory diseases such as asthma has similar effects, leading to increased incidence of vertebral fracture. Iatrogenic Cushing's syndrome is now thought to be the most common cause of secondary osteoporosis. Bone loss is initiated by osteoclastic remodeling, but is compounded by a deficiency of remodeling. The mechanisms by which corticosteroids affect bone remodeling are pleiotropic, and cortisol has both direct and indirect effects on bone cells.

Hypercortisolism has systemic effects on other hormonal axes that indirectly modulate bone turnover. Sex hormones, in particular estradiol and testosterone, are decreased in patients on high doses of steroids [79]. Pharmacological use of glucocorticosteroids also is associated with inhibition of intestinal calcium absorption [2]. Decreased intestinal calcium flux stimulates the parathyroid glands to release PTH, but the role of secondary hyperparathyroidism in glucocorticoid-induced osteoporosis appears to be minor.

Direct effects of glucocorticoids on bone resorption and formation have been measured in multiple studies [17]. Glucocorticoids stimulate osteoclast activity and recruitment *in vitro*: in addition to increasing osteoclast activity [41], glucocorticoids stimulate expression of RANKL by bone stromal cells [124]. Impairment in bone formation is, however, the predominant result of glucocorticoid excess. Osteoblast and osteoclast recruitment are affected, resulting in dysfunctional remodeling and downgrading the maintenance of bone strength [116]. Mice treated with corticosteroids have decreased bone density, decreased serum osteocalcin, decreased cancellous bone area, and trabecular narrowing [117]. These skeletal changes result in diminished bone formation and turnover, along with impaired osteoblastogenesis and osteoclastogenesis. The reduction in osteoblast number and function appears to be due to increased osteoblast apoptosis.

Recently O'Brien et al. showed that glucocorticoid action must be present specifically and locally in the skeleton [83]. Mice transgenic for an osteoblast-specific 11-beta-hydroxysteroid dehydrogenase that locally inactivates the actions of glucocorticosteroids were resistant to osteoblast apoptosis caused by pharmacologic doses of steroids. Interestingly, the bone loss was similar to that in non-transgenic animals, i.e., osteoclast recruitment due to steroids exogenous to the skeleton was unchecked, but bone formation rates were significantly higher. These results show that glucocorticoids have differential effects on osteoclast and osteoblast type cells, both of which contribute to the osteoporotic phenotype consistent with hypercortisolism.

Environmental/Genetic

Paget's Disease (OMIM 602080)

Paget's disease is a primary disease of osteoclasts, with a still controversial etiology best ascribed to subtle interactions of genetic and environmental factors. Clinically Paget's disease manifests as a uni- or multifocal skeletal disease that begins with an intense local bone resorption followed by formation of woven bone. Pagetic osteoclasts are increased in number, are hypernucleated and large (Figure 7.4), and, in contradistinction to osteoclasts in unaffected bone in the same patient, are found to contain paramyxoviral-like inclusions. The clinical syndrome can be silent – simply a radiologist notation of bone sclerosis on a pelvic x-ray – or can be severe with pathologic fractures, bowing of

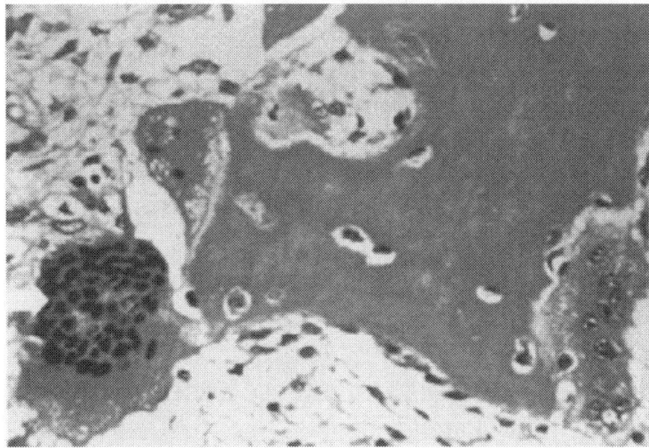

Figure 7.4 Pagetic lesion: The micrograph shows a hypernucleated pagetic osteoclast at the lower left of the field.

long bones, and hearing loss from compression of cranial nerves. Ludwig van Beethoven is thought to have suffered from Paget's disease that led to his unfortunate deafness. Most typical Paget's patients, however, complain of pain from degenerative joint disease, which is exacerbated by mechanical factors due to abnormal loading and weight bearing in the affected bones. In the last century, the incidence of Paget's in the US population has been about 2–3%. There appears to be a decreasing incidence, which correlates with a decreasing prevalence of measles infection in this country over the last half of last century, thought to be the etiologic agent, leaving the paramyxoviral signature in the pagetic osteoclasts [30].

There is a genetic predisposition for Paget's disease. Forty percent of index cases have a first-degree affected relative [65]. Two genetic phenotypes have been documented. The first shows linkage to the RANK protein (TNFSF11A) on chromosome 18. Patients with an 18-bp insertion in the RANK sequence present with early Paget's disease as teenagers, and this may represent a variation of familial expansile osteolysis [65] (see below). This RANK mutation appears to lead to hyperresponsiveness to RANKL, with increased size and nucleation of osteoclasts [93]. The other genetic phenotype is a mutation in the sequestosome 1 gene (SQSTM1). The sequestosome (p62) is an ubiquitin-binding protein that scaffolds signaling molecules in the TNF inflammatory cascade. It is unclear whether Pagetic mutations change availability of ubiquitin for intracellular proteins, perhaps enhancing the inflammatory signal cascade, or affect viral handling within the cell [45].

Gorham-Stout Disease

Gorham-Stout disorder (GSD), or disappearing bone disease, is a monocentric osteolysis, first described in 1955 [37]. (This non-Mendelian disease should be differentiated from another disease, cystic angiomatosis of bone, which also is called Gorham Stout. That syndrome is inherited as an autosomal dominant trait, and is associated with osteosclerosis [94].) The massive osteolysis of GSD is recognized as an aggressive local resorption of bone [25]. There is an angiomatous proliferation of thin-walled vessels in the region of lytic bone, as well as an intracortical fibrosis [67]. The increased osteoclastogenesis is thought to be stimulated by release of local factors. The extreme rarity of GSD has prevented much investigation of its etiology.

Myeloma

The majority of patients with multiple myeloma, a B-cell neoplasm, eventually experience extensive bony destruction that results in hypercalcemia. Myeloma bone disease can present either as osteoporosis, or as discrete bony lesions that lead to pathologic fracture through loss of skeletal integrity (Figure 7.5). Bisphosphonate therapy to repress bone resorption has lately become a cornerstone of myeloma chemotherapy. The lesion of myeloma bone shows increased numbers of active osteoclasts. It has long been known that myeloma cells release factors that induce osteoclast formation and activity, but identification of a specific contributory factor has defied a great deal of effort. Several publications have shown that myeloma stimulates a coordinated increase in bone stromal cell expression of RANKL with a concomitant reduction in osteoprotegerin, leading to osteoclastogenesis [88]. Recombinant osteoprotegerin protein can prevent the bone destruction caused by injection of human melanoma cells into mice [22], indicating at least a secondary role for the RANKL/RANK/OPG axis in the rampant bone lesions of myeloma.

In human disease, elevated serum levels of RANKL along with decreased osteoprotegerin levels have been noted, suggesting that myeloma cells may even secrete this protein [35, 98]. There may be a role, as well, for the DKK1 protein, which is secreted by myeloma cells and prevents Wnt signaling in osteoblasts the Wnt pathway in osteoblasts. Elevated DKK1 levels in bone marrow plasma and in peripheral blood from myeloma patients are associated with focal bone lesions, but this has yet to be linked to osteoclast recruitment or activation [108].

Inherited Disorders of Osteoclasts

Juvenile Paget's Disease (OMIM 239000)

The skeletal lesions of juvenile Paget's disease, or hyperostosis corticalis deformans juvenilis, as described by Bakwin et al. [4], resemble adult Paget's disease with increased skull size, deafness, and expanded and bowed long bones. This rare autosomal recessive disease presents in early childhood with musculoskeletal pain. Affected bones have coarse trabeculations and areas of sclerosis interspersed with osteoporosis. This results in decreased mechanical strength with deformity and increased susceptibility to fracture [16]. Examination of osteoclasts from these patients does not reveal paramyxoviral-like inclusions, and circulating monocytes are clear of viral transcripts [119].

The continuous and intense bone remodeling in juvenile Paget's disease, confirmed by elevated markers of bone turnover, suggests abnormal activation of osteoclasts. Whyte et al.

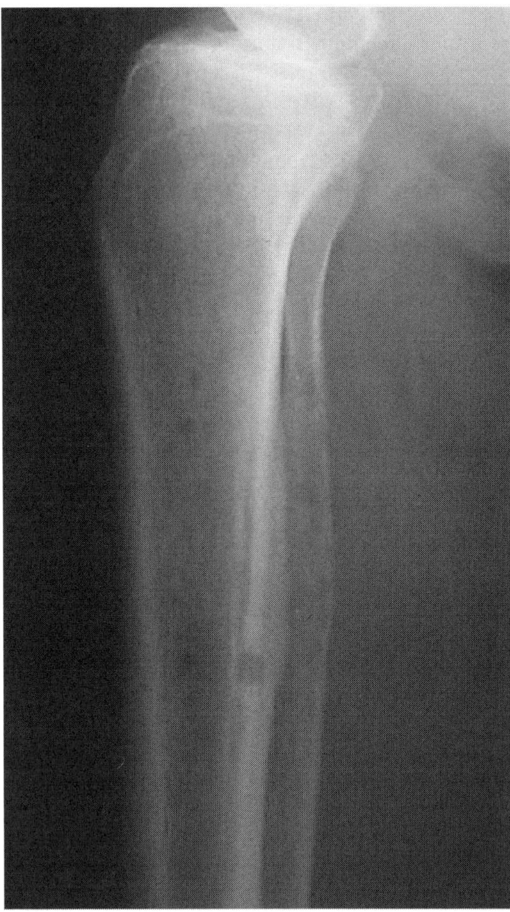

Figure 7.5 Myeloma lytic bone lesions: Myeloma bone disease can present as either diffuse osteoporosis, or as scattered lytic lesions, as shown in the radiograph.

recently linked the disease to a mutation in osteoprotegerin [118]. Using a candidate-gene approach, they considered genes involved in osteoclast activation. They first found the gene locus for RANK to be normal. Because the osteoprotegerin-knockout mouse has accelerated bone remodeling [14], the group focused their search on osteoprotegerin. Both unrelated Navajo patients were found to have a null mutation in osteoprotegerin with an identical breakpoint in chromosome 8; their osteoprotegerin levels were not measurable (Figure 7.6).

A second osteoprotegerin mutation was described in an Iraqi family where three siblings were affected with Juvenile Paget's Disease [23]. The in-frame deletion of three base pairs, com-pared to the 100 kb deletion in the Navajo family [118], resulted in the loss of an aspartate residue, but their osteoprotegerin levels were measurable. The mutant osteoprotegerin, however, was ineffective in suppressing bone resorption.

The mouse osteoprotegerin knockout model replicates the human disease [14]. The skeletal lesion is present early, with a decrease in total bone density and fracture. Interestingly the transgenic mice also exhibit "medial" calcification of the medium and large arteries. This raises the possibility that pathologic calcification of the vasculature involves interplay between cells capable of both generating and resorbing mineral in this unusual location.

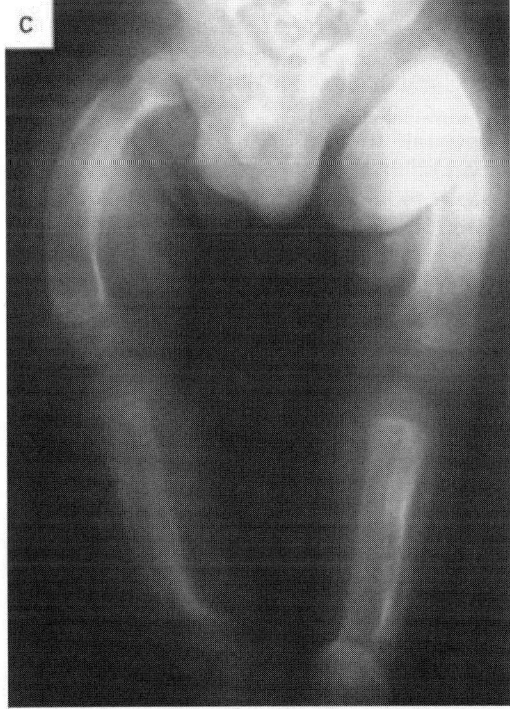
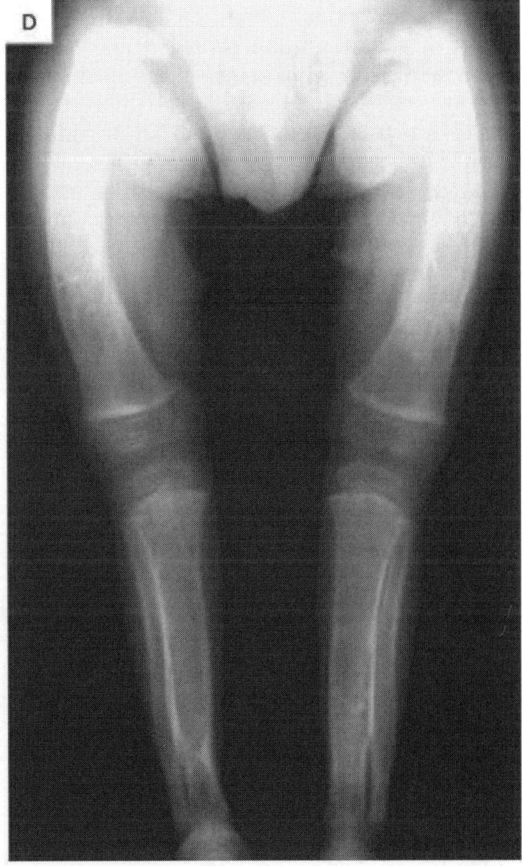

Figure 7.6   Juvenile Paget's disease: Radiographs of a 1-year-old patient from Whyte et al. [121] are shown: the left is the proband's right proximal femur with markedly widened, poorly modeled, and osteopenic bone, with cortical thinning and a coarse trabecular pattern. The radiograph on the right was obtained 27 months after the initiation of calcitonin therapy, demonstrating improvement of bone structure. Copyright 2002 Massachusetts Medical Society. All rights reserved.

Familial Expansile Osteolysis (FEO) (OMIM 174810)

Also known as polyostotic osteolytic dysplasia, familial expansile osteolysis first was described in 1988 in a family from Northern Ireland [84]. This rare autosomal dominant dysplasia shares a focal nature with Paget's disease but appears in the teenage decade. In the focal lesions, osteoclast activity is associated with medullary expansion and painful deformity. The focal lesions, which frequently lead to fracture, are predominantly peripheral. Deafness due to skull dysplasia can be present before puberty.

Linkage studies have shown that the responsible gene in the Irish FEO family was located on chromosome 18 and was due to a mutation in the signal peptide region of the receptor activator of nuclear factor-B (RANK) [47]. Expressing the recombinant mutant RANK in culture showed the mutant protein was resistant to cleavage of the signal peptide; the immature protein causes perturbations in RANK level and results in a total increase in RANK signaling. Thus, FEO is caused by an activating mutation of RANK, leading to hyperactivation of osteoclasts. Why the disease is focal and peripheral remains unclear.

Another expansile disease that was only described in 2000, and is phenotypically distinct from FEO, is expansile skeletal hyperphosphatasia (ESH) [120]. The cases were a mother and daughter who presented with expanding hyperostotic long bones, pain, and early onset deafness. The skeletal lesions, which appear in the appendicular skeleton, are reminiscent in their distribution of Paget's disease, rather than of FEO. Measles virus gene transcripts are not present in cells of monocytic lineage. Whyte et al. identified a mutation in these patients that was identical to the 18-base pair tandem duplication in the RANK signal peptide sequence described in the FEO families [118]. The phenotypic variation between ESH and FEO suggests other genetic or epigenetic factors have a role in remodeling dysplasias.

Polycystic lipomembranous osteodysplasia with sclerosing leukoencephalopathy (PLOSL) (OMIM 221770)

Polycystic lipomembranous osteodysplasia with sclerosing leukoencephalopathy was recognized almost simultaneously in Finland [43] and in Japan [81], but now has been reported globally. This condition, also called Nasu-Hakola disease, presents in midlife with pain after muscle strain has led to the diagnosis of cysts in the epiphyses of long bones. The bone cysts are composed of dysmorphic fatty and collagenous connective tissue. Osteoporotic features are prevalent. Patients in the fourth decade experience neurological symptoms, which, unfortunately, progress to presenile dementia. The genetic etiology is a loss-of-function mutation in the gene encoding the TYRO protein tyrosine kinase-binding protein called DAP12, or in some cases a mutation in the TREM2 adaptor [87, 89]. DAP12 is a transmembrane adaptor protein that associates with the cell surface receptor TREM to form the DAP12-TREM2 complex on natural killer T cells and myeloid cells. The ligand for TREM2 is unknown.

Paloneva et al. showed that peripheral blood mononuclear cells from PLOSL patients that are deficient in DAP12 and TREM2 respond poorly to osteoclastogenic stimuli. This results in a reduced ability to resorb bone *in vitro* [86]. Activation of the DAP12/TREM2 complex appears to be a required co-stimulatory signal during RANKL-induced osteoclast differentiation [58]. This recent work has suggested that the intracellular calcium signal generated by DAP12/TREM2 is necessary for adequate NFAT1 signalling (see Chapter 1); indeed, transgenic knockout of the functional DAP12/TREM2 co-stimulatory receptor resulted in mice with severe osteopetrosis. Interestingly, the evolving understanding in the role of the DAP12/TREM2 pathway in osteoclastogenesis came to light only through investigation of the skeletal lesion associated with this rare genetic disorder.

Rett Syndrome (OMIM 312750)

Rett syndrome is an X-linked dominant disorder recognized in the latter half of last century. Its major problem is an unrelenting progressive encephalopathy that causes severe dementia in girls [42]. Growth retardation is associated with a decreased metabolic rate [80]. There are metatarsal and metacarpal abnormalities in some patients with Rett syndrome [69], as well as a severe osteoporosis [15]. The cause of the osteoporosis is, as yet, unknown, and may be due to problems with osteoclasts, osteoblasts, or coupling. We include Rett syndrome in this chapter because the bone lesion, associated with troublesome fracturing, may cause unregulated osteoclast activity.

Genetic nonsense and missense mutations are found in the gene encoding methyl-CpG-binding protein-2 (Mecp2) [115]. All of the nucleotide substitutions in Rett syndrome involve C to T transitions at CpG hot spots. Transgenic mice expressing the truncated Mecp2 "Rett" protein showed a similar phenotypic neurologic disease, as well as a severe kyphosis, but the skeleton was not specifically examined [99]. The authors of this study suggest that histone H3 is hyperacetylated in this model, possibly leading to abnormal gene expression; however, the effect on bone resorption is not yet understood.

Decreased Osteoclast Activity Resulting in Osteopetrosis

Osteopetrosis is a heterogeneous group of conditions where an impairment in bone resorption leads to accrual of bone mass (Figure 7.7). Classic osteopetrosis is considered a disease of osteoclasts. Walker showed that transplanting the gray-lethal (malignant) osteopetrotic mouse with the bone marrow and spleen of normal littermates cured the osteopetrosis [114]. Indeed, current medical therapy uses marrow transplantation for the classic malignant osteopetrosis: implantation of hematopoietic stem cells containing normal osteoclast precursors

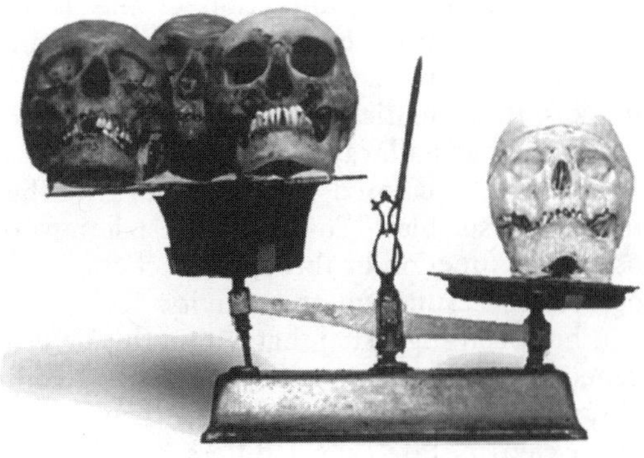

Figure 7.7   The weight of the osteopetrotic skull: A skull from a van Buchem patient is placed in the right pan of the scale. Figure is from [52], Janssens and Van Hul, Molecular genetics of too much bone. Hum Mol Genet 2002; 11:2385–2393, by permission of Oxford University Press.

rescues insufficient bone resorption [28]. In the last ten years, knowledge of spontaneous and engineered genetic mutations has greatly increased understanding of osteopetrotic etiologies, although the cause of many human osteopetroses has not, as yet, been charted.

The phenotype of osteopetrotic disease spans that of completely marbled bones, with a lethal defect of hematopoiesis due to the total absence of a marrow space, to diseases that can be considered advantageous, insofar as the increase in bone mineral promotes a fracture resistant skeleton. The most severe forms of osteopetrosis present early in life with skeletal sclerosis that obliterates the bone marrow compartment and impinges on cranial nerves. Extramedullary hematopoiesis with hepatosplenomegaly rarely rescues the marrow insufficiency; pancytopenia leads to infection, inanition and death. More mild forms of osteopetrosis, or osteosclerosis, can have cranial nerve pathology as well as increased fracture risk. It is likely that the mildest forms of osteoclast dysfunction evade identification because pathologic findings are necessary to initiate diagnosis. Sclerotic bone disease is occasionally noted in other systemic diseases, which may result from changes in osteoclast function. Because information regarding these silent "disorders" is lacking, we will cover only inherited forms of osteopetrosis that lead to clinical disease.

Inherited Diseases Resulting in Dysfunctional Osteoclasts

Osteopetrosis, Malignant (OMIM 259700)

The malignant osteopetroses are autosomal recessive diseases that present in early infancy with macrocephaly, progressive deafness and blindness, extramedullary hematopoiesis, and pancytopenia. It is likely that genetic mutations of many osteoclast functions will be identified in human disease, but so far, mutations in only three proteins that are necessary for osteoclast function have been indexed. These include the osteoclast vacuolar proton pump, the chloride channel-7, and the gray-lethal protein, all necessary for osteoclast function.

Interestingly, the first mutation identified as an etiology for the murine osteopetrotic phenotype op/op, is not associated with human osteopetrosis. The op/op mouse has a deletion in the gene for macrophage colony stimulating factor, or MCSF, which results in an essentially nonfunctioning protein [122]. In the absence of MCSF, hematopoietic stem cells cannot enter the macrophage lineage in the developing mouse, and monocytes, macrophages and osteoclasts are not formed. This leads to lack of tooth eruption and the inability to wean. The op/op mouse dies because of its inability to wean – if the newborn is nursed beyond 2 weeks, osteoclasts appear and the mouse lives. The "rescue" is thought to be due to the ability of secreted vascular endothelial growth factor (VEGF) to support macrophage/osteoclast differentiation and survival [82]. A human analogue of this disease may thus be silent since infants do not eat solid food for many months.

Mutations in the Osteoclast Vacuolar Proton Pump (see also Chapter 3)

The osteoclast proton pump is a vacuolar ATPase [109]. This large molecule has 28 subunits encoded by 13 separate genes that vary in tissue expression. The osteoclast specific subunit, TCIRG1, is a 116-kd subunit [71]. In one series, more than 50% of patients with infantile malignant osteopetrosis had mutations in TCIRG1 [29]. The mutations are extremely variable but uniformly lead to null expression of the proton pump in osteoclasts [60, 105]. Without secretion of acid, osteoclasts cannot resorb bone.

Mutations in the Osteoclast Chloride Channel-7

The process of proton secretion requires that the osteoclast also have a parallel conductance of a negative ion, i.e., a specific chloride channel. In osteoclasts the CLCN7 gene encodes this channel. Disruption of the channel leads to a severe osteopetrosis in mice because osteoclasts were cannot secrete acid and bone is not resorbed. The same defect has also been identified in a patient [59].

Mutation of the Gray-Lethal Gene

The spontaneous GL, or gray-lethal, mutation in mice causes a gray coat color and a severe autosomal recessive osteopetrosis. The osteopetrosis is fully penetrant and lethal, but can be rescued with bone marrow transplantation [113]. The murine gene was cloned and shown to be responsible for the osteopetrosis [19]. The GL protein function is required for osteoclast and melanocyte function, but the protein itself (OMIM 607649) requires further study. One human case has been identified as a GL mutation [19].

Osteopetrosis, Autosomal Dominant, Types I and II

The autosomal dominant osteopetroses are not lethal disorders, but more mild forms due to impaired osteoclastic bone resorption. The grouping is heterogeneous: the conditions in many families are associated with an asymptomatic osteosclerosis. The mild forms of osteopetrosis can cause bone pain and hearing loss, but affected individuals are less susceptible to fracture than persons afflicted with other forms of osteopetrosis. Most interestingly, some forms of osteopetrosis are linked to protection from fracture, as is seen in lesions associated with activating mutations of the LRP5 signal cascade.

As knowledge of murine and human bone resorption and structure increases, it is likely that more mutations will be assigned to this disease category in the future. For instance, high bone density traits have been described in several inbred mouse strains [6]. The high bone density in one of these models is linked to a region on mouse chromosome 11, and is due to a mutation in the 12/15-lipoxygenase enzyme [57]. Pharmacologic inhibition of the 12/15-lipoxygenase improved both bone density and strength in ovariectomized mice. It is not unlikely that mutations that affect the activity of the analogous pathway in humans will be associated with increased bone density – either through osteoblast controlled restriction of osteoclast function or through direct effects on osteoclast recruitment and activity.

It has been suggested that within this heterogeneous grouping there are two distinct radiographic types representing the generalized osteosclerosis [3]. Type I differs mainly from type II in that the increased bone appears to confer fracture protection. We have adhered to the designations of type currently suggested in the literature that also show some differences in serum phosphate (lower in type I) and serum acid phosphatase (markedly increased in type II) [10].

Osteopetrosis, Autosomal Dominant, Type I (OMIM 607634)

Type I osteopetrosis is characterized by pronounced sclerosis of the cranial vault with little increase in vertebral bone. Interestingly, type I confers protection from fracture risk. One form of this disease can be caused by mutations in the low density lipoprotein receptor-related protein 5 (LRP5) gene (OMIM 603506). The first citation was from a research group searching for high bone mass traits. They investigated a family with high bone density that had a heterozygous G-to-T transversion in exon 3 of the LRP5 gene. This mutation resulted in a gly_{171}-to-val change in a predicted beta-propeller module of the LRP5 protein that was observed in all affected individuals [72]. The same mutation was found in a second kindred with high bone density, wide mandibles, and torus palatinus (Figure 7.8) [12]. Interestingly this family, who did not have any symptoms, did note a difficulty in staying afloat while swimming!

The discovery of the mutation in LRP5 and its previously unrecognized relationship to bone remodeling set off a flurry of investigations. Members of the low-density lipoprotein receptor (LDLR) family are cell surface proteins that bind and internalize ligands in the process of receptor-mediated endocytosis. It would appear that the LRP5 pathway through Wnt signaling is functional in osteoblasts, directing osteoblast bone formation. It was quickly noted that another mutation in this protein was associated with an osteopetrotic disease, osteoporosis-pseudoglioma syndrome (OPPG, OMIM 259770). Mutations in LRP5 cause the autosomal recessive disorder, and indeed, heterozygous carriers of OPPG have reduced bone mass compared to age and gender-matched controls [36]. A secreted mutant form of LRP5 appears to reduce bone apposition [36]. Mice with a targeted disruption of LRP5 have low bone density, associated with decreased osteoblast proliferation [54]. It now is accepted that LRP5 is required for optimal Wnt signaling in osteoblasts. The question of how LRP5 affects osteoclasts is now open for discussion. The increased osteoblast activity associated with the LRP5 mutations is not accompanied by concomitant increases in osteoclast activity. Thus, even though the high bone density of this disease may stem from hyperactive osteoblasts, osteoclasts also are affected.

A Belgian family with previously documented type I osteopetrosis was recently shown to have a transversion in the same codon of the LRP5 gene that caused the high-bone-density traits described in the United States [110]. A Sardinian family assigned a diagnosis of van Buchem disease with osteosclerosis of the skull was investigated for mutations in LRP5. Indeed, a novel mutation was found that was also located in the amino-terminal region of the protein [110]. (The skull shown in Figure 7.7 belonged to a patient affected with van Buchem disease (OMIM 607636)). Van Wesenbeck, in reviewing six novel missense mutations in the LRP5 gene, suggested that conditions associated with increased bone density affecting mainly the cortices of long bones and skull are caused by mutations in this gene [110]. There is a phenotypic pleiomorphism, however, with some families having mandible changes and torus palatinus, while others have none. One of the areas that will need attention in the future is the classification of those diseases resulting in endosteal hyperosteosis: are they the result of impaired osteoclast activity, or simply of excessive bone formation?

Osteopetrosis, Autosomal Dominant Type II: Albers-Schönberg Disease (OMIM 166600)

Autosomal dominant osteopetrosis type II is characterized by sclerosis, predominantly involving the vertebrae, the iliac wings, and the base of the skull. In contrast to type I patients, type II patients do have increased fracture frequency [11]. Bone resorption is defective, while bone formation is normal; this is reflected in elevated serum levels of tartrate-resistant acid phosphatase (TRAP) [112]. Why TRAP, which represents osteoclast activity, rises, is unclear: perhaps it represents an attempt by the dysfunctional osteoclast in this disease to increase activity. The elevations in TRAP are helpful in making the diagnosis in families where osteopetrosis type II shows incomplete penetrance: gene carriers have TRAP values that are not different from those of controls [112].

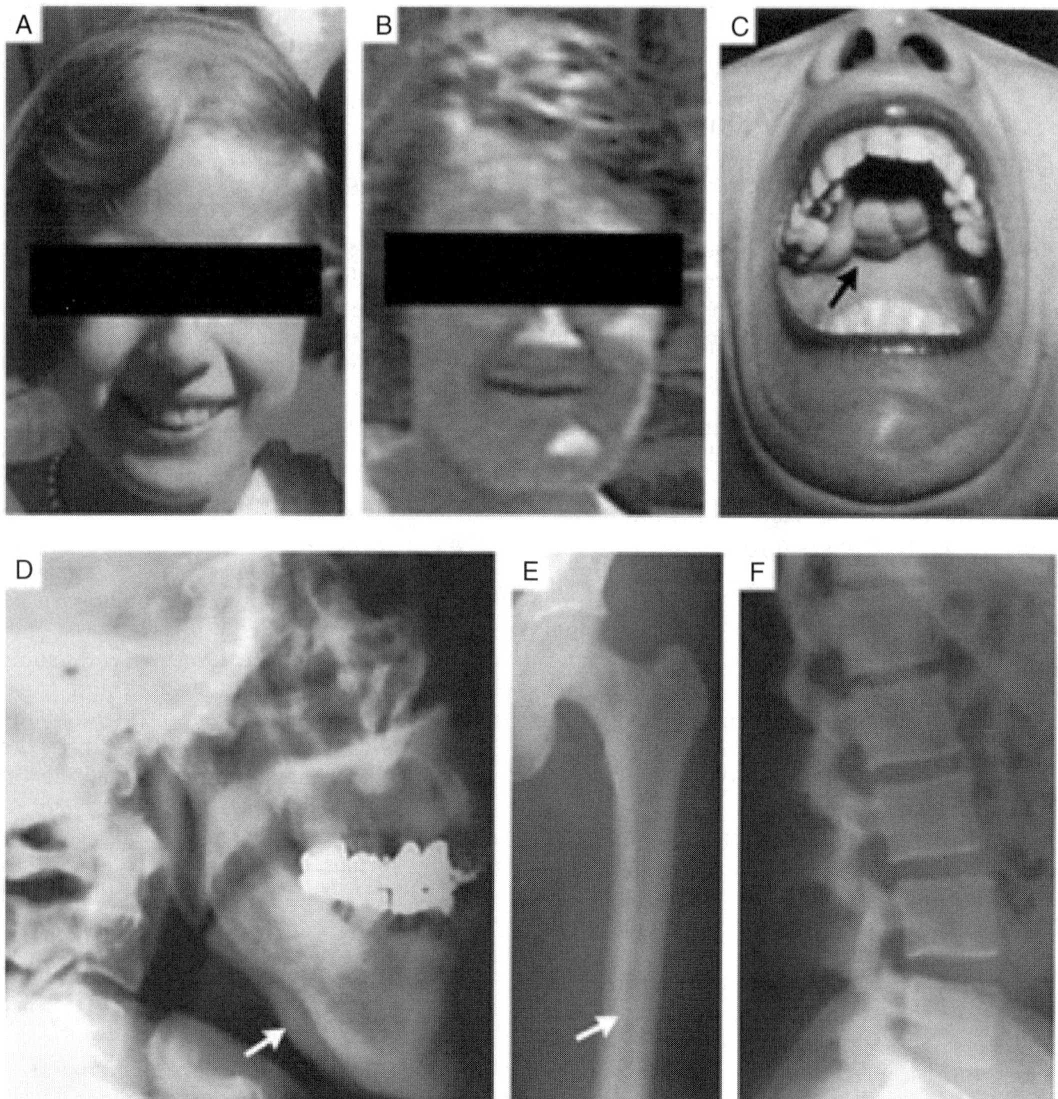

Figure 7.8 Osteosclerosis due to LRP5: "Photographs of an affected member at the ages of 12 years (A) and 45 years (B) show the development of the wide, deep mandible that was characteristic of all affected members of the kindred. A large, lobulated torus palatinus in an affected member (C, arrow) was also characteristic of all affected kindred members. Characteristic radiographic findings included an abnormally thick mandibular ramus (arrow, D); a markedly thickened cortex and narrowed medullary cavity (arrow) in the femur (E), which was otherwise normal; and dense but otherwise normal-appearing vertebrae (F)." Figure used with permission from Boyden et al. [12]. Copyright 2002 Massachusetts Medical Society. All rights reserved.

Benichou et al., studying 42 patients with radiological evidence of type II disease, including the classic sandwich vertebra appearance (or "rugger jersey" spine) found that nearly 80% of patients had fractures [8]. The fractures were slow to heal. Hip osteoarthritis was common, and severe with an increased incidence of osteomyelitis after hip replacement. Increased surgical complications also were experienced by those 50% of patients who required orthopaedic intervention.

The Benichou research team went on to perform a genome wide linkage analysis of an extended French family, localizing the disease to chromosome 16 [7]. The candidate region was then studied in 12 autosomal dominant type II families, and found to contain the CLCN7 gene with at least seven different mutations [21]. It thus appears that this not-so-benign autosomal dominant osteopetrosis is allelic with the CLCN7 mutation that causes the autosomal recessive malignant osteopetrosis. Although not yet proven, it is reasonable to infer that complete absence of chloride transport would cause malignant osteopetrosis, and that the defect in chloride transport in type II "benign" osteopetrosis must be incomplete.

Pycnodysostosis (OMIM 265800)

Pycnodysostosis is an autosomal recessive osteochondrodysplasia characterized by osteosclerosis and short stature, as well as deformity of the skull, maxilla and phalanges, osteosclerosis, and bone fragility. The condition was first described by Marotaux and Lamy who also suggested that Toulouse-Lautre (1864–1901) had the disease [74]. The features of pycnodysostosis are shown in Figure 7.9, from [44]. Gelb et al., on the basis of linkage analysis in a large inbred Arab family, concluded that the affected gene was located on chromosome 1q21 [33]. The gene cathepsin K, a cysteine protease that is predominantly expressed in osteoclasts, is located in this region. This discovery spurred a search for mutations in this gene. Nonsense,

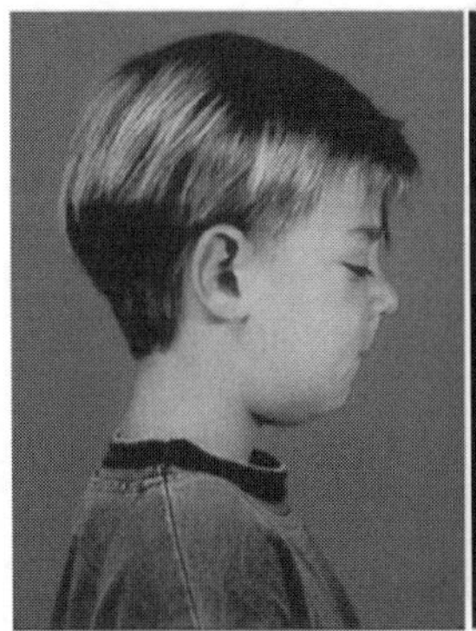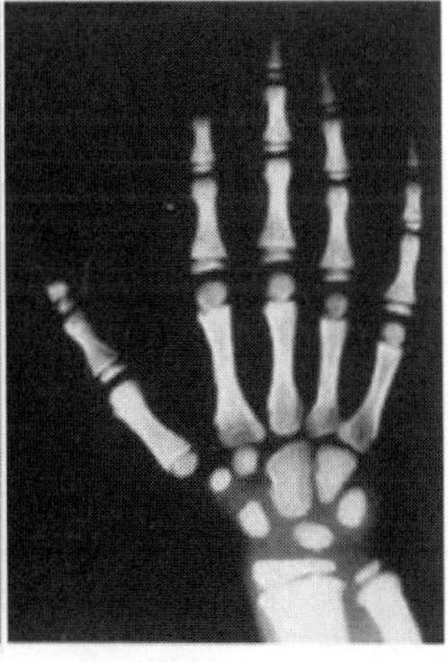

Figure 7.9 Pycnodysostosis: The profile shows a pycnodysostotic 9-year-old boy with a height age of 5 years. Note the prominent forehead and micrognathia. The x-ray shows the generally dense bone and partial loss of several distal phalanges. Figure reproduced from Ho et al. [44], J Bone Miner Res. 1999; 14: 1649–1653, with permission of the American Society for Bone and Mineral Research.

missense, and stop codon mutations in the gene encoding cathepsin K were subsequently found in patients with pycnodysostosis [34]. Indeed, in two siblings with the disease, cathepsin K protein was entirely absent, while the parents, who had no trace of disease, expressed half-normal levels of cathepsin K.

Cathepsin K was first described as cathepsin O [101] and is expressed at its highest levels in musculoskeletal tissues, with the strongest in situ signal in osteoclasts [92]. This protease has potent endoprotease activity against fibrinogen at acid pH, and therefore is effective in degrading extracellular bone matrix under the osteoclast resorption tent. Pycnodysostotic osteoclasts are normal in numbers and in morphology (normal ruffled borders and clear zones) and indeed resorb demineralized bone. The problem occurs in degrading the organic matrix.

Targeted mutation of the cathepsin K in the mouse results in a phenotype consistent with the human disease, showing increased bone density and deformities [38, 64]. Both mice and human phenotypes become more pronounced with age and tend to affect bones that have higher rates of remodeling.

Renal Tubular Acidosis and Carbonic Anhydrase II Deficiency (OMIM 259730)

The syndrome of autosomal recessive osteoporosis associated with renal tubular acidosis was first recognized in 1972 [103]. The disease generally presents in the first two years of life with fracture, but allows for long survival since there are few hematologic disturbances other than a mild anemia. Other features include short stature, mental retardation, dental malocclusion, and visual impairment resulting from optic nerve compression. Electrolyte changes that indicate a hybrid of mild proximal and prominent distal tubular disturbances are a sign of a mild renal tubular acidosis.

The carbonic anhydrases (CAs) are a family of zinc metalloenzymes that, when blocked by sulfonamide inhibitors, produce renal tubular acidosis and PTH-induced release of calcium from bone. Sly et al. [104] postulated that the renal tubular defects were due to an abnormality in carbonic anhydrase II because the disease affected both kidney and brain: CAII is the only CA present in both tissues (although the etiology of cerebral calcifications remains unknown). CAII was shown to be absent in erythrocytes of affected patients [102]. Study of 18 unrelated patients revealed a virtual absence of CA II in erythrocyte hemolysates [104]. Reduced CA II levels were found in obligate heterozygotes.

Carbonic anhydrase II is expressed at high levels in active osteoclasts [61]. The disease has been treated with marrow transplantation. McMahon et al. [77] reported, in a fairly severely affected Irish kindred, that three years after transplantation there was histologic and radiological resolution of osteopetrosis with stabilization of hearing and vision; the transplanted children remained developmentally delayed with beginnings of cerebral calcification and continued to have renal tubular acidosis. Thus bone marrow stem cell replacement cures the osteoclast component of CAII deficiency, but has little effect on the loss of CAII function in renal and cerebral tissues.

A transgenic mouse model where a mutation in CA II was created with N-ethyl-N-nitrosourea produced homozygotes that are runted and have renal tubular acidosis, but interestingly do not have osteopetrosis [70]. There is a great deal of phenotypic heterogeneity in the human disease. Most kindreds are found in the Mediterranean and in the Middle East; the latter families have the greatest degree of mental retardation and metabolic acidosis, but less conspicuous fractures, while other kindred have only mild mental retardation with severe osteopetrotic fracturing [104]. In one family the affected individuals are compound heterozygotes, each inheriting a different mutation from mother and father [96]. The maternal CA II mutation is a missense mutation in exon 3 that substitutes a tyrosine for a histidine. As a result mature enzyme activity is reduced, but not absent. The authors suggest that expression of the remnant enzyme activity has prevented mental retardation in this family.

Camurati-Engelmann Disease (OMIM 131300)

Camurati–Engelmann disease (CED) is an autosomal dominant, progressive diaphyseal dysplasia characterized by hyperosteosis and sclerosis of the diaphyses of long bones. CED patients have severe leg pains, muscular weakness, fatigability, and decreased muscle mass. Other symptoms are exophthalmos, decreased vision,

deafness, and facial paralysis. Radiologically there is thickening of the diaphyseal cortex of the long bones and narrowing of the medullary canal with sclerosis at the skull base. Kinoshita et al. assigned the disease locus to a region where human transforming growth factor-1 gene (TGFB1) is located [56]. TGF-β1 is secreted as a large precursor protein that requires processing to cleave the signal peptide and dimerization. The processed precursor is cleaved into a mature TGF-β1 form with a latency-associated protein that, while linked to the mature growth factor, keeps it inactive by masking TGF-β1 receptor-binding domains [51]. Activation of latent TGF-β1 can be accomplished *in vitro* through heat or chaotropic agents [90]. Three different missense mutations causing CED were expressed *in vitro*; all were shown to disrupt the association of latency-associated protein with TGF-β1, affecting release of the mature TGF-β1 [97].

Osteoclast formation from peripheral blood mononuclear cells of CED patients was enhanced *in vitro* [76]; the activation of osteoclast activity is consistent with clinical reports that show biochemical evidence of increased bone resorption. The increase in osteoclastogenesis was inhibited by a soluble TGF receptor. Total serum TGF-β1 levels were similar in affected and unaffected subjects, but concentrations of active TGF-β1 in conditioned medium of osteoclast cultures were higher in the three CED patients than in the unaffected family member. Interestingly, when exposed to conditioned media from CED fibroblasts, fibroblast growth is suppressed, while osteoblastic cells are growth accelerated [97]. Indeed, the muscle and skeletal pathophysiology in Camurati–Engelmann disease is likely due to differential effects of the TGF activation and response in muscle and skeleton. In the skeleton, the effects of the CED TGF mutation lead to activation of osteoclasts, with a concurrent increase in osteoblast markers due to coupling; the increase in osteoblast activity is also likely a direct effect of TGF-β1 on the osteoblast lineage.

Conclusions

During the last 15 years, understanding of the molecular signals involved in osteoclast recruitment, the pathways necessary for adequate

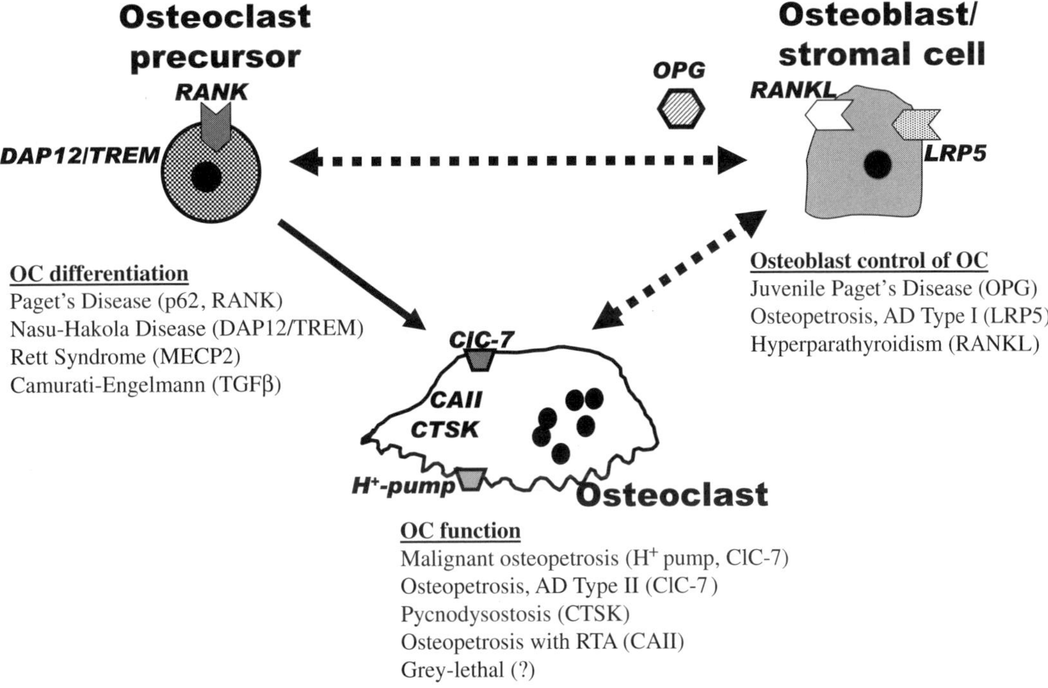

Figure 7.10 Clinical diseases of bone resorption. Specific diseases discussed in this chapter are also delineated in Tables I & II.

osteoclast function, and continued investigation of skeletal pathophysiology, have enlightened our understanding of both common and rare bone diseases. Figure 7.10 presents the known diseases. Further basic and clinical research will surely lead to new disease designations that involve altered remodeling. In turn, new findings are likely to revise understanding of the diseases discussed here.

References

1. Abe E, Marians RC, Yu W, Wu XB, Ando T, Li Y, et al. (2003) TSH is a negative regulator of skeletal remodeling. Cell 115:151–62.
2. Adams JS, Wahl TO, Lukert BP (1981) Effects of hydrochlorothiazide and dietary sodium restriction on calcium metabolism in corticosteroid treated patients. Metabolism 30:217–21.
3. Andersen PE, Jr., Bollerslev J (1987) Heterogeneity of autosomal dominant osteopetrosis. Radiology 164:223–5.
4. Bakwin H, Golden A, Fox S (1964) Familial Osteoectasia with Macrocranium. Am J Roentgenol Radium Ther Nucl Med 91:609–17.
5. Bassey EJ, Rothwell MC, Littlewood JJ, Pye DW (1998) Pre- and postmenopausal women have different bone mineral density responses to the same high-impact exercise. J Bone Miner Res 13:1805–13.
6. Beamer WG, Donahue LR, Rosen CJ, Baylink DJ (1996) Genetic variability in adult bone density among inbred strains of mice. Bone 18:397–403.
7. Benichou O, Cleiren E, Gram J, Bollerslev J, de Vernejoul MC, Van Hul W (2001) Mapping of autosomal dominant osteopetrosis type II (Albers-Schonberg disease) to chromosome 16p13.3. Am J Hum Genet 69:647–54.
8. Benichou OD, Laredo JD, de Vernejoul MC (2000) Type II autosomal dominant osteopetrosis (Albers-Schonberg disease): clinical and radiological manifestations in 42 patients. Bone 26:87–93.
9. Bilezikian JP, Silverberg SJ (2004) Clinical practice. Asymptomatic primary hyperparathyroidism. N Engl J Med 350:1746–51.
10. Bollerslev J, Andersen PE, Jr. (1988) Radiological, biochemical and hereditary evidence of two types of autosomal dominant osteopetrosis. Bone 9:7–13.
11. Bollerslev J, Mosekilde L (1993) Autosomal dominant osteopetrosis. Clin Orthop. 45–51.
12. Boyden LM, Mao J, Belsky J, Mitzner L, Farhi A, Mitnick MA, et al. (2002) High bone density due to a mutation in LDL-receptor-related protein 5. N Engl J Med 346:1513–21.
13. Brown EM, Gamba G, Riccardi D, Lombardi M, Butters R, Kifor O, et al. (1993) Cloning and characterization of an extracellular Ca(2+)-sensing receptor from bovine parathyroid. Nature 366:575–80.
14. Bucay N, Sarosi I, Dunstan CR, Morony S, Tarpley J, Capparelli C, et al. (1998) Osteoprotegerin-deficient

mice develop early onset osteoporosis and arterial calcification. Genes Dev 12:1260–8.

15. Budden SS, Gunness ME (2003) Possible mechanisms of osteopenia in Rett syndrome: bone histomorphometric studies. J Child Neurol 18:698–702.

16. Caffey J (1972) Familial hyperphosphatasemia with ateliosis and hypermetabolism of growing membranous bone; review of the clinical, radiographic and chemical features. Bull Hosp Joint Dis 33:81–110.

17. Canalis E (1996) Clinical review 83: Mechanisms of glucocorticoid action in bone: implications to glucocorticoid-induced osteoporosis. J Clin Endocrinol Metab 81:3441–7.

18. Cenci S, Weitzmann MN, Roggia C, Namba N, Novack D, Woodring J, et al. (2000) Estrogen deficiency induces bone loss by enhancing T-cell production of TNF-alpha. J Clin Invest 106:1229–37.

19. Chalhoub N, Benachenhou N, Rajapurohitam V, Pata M, Ferron M, Frattini A, et al. (2003) Grey-lethal mutation induces severe malignant autosomal recessive osteopetrosis in mouse and human. Nat Med 9:399–406.

20. Chandrasekharappa SC, Guru SC, Manickam P, Olufemi SE, Collins FS, Emmert-Buck MR, et al. (1997) Positional cloning of the gene for multiple endocrine neoplasia-type 1. Science 276:404–7.

21. Cleiren E, Benichou O, Van Hul E, Gram J, Bollerslev J, Singer FR, et al. (2001) Albers-Schonberg disease (autosomal dominant osteopetrosis, type II) results from mutations in the ClCN7 chloride channel gene. Hum Mol Genet 10:2861–7.

22. Croucher PI, Shipman CM, Lippitt J, Perry M, Asosingh K, Hijzen A, et al. (2001) Osteoprotegerin inhibits the development of osteolytic bone disease in multiple myeloma. Blood 98:3534–40.

23. Cundy T, Hegde M, Naot D, Chong B, King A, Wallace R, et al. (2002) A mutation in the gene TNFRSF11B encoding osteoprotegerin causes an idiopathic hyperphosphatasia phenotype. Hum Mol Genet 11:2119–27.

24. Cushing H (1932) The basophil adenomas of the pituitary body and their clinical manifestation. Johns Hopkins Bull 50:137–60.

25. Devlin RD, Bone HG, 3rd, Roodman GD (1996) Interleukin-6: a potential mediator of the massive osteolysis in patients with Gorham-Stout disease. J Clin Endocrinol Metab 81:1893–7.

26. Eghbali-Fatourechi G, Khosla S, Sanyal A, Boyle WJ, Lacey DL, Riggs BL (2003) Role of RANK ligand in mediating increased bone resorption in early postmenopausal women. J Clin Invest 111:1221–30.

27. Ehrlich PJ, Lanyon LE (2002) Mechanical strain and bone cell function: a review. Osteoporos Int 13:688–700.

28. Fischer A, Griscelli C, Friedrich W, Kubanek B, Levinsky R, Morgan G, et al. (1986) Bone-marrow transplantation for immunodeficiencies and osteopetrosis: European survey, 1968–1985. Lancet 2:1080–4.

29. Frattini A, Orchard PJ, Sobacchi C, Giliani S, Abinun M, Mattsson JP, et al. (2000) Defects in TCIRG1 subunit of the vacuolar proton pump are responsible for a subset of human autosomal recessive osteopetrosis. Nat Genet 25:343–6.

30. Friedrichs WE, Reddy SV, Bruder JM, Cundy T, Cornish J, Singer FR, et al. (2002) Sequence analysis of measles virus nucleocapsid transcripts in patients with Paget's disease. J Bone Miner Res 17:145–51.

31. Gagel RF (1997) Multiple endocrine neoplasia type II and familial medullary thyroid carcinoma. Impact of genetic screening on management. Cancer Treat Res 89:421–41.

32. Garnero P, Sornay-Rendu E, Chapuy MC, Delmas PD (1996) Increased bone turnover in late postmenopausal women is a major determinant of osteoporosis. J Bone Miner Res 11:337–49.

33. Gelb BD, Edelson JG, Desnick RJ (1995) Linkage of pycnodysostosis to chromosome 1q21 by homozygosity mapping. Nat Genet 10:235–7.

34. Gelb BD, Shi GP, Chapman HA, Desnick RJ (1996) Pycnodysostosis, a lysosomal disease caused by cathepsin K deficiency. Science 273:1236–8.

35. Glass DA, 2nd, Patel MS, Karsenty G (2003) A new insight into the formation of osteolytic lesions in multiple myeloma. N Engl J Med 349:2479–80.

36. Gong Y, Slee RB, Fukai N, Rawadi G, Roman-Roman S, Reginato AM, et al. (2001) LDL Receptor-Related Protein 5 (LRP5) Affects Bone Accrual and Eye Development. Cell 107:513–23.

37. Gorham LW, Stout AP (1955) Massive osteolysis (acute spontaneous absorption of bone, phantom bone, disappearing bone); its relation to hemangiomatosis. J Bone Joint Surg Am 37-A:985–1004.

38. Gowen M, Lazner F, Dodds R, Kapadia R, Feild J, Tavaria M, et al. (1999) Cathepsin K knockout mice develop osteopetrosis due to a deficit in matrix degradation but not demineralization. J Bone Miner Res 14:1654–63.

39. Greenfield EM, Bi Y, Miyauchi A (1999) Regulation of osteoclast activity. Life Sci 65:1087–102.

40. Greenspan SL, Greenspan FS (1999) The effect of thyroid hormone on skeletal integrity. Ann Intern Med 130:750–8.

41. Gronowicz G, McCarthy MB, Raisz LG (1990) Glucocorticoids stimulate resorption in fetal rat parietal bones in vitro. J Bone Miner Res 5:1223–30.

42. Hagberg B (1995) Rett syndrome: clinical peculiarities and biological mysteries. Acta Paediatr 84:971–6.

43. Hakola HP, Iivanainen M (1973) A new hereditary disease with progressive dementia and polycystic osteodysplasia: neuroradiological analysis of seven cases. Neuroradiology 6:162–8.

44. Ho N, Punturieri A, Wilkin D, Szabo J, Johnson M, Whaley J, et al. (1999) Mutations of CTSK result in pycnodysostosis via a reduction in cathepsin K protein. J Bone Miner Res 14:1649–53.

45. Hocking LJ, Lucas GJ, Daroszewska A, Mangion J, Olavesen M, Cundy T, et al. (2002) Domain-specific mutations in sequestosome 1 (SQSTM1) cause familial and sporadic Paget's disease. Hum Mol Genet 11:2735–9.

46. Hofbauer LC, Khosla S, Dunstan CR, Lacey DL, Spelsberg TC, Riggs BL (1999) Estrogen stimulates gene expression and protein production of osteoprotegerin in human osteoblastic cells. Endocrinology 140:4367–70.

47. Hughes AE, Ralston SH, Marken J, Bell C, MacPherson H, Wallace RG, et al. (2000) Mutations in TNFRSF11A, affecting the signal peptide of RANK, cause familial expansile osteolysis. Nat Genet 24:45–8.

48. Hughes DE, Dai A, Tiffee JC, Li HH, Mundy GR, Boyce BF (1996) Estrogen promotes apoptosis of murine osteoclasts mediated by TGF-beta. Nat Med. 2:1132–6.

49. Ikeda T, Utsuyama M, Hirokawa K (2001) Expression profiles of receptor activator of nuclear factor kappaB ligand, receptor activator of nuclear factor kappaB, and osteoprotegerin messenger RNA in aged and ovariectomized rat bones. J Bone Miner Res 16:1416–25.

50. Iqbal AA, Burgess EH, Gallina DL, Nanes MS, Cook CB (2003) Hypercalcemia in hyperthyroidism: patterns of serum calcium, parathyroid hormone, and 1,25-dihydroxyvitamin D3 levels during management of thyrotoxicosis. Endocr Pract 9:517–21.

51. Janssens K, Gershoni-Baruch R, Guanabens N, Migone N, Ralston S, Bonduelle M, et al. (2000) Mutations in the gene encoding the latency-associated peptide of TGF-beta 1 cause Camurati-Engelmann disease. Nat Genet 26:273–5.

52. Janssens K, Van Hul W (2002) Molecular genetics of too much bone. Hum Mol Genet 11:2385–93.

53. Kanis JA, Delmas P, Burckhardt P, Cooper C, Torgerson D (1997) Guidelines for diagnosis and management of osteoporosis. The European Foundation for Osteoporosis and Bone Disease. Osteoporos Int 7:390–406.

54. Kato M, Patel MS, Levasseur R, Lobov I, Chang BH, Glass DA, 2nd, et al. (2002) Cbfa1-independent decrease in osteoblast proliferation, osteopenia, and persistent embryonic eye vascularization in mice deficient in Lrp5, a Wnt coreceptor. J Cell Biol 157:303–14.

55. Kimble RB, Srivastava S, Ross FP, Matayoshi A, Pacifici R (1996) Estrogen deficiency increases the ability of stromal cells to support murine osteoclastogenesis via an interleukin-1and tumor necrosis factor-mediated stimulation of macrophage colony-stimulating factor production. J Biol Chem 271:28890–7.

56. Kinoshita A, Saito T, Tomita H, Makita Y, Yoshida K, Ghadami M, et al. (2000) Domain-specific mutations in TGFB1 result in Camurati-Engelmann disease. Nat Genet 26:19–20.

57. Klein RF, Allard J, Avnur Z, Nikolcheva T, Rotstein D, Carlos AS, et al. (2004) Regulation of bone mass in mice by the lipoxygenase gene Alox15. Science 303:229–32.

58. Koga T, Inui M, Inoue K, Kim S, Suematsu A, Kobayashi E, et al. (2004) Costimulatory signals mediated by the ITAM motif cooperate with RANKL for bone homeostasis. Nature 428:758–63.

59. Kornak U, Kasper D, Bosl MR, Kaiser E, Schweizer M, Schulz A, et al. (2001) Loss of the ClC-7 chloride channel leads to osteopetrosis in mice and man. Cell 104:205–15.

60. Kornak U, Schulz A, Friedrich W, Uhlhaas S, Kremens B, Voit T, et al. (2000) Mutations in the a3 subunit of the vacuolar H(+)-ATPase cause infantile malignant osteopetrosis. Hum Mol Genet 9:2059–63.

61. Laitala T, Vaananen HK (1994) Inhibition of bone resorption in vitro by antisense RNA and DNA molecules targeted against carbonic anhydrase II or two subunits of vacuolar H(+)-ATPase. J Clin Invest 93:2311–8.

62. Lanyon L, Skerry T (2001) Postmenopausal osteoporosis as a failure of bone's adaptation to functional loading: a hypothesis. J Bone Miner Res 16:1937–47.

63. Laughlin MH, Welshons WV, Sturek M, Rush JW, Turk JR, Taylor JA, et al. (2003) Gender, exercise training, and eNOS expression in porcine skeletal muscle arteries. J Appl Physiol 95:250–64.

64. Lazner F, Gowen M, Pavasovic D, Kola I (1999) Osteopetrosis and osteoporosis: two sides of the same coin. Hum Mol Genet 8:1839–46.

65. Leach RJ, Singer FR, Roodman GD (2001) The genetics of Paget's disease of the bone. J Clin Endocrinol Metab 86:24–8.

66. Lee K, Jessop H, Suswillo R, Zaman G, Lanyon L (2003) Endocrinology: bone adaptation requires oestrogen receptor-alpha. Nature 424:389.

67. Lee S, Finn L, Sze RW, Perkins JA, Sie KC (2003) Gorham Stout syndrome (disappearing bone disease): two additional case reports and a review of the literature. Arch Otolaryngol Head Neck Surg 129:1340–3.

68. Lee SK, Lorenzo JA (1999) Parathyroid hormone stimulates TRANCE and inhibits osteoprotegerin messenger ribonucleic acid expression in murine bone marrow cultures: correlation with osteoclast-like cell formation. Endocrinology 140:3552–61.

69. Leonard H, Thomson M, Glasson E, Fyfe S, Leonard S, Ellaway C, et al. (1999) Metacarpophalangeal pattern profile and bone age in Rett syndrome: further radiological clues to the diagnosis. Am J Med Genet 83:88–95.

70. Lewis SE, Erickson RP, Barnett LB, Venta PJ, Tashian RE (1988) N-ethyl-N-nitrosourea-induced null mutation at the mouse Car-2 locus: an animal model for human carbonic anhydrase II deficiency syndrome. Proc Natl Acad Sci USA 85:1962–6.

71. Li YP, Chen W, Stashenko P (1996) Molecular cloning and characterization of a putative novel human osteoclast-specific 116-kDa vacuolar proton pump subunit. Biochem Biophys Res Commun 218:813–21.

72. Little RD, Carulli JP, Del Mastro RG, Dupuis J, Osborne M, Folz C, et al. (2002) A mutation in the LDL receptor-related protein 5 gene results in the autosomal dominant high-bone-mass trait. Am J Hum Genet 70:11–9.

73. Manolagas SC, Kousteni S, Jilka RL (2002) Sex steroids and bone. Recent Prog Horm Res 57:385–409.

74. Maroteaux P, Lamy M (1965) The Malady of Toulouse-Lautrec. Jama 191:715–7.

75. Marx SJ, Agarwal SK, Heppner C, Kim YS, Kester MB, Goldsmith PK, et al. (1999) The gene for multiple endocrine neoplasia type 1: recent findings. Bone 25:119–22.

76. McGowan NW, MacPherson H, Janssens K, Van Hul W, Frith JC, Fraser WD, et al. (2003) A mutation affecting the latency-associated peptide of TGFbeta1 in Camurati-Engelmann disease enhances osteoclast formation in vitro. J Clin Endocrinol Metab 88:3321–6.

77. McMahon C, Will A, Hu P, Shah GN, Sly WS, Smith OP (2001) Bone marrow transplantation corrects osteopetrosis in the carbonic anhydrase II deficiency syndrome. Blood 97:1947–50.

78. Miura M, Tanaka K, Komatsu Y, Suda M, Yasoda A, Sakuma Y, et al. (2002) A novel interaction between thyroid hormones and 1,25(OH)(2)D(3) in osteoclast formation. Biochem Biophys Res Commun 291:987–94.

79. Montecucco C, Caporali R, Caprotti P, Caprotti M, Notario A (1992) Sex hormones and bone metabolism in postmenopausal rheumatoid arthritis treated with two different glucocorticoids. J Rheumatol 19:1895–900.

80. Motil KJ, Schultz R, Brown B, Glaze DG, Percy AK (1994) Altered energy balance may account for growth failure in Rett syndrome. J Child Neurol 9:315–9.

81. Nasu T, Tsukahara Y, Terayama K (1973) A lipid metabolic disease-"membranous lipodystrophy"-an autopsy case demonstrating numerous peculiar mem-

brane-structures composed of compound lipid in bone and bone marrow and various adipose tissues. Acta Pathol Jpn 23:539–58.

82. Niida S, Kaku M, Amano H, Yoshida H, Kataoka H, Nishikawa S, et al. (1999) Vascular endothelial growth factor can substitute for macrophage colony- stimulating factor in the support of osteoclastic bone resorption. J Exp Med 190:293–8.

83. O'Brien CA, Jia D, Plotkin LI, Bellido T, Powers CC, Stewart SA, et al. (2004) Glucocorticoids act directly on osteoblasts and osteocytes to induce their apoptosis and reduce bone formation and strength. Endocrinology 145:1835–41.

84. Osterberg PH, Wallace RG, Adams DA, Crone RS, Dickson GR, Kanis JA, et al. (1988) Familial expansile osteolysis. A new dysplasia. J Bone Joint Surg Br 70: 255–60.

85. Pacifici R (1996) Estrogen, cytokines, and pathogenesis of postmenopausal osteoporosis. J Bone Miner Res 11:1043–51.

86. Paloneva J, Mandelin J, Kiialainen A, Bohling T, Prudlo J, Hakola P, et al. (2003) DAP12/TREM2 deficiency results in impaired osteoclast differentiation and osteoporotic features. J Exp Med 198:669–75.

87. Paloneva J, Manninen T, Christman G, Hovanes K, Mandelin J, Adolfsson R, et al. (2002) Mutations in two genes encoding different subunits of a receptor signaling complex result in an identical disease phenotype. Am J Hum Genet 71:656–62.

88. Pearse RN, Sordillo EM, Yaccoby S, Wong BR, Liau DF, Colman N, et al. (2001) Multiple myeloma disrupts the TRANCE/ osteoprotegerin cytokine axis to trigger bone destruction and promote tumor progression. Proc Natl Acad Sci USA 98:11581–6.

89. Pekkarinen P, Kestila M, Paloneva J, Terwillign J, Varilo T, Jarvi O, et al. (1998) Fine-scale mapping of a novel dementia gene, PLOSL, by linkage disequilibrium. Genomics. 54:307–15.

90. Piek E, Heldin CH, Ten Dijke P (1999) Specificity, diversity, and regulation in TGF-beta superfamily signaling. Faseb J 13:2105–24.

91. Ralston SH (1997) The Michael Mason Prize Essay 1997. Nitric oxide and bone: what a gas! Br J Rheumatol 36:831–8.

92. Rantakokko J, Aro HT, Savontaus M, Vuorio E (1996) Mouse cathepsin K: cDNA cloning and predominant expression of the gene in osteoclasts, and in some hypertrophying chondrocytes during mouse development. FEBS Lett 393:307–13.

93. Reddy SV, Kurihara N, Menaa C, Roodman GD (2001) Paget's disease of bone: a disease of the osteoclast. Rev Endocr Metab Disord 2:195–201.

94. Reid AB, Reid IL, Johnson G, Hamonic M, Major P (1989) Familial diffuse cystic angiomatosis of bone. Clin Orthop 211–8.

95. Riggs BL, Khosla S, Melton LJ, 3rd (2002) Sex steroids and the construction and conservation of the adult skeleton. Endocr Rev 23:279–302.

96. Roth DE, Venta PJ, Tashian RE, Sly WS (1992) Molecular basis of human carbonic anhydrase II deficiency. Proc Natl Acad Sci USA 89:1804–8.

97. Saito T, Kinoshita A, Yoshiura K, Makita Y, Wakui K, Honke K, et al. (2001) Domain-specific mutations of a transforming growth factor (TGF)-beta 1 latency-associated peptide cause Camurati-Engelmann disease because of the formation of a constitutively active form of TGF-beta 1. J Biol Chem 276:11469–72.

98. Sezer O, Heider U, Zavrski I, Kuhne CA, Hofbauer LC (2003) RANK ligand and osteoprotegerin in myeloma bone disease. Blood 101:2094–8.

99. Shahbazian M, Young J, Yuva-Paylor L, Spencer C, Antalffy B, Noebels J, et al. (2002) Mice with truncated MeCP2 recapitulate many Rett syndrome features and display hyperacetylation of histone H3. Neuron 35: 243–54.

100. Shevde NK, Bendixen AC, Dienger KM, Pike JW (2000) Estrogens suppress RANK ligand-induced osteoclast differentiation via a stromal cell independent mechanism involving c-Jun repression. Proc Natl Acad Sci USA 97:7829–34.

101. Shi GP, Chapman HA, Bhairi SM, DeLeeuw C, Reddy VY, Weiss SJ (1995) Molecular cloning of human cathepsin O, a novel endoproteinase and homologue of rabbit OC2. FEBS Lett 357:129–34.

102. Sly WS, Hewett-Emmett D, Whyte MP, Yu YS, Tashian RE (1983) Carbonic anhydrase II deficiency identified as the primary defect in the autosomal recessive syndrome of osteopetrosis with renal tubular acidosis and cerebral calcification. Proc Natl Acad Sci USA 80: 2752–6.

103. Sly WS, Lang RA, Avioli LV, Haddad J, Lubowitz H, McAlister W (1972) Recessive osteopetrosis: new clinical phenotype. Am J Hum Genet. 24 (Suppl)::34a.

104. Sly WS, Whyte MP, Sundaram V, Tashian RE, Hewett-Emmett D, Guibaud P, et al. (1985) Carbonic anhydrase II deficiency in 12 families with the autosomal recessive syndrome of osteopetrosis with renal tubular acidosis and cerebral calcification. N Engl J Med 313:139–45.

105. Sobacchi C, Frattini A, Orchard P, Porras O, Tezcan I, Andolina M, et al. (2001) The mutational spectrum of human malignant autosomal recessive osteopetrosis. Hum Mol Genet 10:1767–73.

106. Srivastava S, Toraldo G, Weitzmann MN, Cenci S, Ross FP, Pacifici R (2001) Estrogen decreases osteoclast formation by down-regulating receptor activator of NF-kappa B ligand (RANKL)-induced JNK activation. J Biol Chem 276:8836–40.

107. Szulc P, Hofbauer LC, Heufelder AE, Roth S, Delmas PD (2001) Osteoprotegerin serum levels in men: correlation with age, estrogen, and testosterone status. J Clin Endocrinol Metab 86:3162–5.

108. Tian E, Zhan F, Walker R, Rasmussen E, Ma Y, Barlogie B, et al. (2003) The role of the Wnt-signaling antagonist DKK1 in the development of osteolytic lesions in multiple myeloma. N Engl J Med 349:2483–94.

109. Vaananen HK, Zhao H, Mulari M, Halleen JM (2000) The cell biology of osteoclast function. J Cell Sci 113 (Pt 3):377–81.

110. Van Wesenbeeck L, Cleiren E, Gram J, Beals RK, Benichou O, Scopelliti D, et al. (2003) Six novel missense mutations in the LDL receptor-related protein 5 (LRP5) gene in different conditions with an increased bone density. Am J Hum Genet 72:763–71.

111. Vestergaard P, Mosekilde L (2003) Hyperthyroidism, bone mineral, and fracture risk–a meta-analysis. Thyroid 13:585–93.

112. Waguespack SG, Hui SL, White KE, Buckwalter KA, Econs MJ (2002) Measurement of tartrate-resistant acid phosphatase and the brain isoenzyme of creatine

kinase accurately diagnoses type II autosomal dominant osteopetrosis but does not identify gene carriers. J Clin Endocrinol Metab 87:2212–7.

113. Walker DG (1975) Bone resorption restored in osteopetrotic mice by transplants of normal bone marrow and spleen cells. Science 190:784–5.

114. Walker DG (1993) Bone resorption restored in osteopetrotic mice by transplants of normal bone marrow and spleen cells. 1975. Clin Orthop 294:4–6.

115. Wan M, Lee SS, Zhang X, Houwink-Manville I, Song HR, Amir RE, et al. (1999) Rett syndrome and beyond: recurrent spontaneous and familial MECP2 mutations at CpG hotspots. Am J Hum Genet 65:1520–9.

116. Weinstein RS (2001) Glucocorticoid-induced osteoporosis. Rev Endocr Metab Disord 2:65–73.

117. Weinstein RS, Jilka RL, Parfitt AM, Manolagas SC (1998) Inhibition of osteoblastogenesis and promotion of apoptosis of osteoblasts and osteocytes by glucocorticoids. Potential mechanisms of their deleterious effects on bone. J Clin Invest 102:274–82.

118. Whyte MP, Hughes AE (2002) Expansile skeletal hyperphosphatasia is caused by a 15-base pair tandem duplication in TNFRSF11A encoding RANK and is allelic to familial expansile osteolysis. J Bone Miner Res 17:26–9.

119. Whyte MP, Leelawattana R, Reddy SV, Roodman GD (1996) Absence of paramyxo virus transcripts in juvenile Paget bone disease. J Bone Miner Res 11:1041.

120. Whyte MP, Mills BG, Reinus WR, Podgornik MN, Roodman GD, Gannon FH, et al. (2000) Expansile skeletal hyperphosphatasia: a new familial metabolic bone disease. J Bone Miner Res 15:2330–44.

121. Whyte MP, Obrecht SE, Finnegan PM, Jones JL, Podgornik MN, McAlister WH, et al. (2002) Osteoprotegerin deficiency and juvenile Paget's disease. N Engl J Med 347:175–84.

122. Wiktor-Jedrzejczak W, Bartocci A, Ferrante AJ, Ahmed-Ansari A, Sell K, Pollard J, et al. (1990) Total absence of colony-stimulating factor 1 in the macrophage-deficient osteopetrotic (op/op) mouse. Proc Natl Acad Sci USA 87:4828–32.

123. Wu J, Wang XX, Takasaki M, Ohta A, Higuchi M, Ishimi Y (2001) Cooperative effects of exercise training and genistein administration on bone mass in ovariectomized mice. J Bone Miner Res 16:1829–36.

124. Yasuda H, Shima N, Nakagawa N, Yamaguchi K, Kinosaki M, Mochizuki S, et al. (1998) Osteoclast differentiation factor is a ligand for osteoprotegerin/osteoclastogenesis-inhibitory factor and is identical to TRANCE/RANKL. Proc Natl Acad Sci USA 95:3597–602.

8.

Pharmaceuticals for Bone Disease Targeting the Osteoclast

Lorraine A. Fitzpatrick

Introduction

Many pharmaceutical agents target the osteoclast, as this is the cell that resorbs bone leading to bone loss. Recently, important information regarding osteoclast recruitment and function has been discovered, leading to a better understanding of osteoclast biology. Many available agents targeting the osteoclast decrease bone turnover markers, increase bone mineral density (BMD) and prevent fractures.

Bisphosphonate Overview

Pyrophosphates have been used extensively in industry because they inhibit precipitation of calcium carbonates. Pyrophosphates bind avidly to calcium phosphate and impair both the formation of calcium phosphate crystals *in vitro* and in solution. Bisphosphonates display similar physical chemical activity, but resist enzymatic hydrolysis. Bisphosphonates are characterized by two carbon-phosphate (CP) bonds, and specificity is determined by variance in side chains (Figure 8.1). Many bisphosphonates have been tested in humans with respect to their ability to inhibit bone resorption. Etidronate, alendronate, clodronate, ibandronate, pamidronate, tiludronate, and zolendronic acid are available across the world. However, these bisphosphonates possesses physical, chemical, and biological properties that results in different efficacy and toxicity for each one. Bisphosphonates bind to the surface of bone at sites of active remodeling where two distinct molecular mechanisms are thought to be responsible for the ability of bisphosphonates to modify osteoclast function. Non-nitrogen-containing bisphosphonates (etidronate, clodronate, and tiludronate) alter cellular function by being metabolized to cytotoxic ATP-bisphosphonate analogues [44]. The nitrogen-containing bisphosphonates (alendronate, risedronate, ibandronate, and zolendronic acid) inhibit farnesyl pyrophosphatase and other steps in the intracellular mevalonate pathway [5, 48, 75]. As a result, the post-translational modification by prenylation of proteins such as Ras and Rho is impaired, leading to diminished recruitment or differentiation of osteoclast precursors and to osteoclast death. The loss of osteoclast activity results in a decrease in the rate at which new bone remodeling units are activated and a decrease in the amount of bone resorbing activity in each bone remodeling unit. The resulting reduction in bone turnover indirectly decreases osteoblast function and bone formation.

Bisphosphonates are poorly absorbed and can cause esophageal irritation or even ulceration if passage through the esophagus is delayed. As result, instructions for taking medications are complex. Although bisphosphonates are poorly absorbed, approximately 50% of the absorbed amount is taken up by the skeleton. The remainder undergoes renal excretion. In skeletal tissue, bisphosphonates have a long residual half-life.

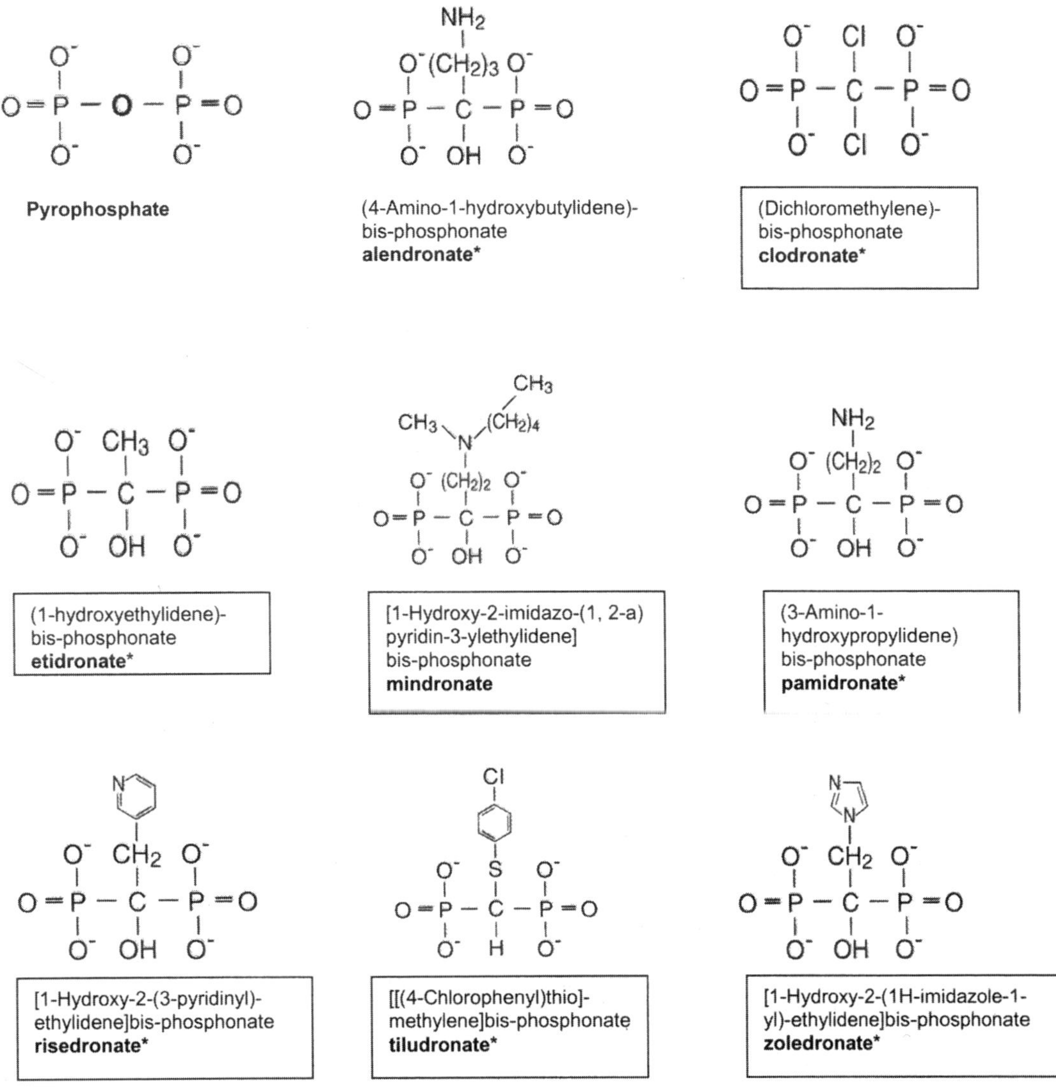

Figure 8.1 Chemical structures of various bisphosphonates.

Differences in structure determine potency, duration of action, side effects, and efficacy.

The pharmacologically active bisphosphonates inhibit bone resorption in organ culture. In the intact animal, bisphosphonates block the degradation of both primary and secondary trabeculae; this results in arrest of the modeling and remodeling of the metaphysis. In growing children, this would be predicted to create a club-shaped bone with a dense metaphysis, a picture similar to that seen in osteopetrotic animals. This effect can be used to estimate the potency of new compounds, and, in rare instances, bisphosphonate administration in high doses has resulted in toxicity in children [79]. Regarding the efficacy of bisphosphonates to inhibit bone resorption, no clear-cut structure and associated effect relationship has emerged regarding the pyro-carbon-phosphate (PCP) structure. Because of their strong affinity for bone mineral, bisphosphonates are deposited in bone and osteoclasts are inhibited when they engulf bisphosphonate-containing bone. Bisphosphonates inhibit the osteoclast function by altering the cytoskeleton and the ruffled border, decreasing acid extrusion and enzyme activity and increasing osteoclast apoptosis. A second target cell is the osteoblast, which secretes an osteoclast recruitment inhibitor that is stimulated by the action of bisphosphonates.

Alendronate

Alendronate is a nitrogen-containing bisphosphonate that was approved by the Food and Drug Administration in 1995 for treatment of osteoporosis in the United States. As a result, it is the most extensively studied bisphosphonate. Alendronate is approved for treatment and prevention of postmenopausal osteoporosis, treatment of osteoporosis in men, treatment of glucocorticoid induced osteoporosis and Paget's disease in men and women.

In two multicenter, dose-ranging studies, the efficacy of continuous oral alendronate therapy in postmenopausal women with osteoporosis was studied [45]. One multicenter study was conducted in the United States, and the other multicenter study recruited women worldwide. These two trials were randomized, double-blind, placebo-controlled studies with identical designs. Women who were 45 to 80 years of age and at least five years post-menopause were enrolled in the study. Enrollment required that the lumbar spine BMD be reduced, with T-scores more than 2.5 standard deviations below peak mass. Women were randomly assigned to receive placebo or 5, 10, or 20 mg of alendronate per day for two years, to be followed by open label therapy during the third year. The protocol was modified to include the third year of double-blind therapy and those subjects receiving 20 mg of alendronate were switched to doses of 5 mg/day for the third year. All women received a daily supplement of calcium carbonate that provided 500 mg of elemental calcium. There were significant increases in BMD of the spine, femoral neck, trochanter, and total body at six months in the alendronate groups and significant losses at all sites in the placebo group. The mean differences in BMD between those women receiving 10 mg of alendronate and those receiving placebo were 8.8% in the spine, 5.9% in the femoral neck, 7.8% in the trochanter and 2.5% in the total body (P < 0.01 for all comparisons). The 10-mg dose of alendronate resulted in BMD increases at all sites during all three years, although the increase in total body BMD during year three was not significant. In the midforearm, a site consisting almost entirely of cortical bone, the 10-mg dose of alendronate

produced increases in BMD that were 2.2% greater than in the placebo group (P < 0.001). During the study, 22 (6.2%) of the 355 women in the placebo group had at least 12 vertebral fractures compared with 17 (3.2%) of the 526 women in the combined alendronate groups (P = 0.03). The relative risk of a new fracture among the women treated with alendronate (all doses pooled) as compared to the placebo group was 0.52 (95% CI, 0.28–0.95). The increased risk among women receiving placebo was found in both multicenter studies. The estimated risk of non-vertebral fractures in women treated with alendronate was 0.79 (95% CI, 0.52–1.22). In this clinical trial setting, alendronate was generally well tolerated with no clinical laboratory evidence of adverse effects that were greater than those found in the placebo group. Similar rates of adverse upper gastrointestinal (GI) effects were noted, and it was only later that it was realized that GI side effects could be an issue, resulting in specialized dosing instructions. The results of several trials were consistent with the prospective epidemiologic studies of the relationship between BMD of the lumbar spine and risk of vertebral fracture. Daily treatment with oral alendronate progressively increased bone mass of the spine, hip, and total body and reduced the risk of vertebral fracture and the progression of vertebral deformities in postmenopausal women with osteoporosis. In a separate study, therapy for one year significantly reduced the incidence of non-vertebral fractures in women with low bone density (T-score <−2.0) [60]. In a prospective study of 2,027 women with pre-existing vertebral fractures, alendronate therapy reduced the incidence of vertebral, hip and wrist fractures by approximately 50% over three years [8]. In this study, women aged 50–81 years with low femoral neck BMD were enrolled in study groups based on the presence or absence of an existing vertebral fracture. Postmenopausal women were randomly assigned to placebo or alendronate and followed for 36 months. The dose of alendronate was initially 5 mg daily and was increased to 10 mg daily at 24 months. Compared with the placebo group, treatment with alendronate significantly increased the average bone mass at the femoral neck (4.1% difference, P < 0.001), at the total hip (4.7%, P < 0.001), and in the posterior-anterior lumbar spine (6.2%, P < 0.001). Follow-up radiographs were obtained in 98% of those in the study at closeout. The risk of new radiographic vertebral fracture was 40% lower in the alendronate groups than in the placebo group and significantly fewer women in the alendronate groups had clinical vertebral fractures (hazard reduction 55%, P < 0.001). There was a significant reduction in hip fractures in the alendronate-treated group compared to the placebo treated women (P = 0.047).

In a younger a group of postmenopausal women, alendronate 5 mg daily for four years prevented the bone loss, but no effect on fracture rate was observed [62]. A trial was conducted to compare daily alendronate (5 to 10 mg/day) to once-weekly dosing of either 35 or 70 mg. In this trial, BMD endpoints were equivalent, although no fracture data are available for the groups receiving weekly doses.

In a two-year double-blind trial, alendronate was tested for its efficacy in men. Some 241 men aged 31–87 years with osteoporosis, one-third with low testosterone levels, were recruited for the trial [57]. The men who received alendronate had a mean increase in BMD of 7.1% the lumbar spine, 2.5% at the femoral neck, and 2.0% for the total body (P < 0.001 for all comparisons to baseline). There were no significant changes in the femoral neck or total body BMD. The incidence of vertebral fractures was lower in the alendronate group than in the placebo group (P = 0.02). Overall, the benefits of alendronate therapy in men with osteoporosis were very similar to those seen for postmenopausal women.

Risedronate

Risedronate is a pyridinyl bisphosphonate approved for the prevention and treatment of osteoporosis in postmenopausal women glucocorticoid induced osteoporosis and Paget's disease. In a randomized, placebo-controlled clinical trial, risedronate demonstrated efficacy for vertebral and non-vertebral fracture prevention [37]. In this trial, 2,458 postmenopausal women younger than 85 years with at least one vertebral fracture at baseline were enrolled. Subjects received oral risedronate (2.5 or 5.0 mg/day) or placebo. All participants received calcium (1,000 mg/day) and vitamin D to normalize 25-hydroxyvitamin D levels. The 2.5 mg/day of risedronate arm was discontinued after one year, and all results refer to the 5-mg/day dosing schedule. Fifty-five per cent of patients in the placebo group and 60% in the treatment group completed the three years of the clinical trial. There were no differences in reasons for patient withdrawal among treatment and placebo groups. A significant reduction of 65% in vertebral fracture risk (P < 0.001) was seen as early as in the first year of treatment. Over the three-year period, there was a 41% reduction in the risk of new vertebral fractures in patients treated with risedronate, compared to women receiving placebo (P = 0.003). The cumulative incidence of nonvertebral fractures over three years of treatment was lowered by 39% compared to women receiving placebo. Over the three years, there was a significant increase in BMD from baseline at the lumbar spine (5.4%), femoral neck (1.6%), and femoral trochanter (3.9%) in the risedronate-treated patients. Significant differences in BMD were notable as early as six months, compared to the placebo group. At the mid-shaft radius, the risedronate group had no change in BMD (0.2%) compared to a significant bone loss of −1.4% in the placebo group (P < 0.05). Markers of bone turnover, which were measured in a subset of subjects, were reflective of these changes and the mechanism of action of risedronate. Bone-specific alkaline phosphatase, a marker of bone formation, declined with risedronate treatment, with a nadir of −35% compared to baseline (median % change) at six months, compared to −12% with the placebo group. At the end of three years, the changes were −33% and −7%, respectively, for risedronate and placebo. When markers of bone resorption were evaluated, the changes were similar. The deoxypyridinoline-creatinine ratio reached a nadir at six months of −38% in the risedronate group compared with −8% in the placebo group and rose by the end of the study to −26% and −1%, respectively.

Overall, adverse events were similar across treatment groups. Digestive symptoms complaints were the most common adverse events that led to discontinuing the study, with 42% of placebo group and 36% of the risedronate group withdrawing. The most common GI events were dyspepsia, abdominal pain, and gastritis, and these events were similar in both treatment and placebo groups. Indeed the risedronate group showed no difference from placebo in the incidence of gastrointestinal tract endoscopy or the rate of abnormal findings on endoscopy.

Bone biopsy samples taken at baseline and at study end showed that bone was normal, without evidence of mineralization problems or marrow abnormalities in risedronate-treated subjects. Histomorphometric analysis demonstrated a 50% reduction in bone turnover and a slight increase in cortical thickness in risedronate treated patients compared to placebo. In both groups, there was an increase in median cortical porosity that may have resulted from the prolongation of the remodeling period.

Overall, this trial demonstrated the efficacy of risedronate in the treatment of women with established postmenopausal osteoporosis. The incidence of both vertebral and nonvertebral fractures was decreased by daily oral risedronate therapy. One of the differences in this trial compared to other anti-resorptives is that the initial criterion for vertebral fracture was based on a vertebral height loss of 15% instead of the more traditional 20% [8, 45]. A re-analysis of the study using the 20% reduction in vertebral fracture criterion was completed and showed similar results.

Risedronate reduced the risk of new vertebral fractures by 41% and reduced the cumulative incidence of non-vertebral fractures by 39% over a three-year period [37, 66]. In women with osteoporosis as defined by low femoral neck BMD who also had a prevalent vertebral fracture, risedronate reduced hip fracture by 60% [55].

The only prospective trial in which hip fracture was the primary endpoint enrolled 9,331 women [55]. Two groups of women were enrolled, one of which was composed of subjects 70 to 79 years old who had osteoporosis as indicated by either a BMD with a femoral neck <T-score −4.0 or femoral neck T-score lower than −3.0, along with at least one risk factor for hip fracture. The other group consisted of women 80 years of age or older who had at least one non-skeletal risk factor for hip fracture, a femoral neck T-score lower than −4.0, or a femoral neck T-score lower than −3.0, plus a hip-axis length of 11.1 cm or greater. Women were randomized to placebo or 2.5 or 5.0 mg/day of risedronate. Complete follow-up data were available for 64% of women (69% of those with confirmed osteoporosis and 58% of those with mainly clinical risk factors). The duration of follow-up was 2.3 years and the mean duration of therapy was 2.0 years. In the analysis of all women, the incidence of hip fracture was 2.8% among the women assigned to risedronate as compared to 3.9% among those assigned to placebo. The incidence of hip fracture in the group of women 70 to 79 years old was 1.9% among those assigned to risedronate and 3.2% among those assigned to placebo (relative risk, 0.6; 95% CI, 0.4–0.9; P = 0.009). In the group of women 80 years of age or older, risedronate had no effect on the incidence of hip fracture. The majority (58%) of the women in this group were recruited solely on the basis of clinical risk factors and only 16% were recruited on the basis of low BMD at the femoral neck. In an analysis of all the women, the incidence of nonvertebral fractures was 9.4% among those assigned to risedronate, as compared to 11.2% among those assigned to placebo (relative risk, 0.8; 95% CI, 0.7–1.0; P = 0.03). Among the women selected primarily on the basis of nonskeletal risk factors, the assigned treatment had no effect on the incidence of nonvertebral fracture. Thus, risedronate prevented hip fractures in elderly women with osteoporosis as determined by low BMD at the femoral neck; interestingly in a very elderly group without criteria for osteoporosis as measured by BMD, risedronate therapy did not prevent hip fractures.

Ibandronate

Oral ibandronate has recently been approved for use in the United States at a dose of 2.5 mg/day, but is not available commercially. Ibandronate has been tested in animal models and found to inhibit bone resorption and improve bone mechanical properties. Ibandronate is an amino bisphosphonate and is more potent than risedronate, alendronate, pamidronate, and clodronate. In a small, phase-one study involving 12 healthy men and 5 postmenopausal women, a single intravenous injection of ibandronate was associated with an increase in lumbar spine BMD of 2% (1 mg) and of 3% (2 mg). The 1-mg dose of ibandronate decreased urinary excretion of the C-terminal portion of type 1 collagen cross-links (CTX) by 200% in men, and the 2-mg dose by 300% after 14 days. CTX excretion continued to decrease up to 30 days after the single ibandronate injection. In a phase II dose-finding study that extended over 12 months, 180 postmenopausal women who had distal forearm T-scores less than 1.5 were randomized to oral ibandronate (0.5, 1.0, 2.5, 5.0 mg/day) or to placebo [63]. A total of 141 patients completed the study and women who received 2.5 or 5.0 mg/day had significant increases in spine and femoral neck BMD, as well as dose-related decrements in biochemical markers of bone turnover. In another study, 125 postmenopausal women with osteoporosis as defined by a T-score < −2.5 received either placebo or intravenous ibandronate (0.25, 0.5, 1.0, or 2.0 mg IV every three months for one year) [73]. Lumbar spine BMD did not change significantly in the placebo group, whereas BMD increased in a dose dependent manner up to 5.2% compared to baseline after 12 months; only the lowest dose of ibandronate (0.25 mg) did not produce significant changes. In addition, total hip BMD increased in the 1- (1.8%) and 2-mg (2.9%) groups. Ibandronate administered intravenously has been tested in a clinical trial with fracture as the primary outcome variable [64]. A total of 2,860 postmenopausal women with a spine BMD T-score less than or equal to −2.0 and at least one vertebral fracture were randomized to receive either placebo or ibandronate (0.5 or 1 mg) intravenously every three months for three years. After three years the BMD of spine increased approximately 5% and that of femoral trochanter BMD by 3.5% from baseline. The incidence of vertebral fracture was too low in both groups to show a significant change due to treatment.

Oral ibandronate has also been studied. In a randomized, placebo-controlled trial, 240 postmenopausal women with osteoporosis received either placebo, daily oral ibandronate (2.5 mg/day) or intermittent oral ibandronate (20 mg every other day for the first 24 days only) [69]. After 12 months, women taking placebo were switched to ibandronate for another 12 months. All patients received calcium 500 mg/day and vitamin D 400 IU/day. BMD was increased by treatment with ibandronate at one year. After two years, women receiving continuous ibandronate had an increase in lumbar spine BMD of 5.6%, while women taking intermittent ibandronate gained 5.5% in lumbar spine BMD. Similarly, women on both forms of ibandronate treatment showed identical BMD gains of 3.4% in the total hip. In a second double-blind randomized trial, 2,946 postmenopausal women with a lumbar spine T-scores <−2.0 and at least one prevalent vertebral fractures received either placebo (n = 982) or oral ibandronate [21]. Women on oral ibandronate received either continuous 2.5 mg/day or intermittent 20 mg every other day for the first 24 days, followed by nine weeks without

treatment (n = 982). In this study, both groups received the same cumulative dose of ibandronate. The primary endpoint was the incidence of new vertebral fractures after three years of treatment. Ibandronate, when administered orally on a daily basis, significantly reduced new vertebral fractures by 62%, and by 50% when using intermittent oral administration. Urinary CTX and serum osteocalcin levels were significantly decreased. In a post hoc subgroup analysis, non-vertebral fractures were reduced by ibandronate in patients with the lowest baseline femoral neck BMD (T-score < −3.0).

The most common adverse reaction observed with intravenous ibandronate is a transient fever that is a common response to intravenous administration of nitrogen containing bisphosphonates. Ibandronate can also cause hypocalcemia as well as decreased serum phosphate. Flu-like symptoms including chills, bone and muscle pain may occur and gastrointestinal discomfort has been reported. In seven patients receiving ibandronate 3 mg intravenously, proteinuria of uncertain clinical significance has been noted [58].

Pamidronate

Pamidronate was the first nitrogen containing bisphosphonate to be studied. Pamidronate is available for the treatment of hypercalcemia of malignancy, for osteolytic lesions in multiple myeloma, to treat metastatic cancer growing in bone, and for Paget's disease. Currently it is not approved for use in osteoporosis. When administered intravenously, pamidronate increased BMD or prevented bone loss in postmenopausal women with osteoporosis when given as an initial dose of 90 mg followed by 30 mg IV every three months [59].

Etidronate

Etidronate was the first bisphosphonate to be studied for treatment of osteoporosis. Continuous administration of etidronate was found to impair mineralization of new bone [38]. For this reason, etidronate was given intermittently following a cyclical regimen (400 mg/d for 14 days every three months). Under these conditions, etidronate appeared to be safe and effective when tested in small clinical trials. In prospective, randomized, placebo-controlled trials, intermittent etidronate therapy produced significant increases in lumbar spine BMD. The trials were not powered to show benefit for fractures, but the results can be interpreted as indicative of a decrease in the risk of vertebral fractures among high-risk patients [72, 77]. At high doses, etidronate impairs mineralization of newly formed bone and may cause bone pain and fractures. For this reason, this older bisphosphonate is not recommended for use in osteoporosis.

Tiludronate

Tiludronate has been administered to postmenopausal women to determine the efficacy and safety of this compound in the treatment of postmenopausal osteoporosis [65]. Two placebo-controlled, randomized, double masked, multicenter, cyclical, intermittent, dose-ranging studies were performed in 1,805 women with low vertebral BMD and prevalent vertebral fractures and in 488 women with low BMD and no prevalent vertebral fracture. Subjects were randomized to tiludronate 50 mg/day, 200 mg/day, or placebo, given orally for the first seven days of each month. A supplement of 500 mg elemental calcium was provided daily from day 8 to the end of the month. Neither study demonstrated a statistical or clinically relevant trend in the incidence of adverse events in the three treatment groups. Tiludronate administered at these two doses in a cyclical, intermittent fashion was not effective in reducing the incidence of vertebral fractures or in increasing spinal BMD.

Clodronate

Several double blind, placebo-controlled studies have shown that clodronate significantly reduces the incidence of both vertebral and non-vertebral fractures in patients with osteolysis caused by breast cancer and myeloma. Controlled studies have also demonstrated the benefit of clodronate in either an oral or intravenous form to increase BMD at the spine and hip in osteoporotic patients [29, 32, 74]. A randomized, placebo-controlled trial with clodronate was conducted that had as its endpoint the reduction of the risk of vertebral fracture [54]. Women with postmenopausal or secondary osteoporosis were recruited if they had BMD in the osteoporotic range (T-score $\leq$ −2.5)

and/or had one prevalent fracture at the time of entry into the study. Subjects received two doses of 400-mg oral clodronate per day or placebo. A total of 593 women with osteoporosis were recruited. In all patients, clodronate administration was associated with a significant increase in mean spine BMD over the 3 year period (4.35% change from baseline with clodronate compared to 0.64% in the placebo group, P < 0.0001). At the hip, clodronate maintained BMD (0.70%) compared to a loss of BMD in the placebo group (−3.03%, P < 0.0001). There were no differences in the treatment effect in the postmenopausal vs. the secondary osteoporosis groups. Distal forearm BMD did not change in either clodronate group. Serum CTX was reduced by a median of 46% in the clodronate-treated group and was significantly lower at all times compared to patients receiving placebo. At the end of the three-year study, the incidence of new fractures in the clodronate-treated patients was 12.7% (RR 0.54; 95% CI, 0.37–0.80), compared to an incidence of 23.3% in the placebo-treated group. The relative risk was more robust in the women with a secondary cause of osteoporosis (RR 0.35; 95% CI, 0.16–0.76 for the latter; RR 0.63; 95% CI 0.40–0.98 in the postmenopausal osteoporosis group). Treatment caused a reduction in the incidence of single and multiple vertebral fractures, with the reduction in vertebral fracture risk noted as early as after one year [54]. The ability of clodronate to reduce fracture risk was independent of traditional risk factors for fracture such as the presence of baseline vertebral fractures, age, corticosteroid use, smoking habits, weight, and BMD determined by ultrasound. Most importantly, the authors suggest that the reduction of fracture risk was independent of baseline BMD.

Zolendronic Acid

Zolendronic acid is the most potent bisphosphonate that has been studied to date. Small doses are required for the inhibition of bone resorption, and long dosing intervals may be used. A phase II study examined the effect of intravenous zolendronic acid on bone density and bone turnover in postmenopausal women with low bone density [67]. A total of 351 postmenopausal women, aged 45 to 80 years, were studied at 24 centers. Women were at least five years postmenopausal and had a BMD at the lumbar spine with a T-score of at least −2.0 and no more than one vertebral fracture at screening. All women received 1 g calcium supplement per day. Women were randomly assigned to receive 16 treatment regimens in a double-blind fashion. Three groups received zolendronic acid by intravenous infusion every three months, at doses of 0.25, 0.5, and 1 mg. Two other groups received the total dose of 4 mg of zolendronic acid either as a single infusion at the beginning of the trial or in divided doses at six-month intervals. A placebo group was included.

At baseline, the mean BMD values in the lumbar spine corresponded to a T-score of −2.9. All groups that received zolendronic acid showed a progressive, statistically significant increase in BMD at the lumbar spine throughout the 12-month study. There were no significant differences among the treatment groups. At 12 months, the mean lumbar spine BMD in the treatment groups was 4.3–5.1% higher than in the placebo group. The BMD at the femoral neck increased progressively throughout treatment, with the femoral neck BMD having increased 3.1 to 3.5% over that of the controls at the end of 12 months (P < 0.001). At the distal radius, BMD of the treated group had increased by 0.8–1.6% at the end of 12 months, whereas in the control group the BMD of the distal radius had decreased by 0.8%. Markers of bone resorption reached a nadir at one month; the median decrease was more than half for serum C-telopeptide and for the urinary N-telopeptide. These decreases were maintained for the next 11 months, while no significant changes were noted in the placebo group. Biopsies of transiliac bone specimens from treated women showed decreases in mineralizing surfaces, in rates of bone formation, in adjusted mineral apposition rates, and in the activation frequency. No changes were noted in cortical bone thickness, porosity, or cancellous bone volume. Likewise, there was no evidence of osteomalacia. Mean serum calcium concentrations were similar to those in the placebo group after three-months. Intact parathyroid hormone (PTH) was measured at baseline and 12 months. The mean value was about 30% higher than at baseline in the group receiving four doses of 1 mg of zolendronic acid. Adverse events were similar in all active treatment groups, but were significantly more common than in controls (45–67% versus 27% in the placebo group). Overall, it may be concluded that when the potent bisphosphonate zolendronic acid was administered intravenously on an intermittent basis, the resultant suppression of biochemical markers of bone turnover and the increases in BMD were similar to those encountered when bisphosphonate is given orally on a daily basis. The lowering of bone turnover due to a single infusion of zolendronic acid is long lasting: it is believed that zolendronic acid promptly becomes bound to bone and is slowly released back into the circulation.

Long-Term Efficacy of the Bisphosphonates

Because bisphosphonates are relatively new antiresorptive agents with a unique mechanism of action, long-term safety concerns have been raised. In an extension of a three-year ("VERT") multinational study [71], subjects were followed for a total of five years. Women who completed the study in the original study centers were entered in an extension study where they continued to receive either risedronate or placebo. Over the two-year extension, risedronate reduced the risk of new vertebral fracture by 59% (95% CI, 19–79%; P = 0.01). Over the five years, risedronate treatment produced significant increases in the lumbar spine BMD (9.3%), with the differences between treated and control groups increasing with time. The proportion of women reporting serious adverse events or withdrawing from the study was similar in both the treatment and control groups. These observations are reassuring regarding the safety and efficacy of five years of treatment.

Recently, the results of 10 years of alendronate treatment of postmenopausal women with osteoporosis have been published [9]. Treatment with alendronate, 10 mg/day, for 10 years produced increases in BMD of 13.7% of the lumbar spine, 10.3% of the trochanter, 5.4% of the femoral neck, and 6.7% of the total proximal femur as compared to baseline values. Importantly, during years 6 through 10, the alendronate treated groups had no significant decline in BMD at any skeletal site. Markers of bone remodeling were reduced to the normal premenopausal range and this effect was sustained through 10 years of treatment. In the group in which medication was discontinued, BMD at the lumbar spine and trochanter did not change significantly after year five, but BMD decreased significantly at the femoral neck and forearm. During the initial three-year study, 6.2% of women in the placebo group had new morphometric vertebral fractures, as compared to 3.2% in the pooled alendronate groups (P = 0.03). The rates of fracture could not be accurately assessed because the date of occurrence within the observational interval was not known. Other difficulties in interpretation of fracture rates are due to the lack of a long-term placebo group. After discontinuation of alendronate, levels of markers of bone remodeling increased within a year, but remained below baseline values. Safety profiles were similar in all three groups, including the incidence of gastrointestinal adverse events. The observed increases in BMD at the lumbar spine during long-term alendronate therapy are consistent with a positive bone balance. The increase in secondary mineralization is a contributing factor to the increase in BMD. The measured levels of bone remodeling markers remained stable and within the premenopausal range during treatment. The long retention time of alendronate in bone may result in recycling of the compound and residual suppression of bone resorption after discontinuation.

How Long Should Bisphosphonate Therapy Be Continued?

Because bisphosphonate is incorporated into bone, a single administration can retain its activity for a long period of time even after drug discontinuation. Controversy exists regarding the appropriate duration of therapy with bisphosphonates. With continuous bisphosphonate use, there has been no waning of efficacy up to 10 years with alendronate [9]. In early postmenopausal women, after two years of treatment with alendronate or risedronate, indices of bone turnover returned towards baseline and bone loss continued at a rate similar to the control group. When alendronate therapy was discontinued after two to five years in older postmenopausal women, BMD remained stable and bone turnover remained suppressed for at least two years [9]. The relationship to fracture efficacy, however, remains less well defined due to the lack of a placebo group in this trial. If

fracture efficacy is not known, it is difficult to make recommendations on the length of treatment. As more potent bisphosphonates become available, this issue will become more difficult to resolve because it is likely that continued suppression of bone turnover may occur long after the drug has been discontinued.

Bisphosphonate Use in Children with Osteoporosis or Genetic Bone Disorders

Children with juvenile osteoporosis have been treated with bisphosphonates. Although the trials are small in size, they point to a small clinical benefit [6, 10]. Several studies have evaluated the effect of bisphosphonates in children with osteogenesis imperfecta [3, 33]. These studies showed that bisphosphonate treatment caused an increase in bone density and reduction of fracture incidence without apparent impairment of skeletal growth. However, a recent case of a child who was overtreated with bisphosphonate and developed profound osteopetrosis was reported [79]. Bisphosphonate treatment should, therefore, be used with caution in children.

Summary of Bisphosphonates

The bisphosphonates are excellent antiresorptive therapies that have been in clinical practice for a number of years. Two orally administered bisphosphonates, alendronate and risedronate, are approved for use in United States. Both of these agents are available for weekly dosing.

Intravenously administered bisphosphonates are currently under investigation. The convenience of intravenous administration, which may be as infrequently as yearly, may provide significant advantage over weekly oral dosing. It is anticipated that compliance would be greatly enhanced by this infrequent administration, however reimbursement issues are unknown. In addition, avascular necrosis of the jaw [53] and renal toxicity [39, 52] have been reported as occurring when certain doses of bisphosphonates have been administered intravenously. For this reason, until data are finalized and regulatory approval is completed, the weekly oral bisphosphonates are recommended. In patients who are intolerant to oral bisphosphonates administration, other antiresorptives may be tried.

Estrogen as an Antiresorptive Agent on Bone

Early cross-sectional studies revealed that BMD decreased with the onset of the menopause. In comparison with age-matched controls, women who undergo premature menopause exhibit a lower bone density in the spine and femur compared to age-matched controls [68]. Bone loss is associated with lower serum levels of estradiol and is most rapid in the years following natural or surgical menopause. This rapid phase of bone loss results in bone loss at rate of 3% per year in the spine and lasts for approximately five years [31]. Thereafter, bone loss slows to a rate of about 0.5–1.0% per year. Estrogen improves activation frequency and preserves bone remodeling, whereas estrogen deficiency decreases the activation of bone remodeling units. The major action of estrogen is to inhibit osteoclasts, which occurs through several different mechanisms. Evidence obtained in avian, rabbit, and human species suggests that estrogen acts directly on the osteoclast by regulating specific genes. RANKL (receptor activator of NFκB ligand) binds to the receptor RANK on the osteoclast surface; this results in the differentiation, activation and increased survival of osteoclasts and leads to an increase in bone resorption [42]. The decoy receptor to RANKL, osteoprotegerin (OPG) is secreted by osteoblasts and reduces RANK–RANKL interactions to inhibit the osteoclast. The fall in estrogen at the time of the menopause decreases the production of OPG; this allows increased RANK–RANKL interactions and increased bone resorption.

Randomized, Placebo-Controlled Trials Using Estrogen: Adherence and Response

One of the important issues regarding prevention or treatment of osteoporosis with estrogen is the number of responders versus nonrespon-

ders to therapy. Estimates of the number of nonresponders vary widely and range from less than 1% to as high as 30%. Difficulties occur because within-person measurement of BMD requires longitudinal measurements. In an analysis of the postmenopausal estrogen/progestin interventions (PEPI) trial, 875 healthy postmenopausal women aged 45–64 years of age were randomized to one of five treatment groups: placebo, conjugated equine estrogens (CEE) 0.625 mg/day; CEE, 0.625 mg/day plus medroxyprogesterone acetate (MPA), 10 mg/day for 12 day/month; CEE 0.625 mg/day plus MPA, 2.5 mg/day; or CEE 0.625 mg/day plus micronized progesterone, 200 mg/day for 12 days/month. Replicate BMD measurements were used to calculate the within-person measurement errors. The investigators also developed several criteria to classify subjects who were actually losing bone. Only subjects who adhered to the prescribed protocol were included in the results analysis. In the first 12 months 2.3% of the subjects lost bone at the total hip. This percentage fell to 0.4% in the next 12–36 months of the study. This indicates that bone loss in women taking hormone therapy is rare [34].

Estrogen and Bone Markers

There are few randomized, placebo-controlled trials that have evaluated the effect of estrogen on biochemical markers of bone turnover. The PEPI trial [34] (see above) tested eight different bone turnover markers and correlated bone markers with BMD of the spine and hip. In the active treatment groups, the mean levels of all bone turnover markers decreased and remained below baseline values throughout the three years of study. In the 54 women assigned to the placebo group, no changes from baseline in the mean levels of any bone turnover marker occurred. With further analysis, the authors suggested that that at baseline, age and bone mass index accounted for 16% and 25% of the variance in the hip and spine BMD, respectively. One of the most sensitive markers was the N-telopeptide of type I collagen (NTX), which accounted for 12% and 8% of the variance at the spine and hip, while the carboxy-terminal telopeptide of type I collagen accounted for 8% and 7% of the variance, respectively. Nevertheless, biochemical markers of bone turnover are not considered useful surrogates for BMD to identify individuals with low BMD who might benefit from treatment [51].

BMD in Postmenopausal Estrogen Progestin Intervention (PEPI) Trial: BMD

In the PEPI trial, BMD measured at baseline, 12 and 36 months were outcome measures of great interest. In the placebo-treated group, there was an average loss of 1.8% and 1.7%, respectively, of lumbar spine and hip BMD at the end of three years. In the active-treatment groups, BMD gains ranged from 3.5% to 5.0% in the lumbar spine and averaged 1.7% in the hip. Among the adherent participants, no significant differences in BMD were noted among the active treatment groups. Women who were older, had lower BMD at baseline, or no history of hormone therapy had larger, more significant gains in BMD compared to younger women, those with higher baseline BMD or those with prior hormone therapy [2].

Other Formulations of Estrogen

Other types of estrogen have been evaluated for their effects on BMD. In one study, 75 women, median age 65 years, received transdermal patches that delivered 0.1 mg/day of estradiol for days 1 to 21 and oral medroxyprogesterone acetate (10 mg/day) for days 11 to 21 of the 28 day cycle [50]. Women had a lumbar spine and femoral neck BMD below the 10th percentile of premenopausal women and greater than one vertebral fracture defined as a decrease in vertebral height of greater than 15%. Eight new fractures occurred in seven women in the estrogen group, compared with 20 fractures in 12 women in the placebo group (relative risk in the estrogen group for a new vertebral fracture, 0.39; 95% CI, 0.16–0.95; P = 0.04). The median percentage change in BMD in the estrogen group was compared to the placebo group. At the lumbar spine, estrogen-treated women experienced a 5.3% change compared to 0.2% in the placebo group. At the femoral trochanter, hormone treated women had a 7.6% increase compared with 2.1% in the placebo group. Histomorphometric evaluation of iliac biopsy samples confirmed the effect of estrogen on bone formation rate expressed on a per bone volume basis. Over a three-year period, the overall increase was 12% above baseline in the lumbar spine BMD in the estrogen-treated group. Measurements of biochemical markers such as serum osteocalcin, serum bone alkaline phosphatase, and urinary hydroxyproline remained depressed [49]. Other studies indicate that transdermal estradiol increased BMD of the spine from 0.8% to 3.7% [28]. Transcutaneous estradiol gel increased BMD approximately 3% in the lumbar spine over the BMD of the placebo group [70].

Ultra-low-dose Estrogen

Several studies have indicated that even in postmenopausal women who are not treated with estrogen, higher serum levels of estradiol are associated with higher BMD and reduced fracture risk, compared with those women within the same cohort with lower serum estradiol levels. Ultra low doses of parental 17-β estradiol administered in the form of a vaginal ring were studied in older women (60 years or older) for a six month period. The ring provided 7.5 μg of estradiol/24 h. Forearm bone density increased by 2.1% in the estradiol users, whereas nonusers lost 2.7%. Bone formation markers decreased in the treatment group, suggesting reduced bone turnover. In this short-term study, there was no evidence of endometrial proliferation as determined by ultrasonography [56].

Recently, a much lower dose of transdermal estradiol was studied than used traditionally. In a randomized, placebo-controlled, blinded trial, 417 postmenopausal women with a BMD z-score < −2.0 were given a transdermal patch that delivered 0.014 mg/day of either estradiol (to increase serum estradiol to 10–15 pg/ml) or placebo. All subjects were treated with 800 mg calcium and 400 IU vitamin D. In this two-year trial, there was a significant increase in lumbar spine BMD of 2.3% in the estradiol-treated group at one year compared with an increase of only 0.5% in the placebo-treated group (P < 0.001). After two years, an increase in the estradiol treated group of 3.0% occurred (P < 0.001 compared to placebo) [27]. At the total hip, the placebo group lost 0.7% of bone at 24 months compared to a gain of 0.8% in the estradiol treated group (P < 0.001). Median fall in CTX was −20% in the estradiol treatment group, with about a 15% fall in markers of bone formation. In this small trial, progestogen was not used, and there were no differences in adverse events in the treatment and placebo groups. Of note, there were no changes in the endometrium, serum lipid levels, or common side effects such as breast tenderness. Other trials have evaluated low-dose estradiol as an alternative to the standard doses of hormone therapy provided in the past [61].

Results from the Women's Health Initiative (WHI)

In clinical trials with estrogen, many of the earlier studies were uncontrolled or contained a flawed control group. The recent publication of the results from the WHI has demonstrated unequivocally that estrogen reduces fracture risk. The use of estrogen alone is currently recommended for women who have undergone hysterectomy. Proven benefits include relief of vasomotor symptoms, of vaginal atrophy, and prevention of osteoporosis. In the WHI, women who had had a hysterectomy received either 0.625 mg/day of conjugated equine estrogen or placebo. The cohort consisted of 10,739 postmenopausal women, aged 50–79 years, and the study was conducted as a randomized, double-blind, placebo-controlled disease prevention trial. The average follow-up was 6.8 years. In a manner similar to that found with combined hormone therapy, there was a reduction in fracture risk with estrogen alone. The hazard ratio of hip fracture on estrogen therapy was 0.61 (nominal 95% CI, 0.41–0.91), for vertebral fracture was 0.65 (nominal 95% CI, 0.42–0.93), and for total fractures was 0.70 (nominal 95% CI, 0.63–0.79). This trial provides strong evidence that conjugated equine estrogen alone reduces the risk of hip, clinical vertebral, and other fractures. The magnitude of reduction was similar to that observed in the WHI combination hormone trial and is consistent with prior observational studies and recent meta-analyses [80].

Interestingly, in the WHI, BMD was only measured in a small subset of women (N = 1,024), who were thought to represent the overall population enrolled in the WHI. The number of women who were osteoporotic was relatively small: 4 % had osteoporosis at the total hip in the hormone therapy group and 6% of women had osteoporosis in the placebo group (defined as a T-score of −2.5). Notwithstanding the small

number of women with osteoporosis, hip fracture was reduced by 33% (HR, 0.67; 95% nominal CI, 0.47–0.96). In a subgroup analysis, hormone therapy decreased the risk of hip fracture by 60% among women who reported a baseline calcium intake of more than 1,200 mg/day. Hazards ratios for total fractures were also lower for all groups who received hormone therapy (HR 0.67; nominal 95% CI, 0.69–0.83). Total hip BMD increased on the average by 1.7% during the first year of hormone therapy and by 3.7% by the end of year 3. After three years of treatment, the difference in favor of hormone therapy reached 4.5% in the lumbar spine and 3.6% in total hip. The WHI hormone therapy trial was the first randomized clinical trial to demonstrate that combination hormone therapy reduced the risk of fractures at the hip, vertebrae, and wrist, even in women who on the basis of BMD did not meet diagnostic criteria for osteoporosis.

Selective Estrogen Receptor Modulators (SERMs) and Postmenopausal Osteoporosis

Although estrogen therapy is approved for prevention of osteoporosis, compliance is low due to adverse effects, especially continued menstrual bleeding. In a recent telephone survey of women who are members of the Kaiser foundation health plan, 62% of those aged 50–55 years and 48% of women 65 years or older discontinued hormone therapy within one year of initiating treatment [25]. Thus, agents that mimic the effect of estrogen on bone, but not on the uterus, were studied.

Tamoxifen

Triphenylethylene compounds were initially evaluated as antitumor agents. Tamoxifen is a partial estrogen agonist with properties of estrogen antagonism. Tamoxifen binds to estrogen receptors and in certain tissues blocks the effect of endogenous estrogen. Tamoxifen antagonizes the growth of estrogen-dependent breast tumor cells and is commonly used in breast cancer patients as an adjuvant therapy. Several studies suggested that tamoxifen may act as a bone antagonist in estrogen-replete premenopausal women. The National Cancer Institute sponsored a trial to test the effect of tamoxifen to prevent breast cancer in high risk subjects. A subset of the trial participants had BMD measurements at baseline, and at one, two, and five years. The primary endpoint of this trial was to prevent breast cancer, and the trial was stopped early because of success in achieving the primary endpoint. Although the number of subjects with BMD measurements at the five-year time point thus was reduced, pre-menopausal women experienced a significant loss of BMD at the hip and spine. Based on limited data, monitoring of BMD in pre-menopausal women using tamoxifen is prudent. In contrast, tamoxifen has a partial protective effect on the skeleton in postmenopausal women [47].

Raloxifene

Raloxifene was developed as an antitumor agent, but its ability to maintain bone density in animal studies led to the implementation of clinical testing. In postmenopausal women, administration of raloxifene decreased bone turnover markers, although to a lesser extent than when they received conjugated equine estrogens. A double-blind, randomized controlled study compared the effects of raloxifene (60 mg per day) to those of a conjugated equine estrogen (0.625 mg/day) [61]. There was a marked decrease in CTX and NTX (59% and 43%, respectively) in the estrogen-treated women, compared to decreases of 23% and 22%, respectively, in raloxifene-treated women. Greater reductions in markers of bone formation such as osteocalcin, bone specific alkaline phosphatase, and C-terminal type I procollagen peptide occurred in the estrogen-treated group. BMD increased in both raloxifene and estrogen treated groups, but the women treated with conjugated equine had a greater increase in BMD after six months. Bone biopsies revealed no distinct histomorphometric differences in static indices. Dynamic indices of bone remodeling were decreased from baseline in the conjugated equine estrogen group, but not in the raloxifene group. Mineralizing surface did not change in either group, suggesting that mineralization was not adversely affected. Bone architecture was also similar in both groups. The Multiple Outcomes of Raloxifene Evaluation (MORE) study was a multicenter, randomized, blinded,

placebo-controlled trial with 7,705 participants aged 31–80 years [24]. At enrollment, the women had to be at least two years postmenopausal with a BMD T-score of less than or equal to −2.5 at the lumbar spine or femoral neck. Participants were randomly assigned to take placebo, raloxifene 60 mg/day, or raloxifene 120 mg/day. In terms of bone turnover markers, osteocalcin decreased by an average of 8.6%, 26.3%, and 31.1% in the placebo, 60-mg/day-raloxifene, and 120-mg/day-raloxifene groups, respectively. Urinary CTX decreased in a similar manner. Women receiving raloxifene had fewer new fractures, whether or not they had a vertebral fracture at the time of study entry. The relative risk of vertebral fracture was 0.7 (95% CI, 0.5–0.8) for the 60 mg/day raloxifene-treated group and 0.5 (95% CI, 0.4–0.7) for the 120 mg/day treated group. After 4 years the reduction in vertebral fracture risk was maintained (RR 0.64 in the 60 mg/day raloxifene-treated group) [22]. As compared to the placebo treated women, women treated with 60 mg/day increased BMD at the femoral neck and spine (by 2.1% and 2.6% respectively).

One of the major side effects in this trial was that women receiving raloxifene had an increased risk of venous thromboembolism (RR 3.1; 95% CI, 1.5–6.2). There was a slight increase in the number of hot flashes and of leg cramps in the raloxifene-treated subjects (hot flashes: 6.4% in the placebo-treated group vs. 9.7% in the 60-mg/day-raloxifene group; leg cramps: 3.7% in the placebo-treated group vs. 7.0% in the 60-mg/day-raloxifene group) [24].

Two identical studies enrolled 1,145 healthy, postmenopausal women worldwide in a parallel, double-blind, placebo-controlled trial. Subjects received placebo, or one of three doses (30, 60, or 150 mg/day) of raloxifene for three years. In the placebo group, there was a −1.32% loss of BMD at the lumbar spine. In the raloxifene-treated groups, there was a respective increase of 0.71%, 1.28%, and 1.20% (30, 60, or 150 mg/d) in BMD at the lumbar spine. Similar changes in BMD were noted at the hip. As with the larger MORE trial, the only significant adverse event was an increase in the number of hot flashes [40].

New Generation SERMs

Levormeloxifene has been evaluated in a phase II clinical trial in which there was a significant increase in lumbar spine BMD. Unfortunately, endometrial thickness increased in the levormeloxifene group and 8 women experienced uterovaginal prolapse. As a result, this SERM is no longer in clinical development [1].

Lasofoxifene is a potent SERM under evaluation for prevention and treatment of postmenopausal osteoporosis. A phase two randomized, double-blind, placebo-controlled study examined the efficacy in bone loss prevention in 190 postmenopausal women. The trial duration was for one year in subjects aged 50–68 years. Subjects received lasofoxifene (0.4, 2.5, and 10 mg/day), or conjugated equine estrogen/medroxyprogesterone (0.6 25/2 .5 mg/day) or placebo. All received calcium and vitamin D daily. All lasofoxifene doses increased lumbar spine and BMD compared with placebo; however, there were no significant differences among groups for hip BMD. Lasofoxifene decreased biochemical markers of bone turnover (P < 0.01) and lowered LDL-cholesterol (P < 0.001). The most commonly reported adverse events associated with lasofoxifene were hot flashes, leg cramps, and leucorrhea [26].

Calcitonin

Calcitonin is a physiologic, endogenous inhibitor of bone resorption. Its inhibition of osteoclast formation and attachment results in bone resorption *in vivo* and *in vitro*. Several studies have evaluated calcitonin as an agent to decrease bone resorption in postmenopausal osteoporosis. Salmon calcitonin has been administered by injection or by nasal spray. A five-year, multicenter clinical trial (the Prevent Recurrence of Osteoporotic Fractures [PROOF] study) determined the long-term safety and efficacy of salmon calcitonin nasal spray in the prevention of vertebral fractures in postmenopausal women with osteoporosis [12]. This double-blind, placebo-controlled trial was conducted in 42 centers in the United States and in five centers in the United Kingdom. Patients were eligible to be included in the study if they were postmenopausal and a lumbar spine BMD T-score of less than or equal to −2. A total of 1,255 women received salmon calcitonin nasal spray at a dose of 100, 200, or 400 IU. All participants received 1,000 mg oral calcium and a multivitamin containing 400 IU vitamin D. Fifty-nine percent of the participants withdrew from the study prematurely, with dropout similar in all dosage groups. A 33% reduction in the relative risk of developing a new vertebral fracture took place in the salmon calcitonin nasal spray 200 IU group compared with the placebo group (RR = 0.67, 95% CI, 0.47–0.97; P = 0.03). In women who had one to five fractures at enrollment, the relative risk was reduced by 35% (P = 0.13) [12]. There were no significant differences in any of the outcomes when the 100 and the 400 IU treatment groups were compared to the placebo group. Compared with placebo, the percentage of participants with nonvertebral fractures was significantly lower in the group who had received 100 IU of salmon calcitonin nasal spray (P < 0.05). This was not true for the groups that had received either 200 or 400 IU. The small number of hip and femoral fractures precluded a meaningful statistical analysis. There was a nonsignificant reduction in the risk of hip fracture in the group that had received 200 IU (RR = 0.5, 95% CI, 0.2–1.6). A significant reduction in hip fractures was recorded in the group that received 100 IU (RR = 0.1, 95% CI, 0.01 to 0.9; P = 0.04), but not in the group that received 400 IU. The risk of fractures of the arm (humerus, radius, ulna, wrist) was significantly reduced in the group that had received the 100 IU dose, but this was not true for the 200 IU or 400 IU groups. Lumbar spine BMD did not change substantially in the placebo group during the course of the study. At years 1 and 2, the BMD of the lumbar spine increased significantly (P < 0.05) in all-calcitonin-treated groups. At the end of year 3, the increase in BMD of the lumbar spine was statistically greater in the 400 IU treatment group only. In the course of five years, lumbar spine BMD in each treatment group increased significantly from baseline every time point measured (P < 0.01). No clinically significant treatment effect on BMD was apparent at the femoral neck or trochanter. There was a statistically significant increase in years one and two in BMD at Ward's triangle in the group that received 200 IU.

Serum C-telopeptide levels decreased significantly from baseline in the groups that had received 200 IU and 400 IU salmon calcitonin by nasal spray. Compared with placebo, serum bone-specific alkaline phosphatase levels decreased significantly in the 200 IU group at each time point (P < 0.05). Serum osteocalcin levels decreased significantly from baseline values, but did not differ from the placebo values. Twenty-six percemt of participants in the 100 IU group, 29% in the 200 IU group, and 34% in the 400 IU group developed antibodies that bind salmon calcitonin with titers >1,000. However, the high titers of antibodies did not alter the effect of salmon calcitonin on the risk reduction of new vertebral fractures.

Adverse effects were similar in the treated and control groups, except for an increase in rhinitis in the calcitonin treatment groups. Rhinitis was defined as nasal congestion, nasal discharge, or sneezing and occurred in 22% of treated participants compared to 15% of the controls (P < 0.01). Headache was reported less frequently in the treated groups compared to the control group.

This five-year clinical trial indicates that 200 IU of salmon calcitonin administered daily by nasal spray significantly reduces the risk of new vertebral fractures by 33–36%. In postmenopausal women with low bone mass or prevalent vertebral fractures, it was surprising that there was no dose response to treatment. Nevertheless, this five-year study demonstrated a sustained effect on reduction of fracture risk at the spine, maintenance of improved BMD, and suppression of bone turnover. This suggests that resistance to the drug did not develop.

Overall, salmon calcitonin nasal spray appears to have been well tolerated. The high rate of dropout (12% per year over the five years) during this trial was disappointing, and it is difficult to anticipate what the outcome might have been had a larger number of subjects completed the trial. One explanation for the dropout rate may be that it was initially not considered ethical to withhold BMD results from the investigator and the participant in a long trial. Two new treatments for osteoporosis were approved in the United States while the trial was under way. Conceivably, the investigators or participants may have perceived the calcitonin spray to be ineffective, which might have caused some participants to drop out of the study prematurely.

The Use of Combination Antiresorptive Therapies

Several studies tested the effects of combination antiresorptive therapies to enhance efficacy further. Harris et al. [37] combined hormone therapy with risedronate in 524 ambulatory postmenopausal women with comparable lumbar spine BMD. Some women received 0.625 mg/day conjugated equine estrogens plus 5 mg/day risedronate, whereas others received 0.625 mg/day conjugated equine estrogens (plus placebo) daily for 12 months. Both the hormone-only and combination risedronate hormone groups produced significant increases from baseline in mean BMD at the lumbar spine, femoral neck, trochanter, midshaft radius, and distal radius. Markers of bone formation and resorption decreased significantly at all time points in both groups. The decrease in bone turnover markers was significantly greater at most time points in the combination therapy group compared to the group receiving hormone alone. Differences between treatment groups were relatively small and of uncertain clinical significance. The major limitation of the study was the short duration and the lack of a group that received risedronate only.

In another study of combination therapy, 573 postmenopausal women were given 0.625 mg/day of estrogen combined with medroxyprogesterone (2.5 mg/day), alendronate (10 mg/day), or a combination of hormone therapy plus alendronate. Bone mass of the entire cohort was categorized as osteopenic by the World Health Organization criteria; and among this cohort, 34% had osteoporosis. At the end of three years, total hip BMD showed a mean increase of 5.9% with combination alendronate and hormone therapy, an increase of 4.2% with alendronate alone and an increase of 3.0% with hormone alone (all P < 0.001). BMD remained level in the placebo group that was given calcium and vitamin D. At 36 months, women treated with combination therapy exhibited significantly greater increase in total hip and lumbar spine BMD than those on either alendronate or hormone therapy alone. At the posterior anterior lumbar spine, BMD increased 10.4% in the combination group, 7.7% in the alendronate group, 7.1% in the hormone therapy group, and 1.1% in the placebo group. It thus seems that combination therapy yielded greater improvements in BMD at the spine and total hip than treatment with either hormone therapy or alendronate alone. The study is important because the cohort of women were approximately a decade older than the subjects in the WHI that excluded women older than 79 years of age. Interestingly, therapy with alendronate alone was superior to hormone therapy, and combination therapy with both was superior to either one alone [35].

In a three-year, double-blind, placebo-controlled trial, women were randomized to receive alendronate (10 mg/day, n = 92), conjugated equine estrogen (0.625 mg/day, n = 143), alendronate and conjugated equine estrogen (n = 140), or placebo (n = 50) [34]. Women who received estrogen during the first two years and then were switched to placebo showed significant losses in BMD at the spine (−4.5%), total hip (−1.8%), femoral neck (−2.4%), and trochanter (−2.7%). Patients in the alendronate and combination therapy groups that were switched to placebo in year 3 showed no significant changes in BMD at any skeletal site. Women who continued taking combination therapy with alendronate and conjugated equine estrogens for the third year had a spine BMD that was 11.3% higher and a hip BMD that was 6.6% higher than placebo recipients. The accelerated rate of bone loss after discontinuation of hormone therapy has been confirmed in other studies. It is interesting to note that women who took placebo with calcium supplementation for three years maintained bone mass at the hip and spine.

The Use of Combination Anabolic and Antiresorptive Therapies

The question of efficacy and safety of combination therapy with antiresorptive and anabolic agents is frequently raised. An initial study that looked only at bone markers indicated that the combination of a bisphosphonate such as alendronate and of PTH, an anabolic agent, would have an additive effect [14]. Recently, several studies have been published that combine PTH with a bisphosphonate, estrogen, or SERM. Both PTH (1–34) and PTH (1–84) stimulate bone formation, in contrast to the antiresorptive agents that target the osteoclast. The actual findings in these studies were surprising, as using a bisphosphonate in combination with an anabolic agent was predicted to produce a larger increase in BMD than in either agent alone.

In a randomized, multicenter, double-blind clinical trial, therapy with rhPTH(1–84), alen-

dronate alone or the two in combination were studied [7]. Postmenopausal women, aged 55–85 years with a BMD T-score of −2.5, or a T-score of −2.0 with an additional risk factor (age >65 years, vertebral or nonvertebral fracture, or maternal history of fracture) were enrolled. Women who had previously been treated with bisphosphonate for more than one year were not excluded. All subjects were given 500 mg elemental calcium and 400 IU of vitamin D. A total of 238 women were randomly assigned to PTH(1–84) (n = 119), alendronate 10 mg/day (n = 60), or a combination of these agents (N = 59). Matching placebos were provided to the patients on monotherapy. Changes in the BMD of the lumbar spine in the PTH alone and the combination of PTH and alendronate groups were similar (6.3 and 6.1%, respectively) at 12 months. There was no statistical difference between these data and the 4.6% change in BMD of the lumbar spine in the group that received only alendronate. At the total hip and femoral neck sites, BMD remained unchanged in the group given only PTH. However, an increase in BMD at these sites occurred in the subjects on combination therapy or on alendronate alone. The increase in the total hip BMD on the combination therapy was statistically significant. At the distal radius, there was a statistically significant decrease in the PTH treated group and this effect was attenuated by the addition of alendronate. To evaluate volumetric density in these subjects, quantitative computer tomography was performed. The combined trabecular and cortical volumetric density of the lumbar spine revealed a finding similar to that found in the areal results. In the trabecular component of the lumbar spine, there was a significant increase in volumetric density of the lumbar spine in all groups, but the increase in the PTH treated group was approximately twice that found in the combination group. The amount of increase in volumetric density of the trabecular lumber spine was similar in the two groups that received either alendronate alone or a combination of the two agents. In all groups, the patterns of volumetric density were similar at the femoral neck. In the patients treated with PTH alone, cortical bone volumetric density increased significantly at the total hip (3.5%) and femoral neck (3.4%); this effect was mitigated by alendronate, suggesting that the antiresorptive may prevent bone formation due to PTH.

Finkelstein et al. [30] studied 83 men between 46 and 85 years of age with low BMD (T-score less than 2). The men were stratified into blocks on the basis of age (<65 years of age or >65 years of age) and according to BMD of the spine. Subjects received alendronate (10 mg/day), PTH (40 µg/day injected subcutaneously), or both. Alendronate was given for six months prior to the initiation of PTH therapy. The study was not double blind, because the IRB considered it unethical to administer placebo injections for two years. Calcium intake was ~1,000 mg/day through diet or supplementation and all subjects received 400 IU/day of vitamin D. The baseline characteristics of the 73 men included in the intention-to-treat analysis were similar among all treatment groups. BMD at the posterior anterior spine increased more in men treated with PTH alone than in those treated with alendronate alone or with a combination of the two. This was true even though the period of active PTH treatment was six months shorter when given alone. The BMD at the posterior anterior spine increased more with combination therapy than with alendronate alone (P < 0.001). At the femoral neck, BMD increased more in the PTH (9.7%; 95% CI 6.2–13.4) than in the alendronate group (3.2%; 95% CI 1.5–4.8) (P < 0.001) or the combined therapy group (6.2%; 95% CI 4.0–8.4) (P = 0.01). The BMD at the total hip increased more in the PTH (6.4%; 95% CI 3.6–9.1) than in the alendronate group (4.8%; 95% CI 3.3–6.3). Density at the total hip changed to the same degree in the alendronate and the combined therapy groups. The BMD at the radial shaft increased slightly in the alendronate (1.0%; 95% CI 0.2–1.8) and in the combined therapy groups (1.0%; 95% CI −0.1–2.1), but decreased slightly in the PTH treated group (−0.8%; 95% CI −2.3–0.6). Total body BMD did not differ in the three treatment groups.

Black et al. [7] reported similar data showing a negative effect of alendronate on PTH-induced bone formation in postmenopausal women. Alendronate administration diminished the PTH-associated increase in serum total alkaline phosphatase levels normally associated with PTH induction of osteoblastic activity. The finding that alendronate reduced the ability of PTH to increase the activity of serum alkaline phosphatase and reduced the effect on BMD at the spine and femoral neck suggests that the effect of PTH depends, at least in part, on its ability to reduce bone resorption.

These two studies [30, 7] indicate that with regard to trabecular bone at the spine, treatment by PTH alone is better than combination therapy of PTH and alendronate, either choice of which is better than alendronate alone. This contradicts the hypothesis that alendronate and PTH would have additive or synergistic effects. In men who were treated for a longer period of time [30], PTH therapy alone was the most effective treatment. Khosla [41] proposed that the overall inhibition of bone turnover by alendronate impairs the anabolic activity of PTH. There is little evidence that PTH can cause the pool of pre-osteoblastic cells to expand. If bone turnover and, therefore, bone formation is reduced, PTH may be less effective. Alternatively, alendronate may inhibit the osteoblast, preventing PTH from exerting its anabolic effect.

Combining PTH treatment with gonadal hormone replacement therapy (HRT) showed markedly different results. In one study, women who had been on HRT for at least two years were divided randomly into two groups. The first group remained on HRT and received daily PTH (1–34) (25 µg/day, subcutaneously) for three years, while the second group remained on HRT alone. Subjects in the combination therapy group increased their bone mass by 13.4% in the lumbar spine, 4.4% in the total hip, and 3.7% in the total body. After discontinuation of PTH, bone density measurements remained stable for one year. Vertebral fractures were reduced in the women on the combination PTH plus HRT therapy compared to women who did not get PTH (P < 0.02) [13]. In a smaller study (n = 17 per group), women received estrogens for one year and then were randomly assigned to receive either human PTH (1–34) plus estrogen or remain on estrogen alone. During the early months of PTH treatment, osteocalcin levels increased significantly; this had not been true in patients treated with a combination of alendronate and PTH. Bone mass in the lumbar spine increased continuously throughout the study in the PTH-treated group. At the end of three years of treatment, vertebral bone mass had increased by 13% in the PTH treated group and had not significantly declined in the group treated with hormone therapy alone. There was only a modest increase of 2.7% in the total hip for the PTH-treated patient and no significant decline in the hormone-treated group [46].

In a head-to-head study, Ettinger et al. [23] compared alendronate, raloxifene, and their combination with PTH on BMD in post-menopausal women aged 60 to 87 years with a prior lumbar spine or total hip BMD T-score of −2.0 on entry. Before the study, subjects had been regularly receiving alendronate (10 mg/day) or raloxifene (60 mg/day) for 18–36 months. All women received daily self-administered subcutaneous injections of teriparatide (rhPTH1–34), 20 µg/day, 1,000 mg calcium, and 400 IU of vitamin D. After one month of teriparatide treatment, both groups of women had statistically significant increases in median osteocalcin, PINP, and bone alkaline phosphatase levels. At 3 and 6 months, lumbar spine BMD increased 2.1% and 5.2%, respectively, relative to baseline in the group that had been on raloxifene. This was not true for the group that had been receiving alendronate. After 6 months, increases in BMD were similar in all groups. At 18 months, the lumbar spine BMD had increased 10.2% in the group that had been on raloxifene. It had increased only 4.1% in the group that had been on alendronate. Early changes in total hip BMD also differed: at 6 months, the raloxifene-treated group showed little change, whereas hip BMD decreased significantly in the alendronate group (−1.8%; P = 0.0002).

This study highlights differences in the mechanisms of action by raloxifene and alendronate, which may be related to the low availability of target cells for the anabolic actions of teriparatide. After two to three years of alendronate treatment, histomorphometric analyses of bone biopsy specimens indicated that bone activation frequency and mineralizing surfaces decreased by 90% compared to baseline [11]. Consequently, few osteoblasts or pre-osteoblasts are available for teriparatide to act on. An alternative explanation is that alendronate reduced the PTH-induced increase in bone resorption and thus prevented the osteoclast-dependent release of cytokines that stimulate bone formation. Raloxifene may cause less suppression of bone turnover, and thus allow osteoblast, pre-osteoblast and stromal target cells to remain available as target cells for the anabolic actions of PTH. The finding that lumbar spine BMD and bone turnover markers were not correlated in the subjects treated previously with alendronate supports the concept that changes in the remodeling rates and in mineralization are responsible for obscuring the anabolic effects of PTH.

Meta-analysis of Antiresorptive Therapies

A series of meta-analyses were recently published that utilized the Cochrane Collection system to evaluate the changes in BMD and fracture risk associated with antiresorptive therapies [15, 20]. The methodology is described in detail in the first paper of the series [15] and the summary [20] cautions the reader that these data should not be used as head-to-head comparisons among antiresorptive agents.

Eleven trials evaluated the effect of alendronate for at least one year [16]. BMD changes varied positively with both dose and time of alendronate administration. After three years of treatment with 10 mg/day of alendronate or more, the pooled estimate of the difference in percentage change between alendronate and placebo was 7.48% (95% CI, 6.12–8.85) for the lumbar spine (2–3 years), 5.60% (95% CI, 4.80–6.39) for the hip (3–4 years), and 2.08% (95% CI, 1.53–2.63) for the forearm (2–4 years). The effects on BMD were similar in the prevention and treatment trials. The pooled relative risk for vertebral fractures in subjects given 5 mg/day or more of alendronate was 0.52 (95% CI, 0.43–0.65). The relative risk of nonvertebral fractures in patients given 10 mg/day or more of alendronate was 0.51 (95% CI, 0.38–0.69). The relative risk of adverse events was pooled from data reported from nine trials: the relative risk leading to discontinuation of alendronate was 1.15 (95% CI 0.93–1.42) largely due to gastrointestinal side effects. Although these relative risks for adverse events are low, they may not apply to the general population, which on average may be less healthy than participants in a clinical trial setting.

For risedronate, a total of nine randomized, placebo-controlled clinical trials in post-menopausal women were reviewed [17]. The increase in BMD at the lumbar spine, femoral neck, and combined forearm was generally larger for the 5-mg/day dose than seen for cyclic administration or for lower doses. The pooled estimate of the difference in percentage change in BMD between 5 mg/day of risedronate and placebo after the final year of treatment (1.5–3 years) was 4.54% (95% CI, 4.12–4.97) for the lumbar spine, and 2.75% (95% CI, 2.32–3.17) at the femoral neck. The pooled relative risk for vertebral fractures in postmenopausal women given 2.5 mg or more of risedronate was decreased to 0.64 (95% CI, 0.54–0.77). The pooled relative risk of non-vertebral fractures in patients given risedronate was also decreased to 0.73 (95% CI, 0.61–0.87). In the eight trials that provided information about adverse events and discontinuation, no treatment effect was noted [77].

For HRT, 57 randomized placebo trials lasting more than one year (calcium/vitamin D as placebo) were reviewed [78]. Seven trials included fracture risk. HRT had a consistent effect on BMD at all sites, with the largest effect noted at the lumbar spine. The difference between HRT and control in the percent change in bone density at two years was 6.76% (95% CI, 5.83–7.89; 21 trials) at the lumbar spine and 4.53% (95% CI, 3.68–5.36; 14 trials) and 4.12% (95% CI, 3.45–4.80; 9 trials) at the forearm and femoral neck, respectively. The effects of combined estrogen and progestogen therapy were similar to unopposed estrogen, but consistently larger, from 1% to 3%, after two years of therapy [78]. No differences were noted when the data were analyzed by the type of estrogen preparation. Although the relative risk for vertebral and non-vertebral fractures was estimated, this estimate has been supplanted by the data obtained from the WHI (see above).

Seven trials with raloxifene were included for meta-analysis. Raloxifene resulted in positive effects on the percentage change in BMD, which increased over time and was independent of dose. There was an increased impact on BMD with longer duration of use of raloxifene, but no impact of dose. Data from one large dominating trial suggested a reduction in vertebral fractures with a relative risk of 0.60 (95% CI, 0.50–0.70, P < 0.01). Raloxifene slightly increased rates of withdrawal from therapy as a result of adverse effects in three trials that were evaluated (RR 1.15, 95% CI, 1.00–1.33, P = 0.05). For other adverse events, four trials were evaluated. There was a significant increase in deep venous thrombosis in the raloxifene arm, as noted in the results from the MORE trial (3.51; 95% CI, 1.44–8.56, P = <0.01) [18].

A number of randomized trials suggested that calcitonin could prevent loss of BMD of the spine in late postmenopausal women. Due to the wide variability in the daily doses used, the authors used total weekly doses as the basis for comparison. Of 30 trials, all but two utilized salmon calcitonin [19]. Nine trials had a greater

than 20% loss to follow up and the largest trial, PROOF, had an almost 60% loss to follow up. For bone density of the lumbar spine, the pooled weekly dose of 250 to 2,800 IU per week resulted in significant increase in the weighted mean difference of 3.74% (95% CI, 2.04–5.43, P < 0.01, n = 2,260, 24 trials). The combined forearm showed a similar effect, with a difference of 3.02% (95% CI, 0.98–5.07, P < 0.01, n = 468, 9 trials). At the femoral neck, the pooled weighted mean difference showed a statistically nonsignificant trend toward benefit, 3.80% (95% CI, 0.32–7.91, P = 0.07, 9 trials, n = 513).

These meta-analyses provide precise pooled estimates of the magnitude of treatment effects for many antiresorptive therapies. Rigorous criteria were used to assess inclusion of the clinical trials in the analysis. Data are provided in Tables 8.1 and 8.2, but inferences and comparisons among the various therapies should not be drawn, as the confidence intervals around the treatment effects vary considerably and different patient populations and methodologies were employed in the various trials. For an individual patient, other factors weigh in on treatment selection such as side effects, cost, and convenience. These values and preferences may drive treatment decisions.

Conclusion

Currently, approximately 10 new compounds in phase II clinical trials are under investigation for the treatment of bone loss. In addition to the newer bisphosphonates and SERMs discussed above, other therapies that target the osteoclast have been developed. Several compounds that are now in preclinical or early clinical trials may be found useful to reduce osteoclast-mediated bone resorption. One such agent is an estrogen-related synthetic ligand that has non-genotropic effects on bone, thereby by-passing the reproductive organs. In animal studies, estren (4-estren-3α,17-diol) did not induce transcriptional activity in reproductive tissues of female mice, but inhibited etoposide-induced apoptosis in isolated osteoblasts and increased apoptosis of osteoclasts. In the estren-treated mice, the ovariectomy-induced bone loss was reduced and bone strength was restored, at least in part. These mechanism-specific ligands may provide

Table 8.1. Magnitude of Effect on Vertebral Fractures

Intervention	No. of Trials/Patients	Relative Risk (95% CI)	Relative Risk, P-value	Heterogeneity, P-value
Calcium	5 (576)	0.77 (0.54–1.09)	0.14	0.40
Vitamin D	8 (1130)	0.63 (0.45–0.88)	<0.01	0.16
Alendronate (5–40 mg)	8 (9360)	0.52 (0.43–0.65)	<0.01	0.99
Etidronate (400 mg)	9 (1076)	0.63 (0.44–0.92)	0.02	0.87
Risedronate	5 (2604)	0.64 (0.54–0.77)	0.01	0.89
Calcitonin[a]	1 (1108)	0.79 (0.62–1.00)	0.05	n/a
Raloxifene	1 (6828)	0.60 (0.50–0.70)	0.01	n/a
HRT	5 (3117)	0.66 (0.41, 1.07)	0.12	0.86
Fluoride (4 yr)	5 (646)	0.67 (0.38, 1.19)	0.17	0.01

[a] Due to the potential for publication bias, we are presenting the estimate for the larger RCT estimate from the PROOF trial. The pooled estimate for calcitonin from the PROOF trial and the three smaller studies combined is 0.46 (95% CI 0.25–0.87, P = 0.02, n = 1,404).
Reproduced with permission from Cranney A, Guyatt G, Griffith L, Wells G, et al. (2002) Summary of meta-analyses of therapies for postmenopausal osteoporosis. Endocrine Reviews 23(4):570–578. Copyright 2002, The Endocrine Society.

Table 8.2. Magnitude of Effect on Nonvertebral Fractures

Intervention	No. of Trials/Patients	Relative Risk (95% CI)	Relative Risk, P-value	Heterogeneity, P-value
Calcium	2 (222)	0.86 (0.43, 1.72)	0.66	0.54
Vitamin D	6 (6187)	0.77 (0.57, 1.04)	0.09	0.09
Etidronate	7 (867)	0.99 (0.69, 1.42)	0.97	0.94
Alendronate (5 mg)	8 (8603)	0.87 (0.73, 1.02)	0.09	0.31
Alendronate (10–40 mg)	6 (3723)	0.51 (0.38, 0.69)	<0.01	0.88
Raloxifene	2 (6961)	0.91 (0.79, 1.06)	0.24	0.43
Calcitonin[a]	1 (1245)	0.80 (0.59, 1.09)	0.16	n/a
Risedronate	7 (12958)	0.73 (0.61, 0.87)	<0.01	0.81
HRT	6 (3986)	0.87 (0.71, 1.08)	0.10	0.57
Fluoride	5 (950)	1.46 (0.92, 2.32)	0.11	0.06

[a] Due to the potential for publication bias, we are presenting the estimate for the larger RCT estimate from the PROOF trial. The pooled estimate for calcitonin from the PROOF trial and the three smaller studies combined is 0.52 (95% CI 0.22–1.23, P = 0.14, n = 1,481).
Reproduced with permission from Cranney A, Guyatt G, Griffith L, Wells G, et al. (2002) Summary of meta-analyses of therapies for postmenopausal osteoporosis. Endocrine Reviews 23(4):570–578. Copyright 2002, The Endocrine Society.

advantages over the more traditional estrogen-like compounds [43].

Cathepsin K is a cysteine protease that is highly expressed in osteoclasts and degrades bone matrix proteins, including collagen. Mutations of the gene that regulates cathepsin K result in mouse models consistent with phenotypic features of pcynodysostosis with increased bone density. Several areas are targeted on this pathway, since loss of cathepsin K function results in a decrease in osteoclast-mediated bone resorption. In addition, estrogen down-regulates cathepsin K expression, resulting in bone loss after the menopause [76].

Other agents interfere with physiologic pathways responsible for the differentiation, activation and survival of the osteoclast. The receptor activator of NFκB (RANK) is found on the osteoclast and is a specific mediator of osteoclast differentiation, function and survival. The ligand (RANKL) is secreted by the osteoblast and the binding of RANK to RANK ligand results in an increase in the number and activity of osteoclasts. Osteoprotegerin (OPG) is a decoy receptor that interferes with the binding of RANK ligand to its receptor RANK. Interference with any steps of this pathway results in decreased activity and differentiation of osteoclasts. Data from a recent phase 1 trial that tested an antibody to RANK ligand in postmenopausal women have shown a rapid, dose-dependent decrease in urinary

NTX/creatinine and serum NTX in healthy women [4].

Other targets directed toward the osteoclast include the alpha v beta 3 integrins that are responsible for the attachment of osteoclasts to bone, or interference with the GM-CSF differentiation pathway. Several compounds block osteoclast function or activity by interfering with the actin ring at the site of osteoclast attachment to bone.

References

1. Alexandersen P, Riis BJ, Stakkestad JA, Delmas PD, Christiansen C (2001) Efficacy of levormeloxifene in the prevention of postmenopausal bone loss and on the lipid profile compared to low dose hormone replacement therapy. JCEM 86:755–60.
2. Anonymous (1996) Effects of hormone therapy on BMD: results from the postmenopausal estrogen/progestin interventions (PEPI) trial. The writing group for the PEPI. Journal of the American Medical Association 276:1389–96.
3. Astrom E, Soderhall S (2002) Beneficial effect of long-term intravenous bisphosphonates treatment of osteogenesis imperfecta. Arch Dis Child 86:356–64.
4. Bekker PJ, Holloway DL, Rasmussen AS, Murphy R, et al. (2004) A single-dose placebo-controlled study of AMG 162, a fully human monoclonal antibody to RANKL, in postmenopausal women. JBMR 19:1059–66.
5. Bergstrom JD, Bostedor RG, Masarachia PJ et al (2000) Alendronate is a specific, nanomolar inhibitior of farnesyl diphosphate synthase. Arch Biochem Biophys 373:231–41.
6. Bianchi ML, Cimaz R, Bardare M, et al. (2000) Efficacy and safety of alendronate for the treatment of osteoporosis in diffuse connective tissue diseases in children: a prospective multicenter study. Arthritis Rheum 43: 1960–6.
7. Black DM, Greenspan SL, Ensrud KE, Palermo L, et al. (2003) The effects of PTH and alendronate alone or in combination in postmenopausal osteoporosis. NEJM 349(13):1207–15.
8. Black DM, Cummings SR, Karpf DB, Cauley JA, et al. (1996) Randomised trial of effect of alendronate on risk of fracture in women with existing vertebral fractures. The Lancet 348:1535–41.
9. Bone HG, Hosking D, Devogelaer JP, Tucci JR, et al. (2004) Ten years' experience with alendronate for osteoporosis in postmenopausal women. NEJM 350(12): 1189–99.
10. Brumsen C, Hamdy NA, Papapoulos SE (1997) Long-term effects of bisphosphonates on the growing skeleton. studies of young patients with severe osteoporosis. Medicine (Baltimore) 76:2166–83.
11. Chavassieux PM, Arlot ME, Reda C, Wei L, et al. (1997) Histomorphometric assessment of the long-term effects of alendronate on bone quality and remodeling in patients with osteoporosis. J Clin Invest 100:1475–80.
12. Chesnut CH, III, Silverman S, Andriano K, et al. (2000) A randomized trial of nasal spray salmon calcitonin in postmenopausal women with established osteoporosis: The prevent recurrence of osteoporotic fractures study. American Journal of Medicine 109:267–76.
13. Cosman F, Nieves J, Woelfert L, et al. (2001) PTH added to established hormone therapy: effects on vertebral fracture and maintenance of bone mass after PTH withdrawal. JBMR 16(5):925–32.
14. Cosman F, Nieves J, Woelfert L, et al. (1998) Alendronate does not block the anabolic effect of PTH in postmenopausal osteoporotic women. JBMR 13(6):1051–5.
15. Cranney A, Tugwell P, Wells G, Guyatt G, et al. (2002) Systematic reviews of randomized trials in osteoporosis: introduction and methodology. Endocrine Reviews 23(4):497–507.
16. Cranney A, Wells G, Willan A, Griffith L, et al. (2002) Meta-analysis of alendronate for the treatment of postmenopausal women. Endocrine Reviews 23(4): 508–16.
17. Cranney A, Tugwell P, Adachi J, Weaver B, et al. (2002) Meta-analysis of risedronate for the treatment of postmenopausal osteoporosis. Endocrine Reviews 23(4): 517–23.
18. Cranney A, Tugwell P, Zytaruk N, Robinson V, et al. (2002) Meta-analysis of raloxifene for the prevention and treatment of osteoporosis. Endocrine Reviews 23(4):524–8.
19. Cranney A, Tugwell P, Zytaruk N, Robinson V, et al. (2002) Meta-analysis of calcitonin for the treatment of postmenopausal osteoporosis. Endocrine Reviews 23(4):540–51.
20. Cranney A, Guyatt G, Griffith L, Wells G, et al. (2002) Summary of meta-analyses of therapies for postmenopausal osteoporosis. Endocrine Reviews 23(4): 570–8.
21. Delmas PD, Recker RR, Chestnut CH, et al. (2004) Daily and intermittent oral ibandronate normalize bone turnover and provide significant reduction in vertebral fracture risk: results from the BONE study. Osteoporosis International 15:792–8.
22. Eastell R, Adachi J, Harper K, Sarkar S, Delmas PD, Ensrud K, et al. (2000) The effects of raloxifene on incident vertebral fractures in postmenopausal women with osteoporosis: 4-year results from the MORE trial. JBMR 15:S229.
23. Ettinger B, San Martin J, Crans G, and Pavo I (2004) Differential effects of teriparatide on BMD after treatment with raloxifene or alendronate. JBMR 19(5):745–51.
24. Ettinger B, Black DM, Mitlak BH, Knickerbocker RK, Nickelsen T, Genant HK, et al. (1999) Reduction of vertebral fractures in postmenopausal women with osteoporosis treated with raloxifene: results from a 3-year randomized trial. JAMA 282:637–45.
25. Ettinger B, Pressman A, Silver P (1999) Effect of age on reasons for initiation and discontinuation of hormone replacement therapy. Menopause 6:289.
26. Ettinger M, Schwartz E, Emkey R, Moffett AF, et al. Lasofoxifene, a next generation selective estrogen receptor modulator (SERM), in the prevention of bone loss in postmenopausal women. The Endocrine Society's 86th Annual Meeting, New Orleans, LA, June 14–19, 2004: Abstract S35–2.
27. www.fda.gov

28. Field CS, Ory SJ, Wahner HW, Herrmann RR, et al. (1993) Preventive effects of transdermal 17 beta-estradiol on osteoporotic changes after surgical menopause: a two-year placebo-controlled trial. Am J Obstet Gynecol 168:114–21.

29. Filipponi P, Cristallini S, Rizzello E, Policani G, et al. (1996) Cyclical intravenous clodronate in post-menopausal osteoporosis: results of a long-term clinical trial. Bone 18:179–84.

30. Finkelstein J, Hayes A, Hunzelman J, et al. (2003) The effects of PTH, alendronate, or both in men with osteoporosis. NEJM 349(13):1216–26.

31. Gallagher JC (2001). Role of estrogens in the management of postmenopausal bone loss. Rheum Dis Clin North Am 27:143–62.

32. Giannini S, D'Angelo A, Sartori L. Passeri G, et al. (1996) Continuous and cyclical clondronate therapies and bone density in postmenopausal bone loss. Obstet Gynecol 88:431–6.

33. Glorieux FH, Bishop NJ, Plotkin H, et al. (1998) Cyclic administration of pamidronate in children with severe osteogenesis imperfecta. NEJM 339:947–52.

34. Greendale GA, Wells B, Marcus R, Barrett-Connor E (2000) How many women lose BMD while taking hormone replacement therapy? Results from the post-menopausal estrogen/progestin interventions trial. Arch Intern Med 160:3065–71.

35. Greenspan SL, Resnick NM, and Parker RA (2003) Combination therapy with hormone replacement and alendronate for prevention of bone loss in elderly women. JAMA 289(19):2525–33.

36. Greenspan SL, Emkey RD, Bone HG, Weiss SR, et al. (2002) Significant differential effects of alendronate, estrogen, or combination therapy on the rate of bone loss after discontinuation of treatment of post-menopausal osteoporosis. Ann Intern Med 137:875–83.

37. Harris ST, Watts NB, Genant HK, McKeever CD, et al. (1999) Effects of risedronate treatment on vertebral and nonvertebral fractures in women with postmenopausal osteoporosis. JAMA 282(14):1344–52.

38. Heaney RP, Saville PD (1976). Etidronate disodium in postmenopausal osteoporosis. Clin Pharm Therap 20: 593–604.

39. Ibrahim A, Scher N, Williams G, Sridhara R, et al. (2003) Approval summary for zoledronic acid for treatment of multiple myeloma and cancer bone metastases. Clinical Cancer Research. 9(7):2394–9.

40. Johnston CCJr, Bjarnason NH, Cohen FJ, Shah A, Lindsay R, Mitlak BH, et al. (2000) Long-term effects of raloxifene on BMD, bone turnover, and serum lipid levels in early postmenopausal women: three-year data from 2 double-blind, randomized, placebo-controlled trials. Arch Intern Med 160:3444–50.

41. Khosla S (2003) PTH plus alendronate – a combination that does not add up. NEJM 349(13):1277–9.

42. Kostenuik PJ and Shalhoub V (2001) Osteoprotegerin: a physiological and pharmacological inhibitor of bone resorption. Current Pharmaceutical Design 7(8):613–35.

43. Kousteni S, Han L, Chen J, Almeida M, Plotkin LI, et al. (2003) Kinase-mediated regulation of common transcription factors accounts for the bone-protective effects of sex steroids. Journal of Clinical Investigation 111(11):1651–64.

44. Lehenkari PP, Kellinsalmi M, Napankangas JP, et al. (2002) Further insight into mechanism of action of clodronate: inhibition of mitochondrial ADP/ATP translocase by a nonhydrolyzable, adenine-containing metabolite. Mol Pharmacol 61:1255–62.

45. Lieberman UA, Weiss SR, Bröll J, Minne HW, et al. (1995) Effect of oral alendronate on BMD and the incidence of fractures in postmenopausal osteoporosis. NEJM 333(22):1437–43.

46. Lindsay R, Nieves J, Formica C, et al. (1997) Randomised controlled study of effect of PTH on vertebral-bone mass and fracture incidence among postmenopausal women on oestrogen with osteoporosis. The Lancet 350:550–5.

47. Love RR, Mazess RB, Barden HS, Epstein S, Newcomb PA, Jordan VC, et al. (1992) Effects of tamoxifen on BMD in postmenopausal women with breast cancer. NEJM 326:852–6.

48. Luckman SP, Hughes DE, Coxon FP, et al. (1998) Nitrogen-containing bisphosphonates inhibit the mevalonate pathway and prevent post-translational prenylation of GTP-binding proteins, including Ras. JBMR 13:581–9.

49. Lufkin EG, Riggs LB (1996) Three-year follow up on effects of transdermal estrogen. Ann Intern Med 125(1):77.

50. Lufkin EG, Wahner HW, O'Fallon WM, Hodgson SF, et al. (1992) Treatment of postmenopausal osteoporosis with transdermal estrogen. Ann Intern Med 117(1):1–9.

51. Marcus R, Holloway L, Wells B, Greendale G, James MK, Wasilauskas C, et al. (1999) The relationship of biochemical markers of bone turnover to bone density changes in postmenopausal women: results from the postmenopausal estrogen/progestin interventions (PEPI) trial. JBMR 14:1583–95.

52. Markowitz GS, Appel GB, Fine PL, Fenves AZ, et al. (2001) Collapsing focal segmental glomerulosclerosis following treatment with high-dose pamidronate. Journal of the American Society of Nephrology 12(6): 1164–72.

53. Marx RE (2003) Pamidronate (Aredia) and zoledronate (Zometa) induced avascular necrosis of the jaws: a growing epidemic. Journal of Oral & Maxillofacial Surgery 61(9):1115–17.

54. McCloskey E, Selby P, Davies M, Robinson J, et al. (2004) Clodronate reduces vertebral fracture in women with postmenopausal or secondary osteoporosis: results of a double-blind, placebo-controlled 3-year study. JBMR 19(5):728–36.

55. McClung MR, Geusens P, Miller PD, Zippel H, et al. (2001) Effect of risedronate on the risk of hip fracture in elderly women. NEJM 344(5):333–40.

56. Naessen T, Berglund L, Ulmsten U (1997) Bone loss in elderly women prevented by ultralow doses of parenteral 17 beta-estradiol. Am J Obstet Gynecol 177:115–19.

57. Orwoll E, Ettinger M, Weiss S, Miller P, et al. (2000) Alendronate for the treatment of osteoporosis in men. NEJM 343:604–10.

58. Pecherstorfer M, Ludwig H, Schlosser K, et al. (1996) Administration of the bisphosphonate ibandronate (BM 21.0955) by intravenous bolus injection. JBMR 11(5):587–93.

59. Peretz A, Body JJ, Dumon JC, et al. (1996) Cyclical pamidronate infusions in postmenopausal osteoporosis. Maturitas 25:69–75.

60. Pols HA, Felsenberg D, Hanley DA, et al. (1999) Multinational, placebo-controlled, randomized trial of

the effects of alendronate on bone density and fracture risk in postmenopausal women with low bone mass: results of the FOSIT study. Osteoporosis International 9: 461–8.

61. Prestwood KM, Gunness M, Muchmore DB, Lu Y, Wong M, Raisz LG (2000) A comparison of the effects of raloxifene and estrogen on bone in postmenopausal women. JCEM 85:2197–202.

62. Ravn P, Weiss SR, Rodriquez-Portales JA, McClung MR, et al. (2000) Alendronate in early postmenopausal women: effects on bone mass during long-term treatment and after withdrawal. JCEM 85(4):1492–7.

63. Ravn P, Clemmesen B, Riis BJ, Christiansen C (1996) The effect on bone mass and bone markers of different doses of ibandronate: a new bisphosphonate for prevention and treatment of postmenopausal osteoporosis: a 1-year, randomized, double-blind, placebo-controlled dose-finding study. Bone 19(5):527–33.

64. Recker RR, Stakkestad JA, Felsenberg D, et al. (2000) A new treatment paradigm: quarterly injections of ibandronate reduce the risk of fractures in women with postmenopausal osteoporosis: results of 3-year trial. Osteoporosis International 11(Suppl. 2):S209.

65. Reginster JY, Christiansen C, Roux C, et al. (2001) Intermittent cyclic tiludronate in the treatment of osteoporosis. Osteoporosis International 12(3):169–77.

66. Reginster JY, Minne HW, Sorensen O, Hooper M, Roux C, Brandi ML, et al. (2000) Randomized trial of the effects of risedronate on vertebral fractures in women with established postmenopausal osteoporosis. Osteoporosis International 11:83–91.

67. Reid IR, Brown JP, Burckhardt P, Horowitz Z, et al. (2002) Intravenous zoledronic acid in postmenopausal women with low BMD. NEJM 346(9):653–61.

68. Richelson LS, Wahner HW, Melton LJ, III, Riggs BL (1984) Relative contributions of aging and estrogen deficiency to postmenopausal bone loss. NEJM 311: 1273–5.

69. Riis BJ, Ise J, Von Stein T, et al. (2001) Ibandronate: a comparison of oral daily dosing versus intermittent dosing in postmenopausal osteoporosis. JBMR 16(10): 1871–8.

70. Riis BJ, Thomsen K, Strom V, Christiansen C (1987) The effect of percutaneous estradiol and progesterone on postmenopausal bone loss. Am J Obstet Gynecol 156: 61–5.

71. Sorensen OH, Crawford GM, Mulder H, Hosking DJ, et al. (2003) Long-term efficacy of risedronate: a 5-year placebo-controlled clinical experience. Bone 32: 120–6.

72. Storm T, Thamsborg G, Steiniche T, et al. (1990) Effect of intermittent cyclical etidronate therapy on bone mass and fracture rate in women with postmenopausal osteoporosis. NEJM 322:1265–71.

73. Thiébaud D, Burckhardt P, Kriegbaum H, et al. (1997) Three monthly intravenous injections of ibandronate in the treatment of postmenopausal osteoporosis. The American Journal of Medicine 103:298–307.

74. Valimaki M, Laitinen K, Patronen A, Puolijoki H, et al. (2002) Prevention of bone loss by clondronate in early postmenopausal women with vertebral osteopenia: a dose-finding study. Osteoporosis International 13: 937–47.

75. VanBeek E, Pieterman E, Cohen L, et al. (1999) Nitrogen-containing bisphosphonates inhibit isopentenyl pyrophosphate isomerase/farnesyl pyrophosphate synthase activity with relative potencies corresponding to their antiresorptive potencies in vitro and in vivo. Biochem Biophys Res Commun 255:491–4.

76. Votta BJ, Levy MA, Badger A, Bradbeer J, et al. (1997) Peptide aldehyde inhibitors of cathepsin K inhibit bone resorption both in vitro and in vivo. JBMR 12:1396–406.

77. Watts NB, Harris ST, Genant HK, et al. (1990) Intermittent cyclical etidronate treatment of postmenopausal osteoporosis. NEJM 323(2):73–9.

78. Wells G, Tugwell P, Shea B, Guyatt G, et al. (2002) Meta-analysis of the efficacy of hormone replacement therapy in treating and preventing osteoporosis in postmenopausal women. Endocrine Reviews 23(4):529–39.

79. Whyte MP, Wenkert D, Clements KL, McAllister WH, Mumm S (2003) Bisphosphonate-induced osteoporosis. NEJM 349(5):457–63.

80. The Women's Health Initiative Steering Committee (2004) Effects of conjugated equine estrogen in postmenopausal women with hysterectomy. JAMA 291(14): 1701–12.

9.

Skeletal Complications of Malignancy: Central Role for the Osteoclast

Gregory A. Clines, John M. Chirgwin, and Theresa A. Guise

Introduction

Skeletal complications of malignancy are diverse and include hypercalcemia of malignancy, bone metastases, and oncogenic osteomalacia [78]. Of these syndromes, bone metastases are most common, followed by hypercalcemia of malignancy. Although the pathophysiology of these skeletal complications of cancer is diverse, it is clear that the osteoclast is a major player in the development and progression of both malignant hypercalcemia and bone metastases. As a result of the widespread treatment with bisphosphonates, hypercalcemia of malignancy is much less prevalent than it was 10 years ago and new therapies for bone metastases have become the focus of current research. Furthermore, cancer survival has increased as a result of advances in treatment. Because of the longer lifespan of cancer patients, a new skeletal complication of malignancy, referred to as cancer-treatment-induced bone loss, is likely to be the most common skeletal complication of malignancy in the coming years. Similar to hypercalcemia and bone metastases, the pathophysiology of this complication of cancer also intimately involves the osteoclast. Oncogenic osteomalacia remains relatively rare and will not be addressed in this chapter.

Hypercalcemia of Malignancy

Malignancy is the most common cause of hypercalcemia in the hospitalized patient, and malignancy-associated hypercalcemia is one of the more common paraneoplastic syndromes. Up to 30% of patients with cancer may develop hypercalcemia during the course of their disease [75, 78]. Hypercalcemia of malignancy may be due to (1) factors, secreted by tumors, that act systemically on target organs of bone, kidney, and intestine to disrupt normal calcium homeostasis; (2) local factors secreted by tumors in bone, either metastatic or hematological, which directly stimulate osteoclastic bone resorption; and (3) coexisting primary hyperparathyroidism.

The first two of these situations should be viewed as constituting the opposite ends of a continuous spectrum, rather than as completely unrelated pathologies. Clearly the pathophysiology of hypercalcemia in patients with solid tumors and no bone metastases at one end of the spectrum, and myeloma associated with extensive local bone destruction adjacent to the tumor cells at the other, is very different. However, in between these extremes are hypercalcemic patients with squamous cell carcinomas in whom hypercalcemia may occur, accompanied by not very extensive, osteolytic bone metastases, and hypercalcemic patients with advanced breast carcinoma in whom hypercalcemia almost never occurs unless osteolytic bone destruction is extensive. Separating hypercalcemia into categories on the assumption that the underlying mechanisms are distinct is not entirely satisfactory because the same mediator molecule may be of local or systemic origin. However, if tumor burden is extensive, enough mediators may be generated by the tumors to have both local and systemic effects. This review will categorize the effects of cancer on bone, but in a significant proportion of cancer patients, i.e., those in the middle of this spectrum, the effects on bone are due to both humoral and local mediators.

Humoral Mediators of Hypercalcemia of Malignancy

Parathyroid Hormone-related Protein

Hypercalcemia has been associated with malignancy since the development of serum calcium assays in the 1920s. Only in 1941, however, did Fuller Albright advance the hypothesis that PTH is ectopically produced by certain tumors. Over the subsequent five decades investigators determined that PTH was not, in fact, the cause for most cases of humoral hypercalcemia of malignancy (HHM), but that a "PTH-like factor" was responsible. In 1987 this PTH related-protein (PTHrP) was isolated from human lung cancer [131], breast cancer [24], and renal cell carcinoma [190], and was cloned shortly thereafter [194].

PTHrP shares 70% sequence homology with PTH over the first 13 amino acids at the N-terminus. Beyond the initial amino-terminal sequence the protein is unique and shows no further sequence homology with PTH. The PTHrP protein is larger than PTH and three distinct isoforms of 139, 141, and 173 amino acids have been identified. Similarly, the human PTHrP gene is much larger and more complex than the PTH gene, spanning 15 kb of genomic DNA with nine exons and three promoters. These differences not withstanding, both PTH and PTHrP bind to a common PTH/PTHrP receptor [1, 66] and share similar biological activities [86].

PTHrP has been detected in a variety of tumor types as well as in normal tissue. The widespread expression of PTHrP in normal tissue was the first evidence that the hormone had a role in normal physiology. In addition to its PTH-like effects, PTHrP plays a role in the (1) regulation of cartilage differentiation and bone formation [129]; (2) the growth and differentiation of skin [219], mammary gland [221], and teeth [149]; (3) cardiovascular function [175]; (4) transepithelial calcium transport in mammary epithelia and placenta [108, 220]; (5) relaxation of smooth muscle in uterus, bladder, arteries, and ileum [15, 150, 198, 223]; and (6) host immune function [61, 62]. The normal functions of PTHrP have been extensively reviewed elsewhere [191]. Normal subjects do not have detectable circulating levels of PTHrP – this suggests that, in the tissues where it is produced, PTHrP acts locally as a regulator or cytokine.

Approximately 80% of hypercalcemic patients with solid tumors have detectable or increased plasma concentrations PTHrP [23]. In cancer, PTHrP has these additional functions: (1) mediating hypercalcemia; (2) aiding in the development and progression of osteolytic bone metastasis (see below); (3) regulating cancer cell growth [112, 119]; and (4) acting as a cell survival factor [28].

Modulation of PTHrP Effects by Other Tumor-associated Factors

Cytokines and comparable tumor-associated factors modulate the actions of PTH and PTHrP in similar fashions. Both PTH and PTHrP induce a comparable degree of hypercalcemia, as well as increases in osteoclastic bone resorption, more committed marrow mononuclear osteoclast precursors, and mature osteoclasts [206]. However, the multipotent osteoclast precursors, the granulocyte/macrophage colony-forming units, were not stimulated. IL-6 potentiated the hypercalcemia and bone resorption mediated by PTHrP *in vivo* by stimulating production of early osteoclast precursors [41]. Likewise, TGFα has been shown to enhance the hypercalcemic effects of PTHrP in an animal model of malignancy-associated hypercalcemia [81] and to modulate the renal and bone effects of PTHrP. Sato et al. [172] demonstrated that IL-1α and PTHrP may have synergistic effects *in vivo*, and others have shown that IL-1 may modulate the renal effects of PTHrP [202]. Finally, Uy et al. [207] have demonstrated that tumor necrosis factor-α (TNFα) enhanced the hypercalcemic effect of PTHrP by increasing the pool of committed osteoclast progenitors with a subsequent increase in osteoclastic bone resorption. Bone formation parameters indicate that TNFα did not inhibit the new bone formation stimulated by PTHrP in nude mice.

Such tumor-associated factors also appear to be important regulators of PTHrP expression and secretion by tumors [78]. EGF has been shown to stimulate PTHrP expression in a keratinocyte and a mammary epithelial cell line, whereas TGFα enhanced PTHrP expression in a human squamous cell carcinoma of the lung. Interleukin-6, TNF, IGF-I, and IGF-II increased the production of PTHrP *in vitro* by a human squamous cell carcinoma. TGFβ, which is abundant in bone, is released in active form by resorbing bone, and is expressed by some breast cancers and cancer-associated stromal cells, has been shown to enhance secretion and stabilization of PTHrP message in renal and squamous cell carcinomas. The role of TGFβ in the regulation of PTHrP will be discussed below.

PTHrP in Hypercalcemia Associated with Breast Cancer

The role of PTHrP in breast cancer-associated hypercalcemia deserves special consideration. Breast cancer affects bone predominantly through metastatic mechanisms, typically leading to lytic deposits in the skeleton. Approximately 10% of women with breast cancer will at some point in their disease have hypercalcemia. The association of hypercalcemia with extensive osteolytic lesions in breast cancer is so strong that the presentation of hypercalcemia without bone metastases suggests coexistence of primary hyperparathyroidism [53]. It was therefore long held that breast cancer-associated hypercalcemia is the result of excessive resorption of bone around tumor deposits. However, clinical studies [154] failed to demonstrate any relationship between extent of bone metastasis and serum calcium levels. Conversely, studies exploring the potential role for a humoral mediator of hypercalcemia in breast cancer have clearly demonstrated altered renal handling of calcium and phosphate, as well as an increase in nephrogenous camp. This suggests that at least some of hypercalcemic breast cancer patients have a circulating factor with PTH-like properties. The identification of PTHrP as this factor is hardly surprising when it is recalled that PTHrP may play an important role in normal breast physiology. In the case of breast cancer, PTHrP appears to have both paracrine and endocrine functions.

PTHrP was detected by immunohistochemical staining in 60% of 102 invasive breast tumors that had been removed from normocalcemic women. It is not found in normal breast tissue [186]. At least four other studies have confirmed these percentages [21, 22, 104, 114]. One of these reported the presence of immunoreactive PTHrP within the cytoplasm of lobular and ductal epithelial cells in normal and fibrocystic breast tissues [114]. Furthermore, 65–92% of hypercalcemic breast cancer patients (with or without bone metastases) had plasma PTHrP concentrations at a level similar to that in patients whose hypercalcemia was the result of nonbreast tumors [21, 74]. Thus, PTHrP is an important mediator of hypercalcemia in breast cancer. It is also a major mediator of bone destruction in breast cancer that has metastasized to bone (see also below).

PTHrP in Hypercalcemia Associated with Hematologic Malignancies

Hypercalcemia associated with hematologic malignancies results both from systemically produced tumor factors such as $1,25\text{-}(OH)_2D_3$ (discussed below), and from locally produced cytokines, such as IL-6, IL-1, and lymphotoxin or TNFβ, that have their origin in bone tumors. PTHrP has recently been shown to be an important pathogenetic factor in the development of hypercalcemia in some patients with hematologic malignancies. In a clinical study of 76 patients with various hematological malignancies, 50% of the fourteen hypercalcemic patients had significant increases in plasma PTHrP concentrations [109]. Of these, five had non-Hodgkin's lymphoma, one had Hodgkin's disease, and one had multiple myeloma. The serum $1,25\text{-}(OH)_2D_3$ concentrations were low in the patients with non-Hodgkin's lymphoma patients whose plasma PTHrP concentrations were increased. Also of interest is that plasma PTHrP concentrations were increased in several normocalcemic patients with non-Hodgkin's lymphoma, Hodgkin's lymphoma, multiple myeloma, and Waldenstrom's macroglobulinemia [177]. Using a sensitive two-site immunoradiometric assay, other investigators have noted increased plasma PTHrP concentrations in patients with adult T-cell leukemia and B-cell lymphoma [92]. Finally, in separate studies, plasma concentrations of PTHrP similar to those in HHM were encountered in two of four hypercalcemic patients with non-Hodgkin's lymphoma, in three of nine with myeloma, and in a patient with myeloid blast crisis of chronic myeloid leukemia [54, 178]. Thus, the humoral mediators in the hypercalcemia associated with hematological malignancies include both 1,25-$(OH)_2D_3$ and PTHrP.

1,25-dihydroxyvitamin D

Under normal physiologic conditions, serum calcium and 1,25-$(OH)_2D_3$ concentrations bear an inverse relationship to one another. In hypercalcemia, serum 1,25-$(OH)_2D_3$ concentrations are suppressed unless there is persistent stimulation of 1α-hydroxylase activity from an autonomous source of PTH, as in primary hyperparathyroidism. Other than that the failure of 1,25-$(OH)_2D_3$ to go down as calcium goes up indicates abnormal regulation of 1,25-$(OH)_2D_3$ synthesis and suggests that 1,25-$(OH)_2D_3$ may be produced extrarenally, as is the case in granulomatous disease. In that condition, activated macrophages within the granuloma synthesize 1,25-$(OH)_2D_3$ [2, 71, 125]. Similarly, 1,25-$(OH)_2D_3$ seems to be the major factor causing hypercalcemia in Hodgkin's disease, non-Hodgkin's lymphoma, and other hematological malignancies [177, 178]. The mechanism is similar to that observed in granulomatous disease. In this scenario, hypercalcemic patients have increased plasma 1,25-$(OH)_2D_3$ concentrations, even though their plasma PTH levels and urinary cAMP output are low to normal [164]. There is no bone involvement. Lymphoma patients exhibit an increase in urinary calcium excretion [164], as well as in intestinal calcium absorption, as measured with the aid of radiocalcium [19]. Increased 1,25-$(OH)_2D_3$ concentrations were also noted in 12 of 22 hypercalcemic patients with non-Hodgkin's lymphoma. In addition, 71% of 22 normocalcemic patients with non-Hodgkin's lymphoma were hypercalciuric, and 18% had increased serum 1,25-$(OH)_2D_3$ concentrations. These findings led the investigators to conclude the dysregulated 1,25-$(OH)_2D_3$ production is common in patients with diffuse large cell lymphoma [178]. The low serum PTH and urinary cAMP concentrations indicate that neither PTH nor PTHrP mediates the hypercalcemia in this setting. Prostaglandin concentra-tions tend to be low and indomethacin therapy did not seem to lower plasma calcium [54].

Thus, the mechanisms responsible for hypercalcemia in lymphoma are multifactorial, including an increase in intestinal calcium absorption and in osteoclastic bone resorption. Many of the patients also had altered renal function; this suggests that impaired renal calcium clearance may contribute to the hypercalcemia. It is likely that in lymphoma, as in granuloma, the diseased tissue hydroxylates 25-hydroxyvitamin D to the active 1,25-$(OH)_2D_3$. 1α-Hydroxylase activity has been demonstrated in human T-cell lymphotrophic virus type-I-transformed lymphocytes, as well as in other extrarenal tissues [51, 230]. None of the patients with 1,25-$(OH)_2D_3$-mediated hypercalcemia had granulomatous disease. Their hypercalcemia was often reduced as a result of medical or surgical therapy that led to a decrease in their serum 1,25-$(OH)_2D_3$ concentration. Recurrence of disease is associated with recurrent hypercalcemia and increased plasma 1,25-$(OH)_2D_3$ concentrations [127].

Parathyroid Hormone (PTH)

For many years after Fuller Albright's observations in 1941 malignancy-associated hypercalcemia was attributed to PTH produced by an ectopic tumor. It is now clear that in the majority of cases of HHM, PTHrP is the ectopically produced factor. There have been rare cases, however, when the hypercalcemia was due to authentic, tumor-produced PTH. Ectopic PTH production has been documented in small cell carcinoma of the lung [229], in squamous cell carcinoma of the lung [142], in ovarian cancer [143], in widely metastatic primitive neuroecto-dermal tumor [189], in papillary adenocarci-noma of the thyroid [90], and in thymoma [160]. Molecular analysis of the ovarian carcinoma revealed both DNA amplification and rearrangement in the upstream regulatory region of the PTH gene. Interestingly, the primitive neuroectodermal tumor produced both PTH and PTHrP that resulted in severe hypercalcemia. These patients did not have coexisting primary hyperparathyroidism, because their parathyroid glands were normal on neck exploration or autopsy. Nevertheless, ectopic production of PTH is rare. Indeed most patients with malignancy-associated hypercalcemia have low plasma PTH concentrations [188]. Therefore hypercalcemia of malignancy where the serum PTH concentration is normal or increased is most often the result of hyperparathyroidism.

Other Tumor-associated Factors

There is accumulating evidence that solid tumors may produce other humoral factors, alone or in combination with PTHrP, that can stimulate osteoclastic bone resorption and cause hypercalcemia [162]. These factors include IL-1, IL-6, TGFα, tumor necrosis factor (TNF) and granulocyte colony-stimulating factor (G-CSF). Administration of IL-1 to mice causes a mild hypercalcemia [17, 168], which can be effectively blocked by the IL-1 receptor antagonist [77]. Mice bearing Chinese hamster ovarian tumors transfected with the cDNA for IL-6 develop mild hypercalcemia [11], as do mice that bear renal carcinoma that co-secreted IL-6 and PTHrP [216]. Patients with humoral hypercalcemia of malignancy have high serum concentrations of IL-6 [5, 205].

Human TGFα and TNFα stimulate osteoclastic bone resorption *in vitro* and cause hypercalcemia *in vivo* [8, 89, 224]. In mice, TNFα causes hypercalciuria, without an increase in nephrogenous cAMP, and increases osteoclastic bone resorption [96]. As noted in the previous section, some of these factors modulate the end-organ effects of PTHrP on bone and kidney. In some instances, factors such as TGFα, IL-1, IL-6, and TNF enhance the hypercalcemic effects of PTHrP [41, 81, 207]. The ability of IL-6 to enhance PTHrP-mediated hypercalcemia appears to be due to increased production of the early osteoclast precursors, granulocyte macrophage colony forming units. IL-6, along with the production of more committed osteoclast precursors, stimulates PTHrP, thereby enhancing hypercalcemia [41].

Prostaglandins of the E series are powerful stimulators of bone resorption [103], although their role in bone destruction associated with malignancy remains unclear [135]. Some of the effects of cytokines on bone may be mediated by prostaglandins. Indomethacin, a prostaglandin synthesis inhibitor, has been shown to block part of the osteoclast-stimulatory effects of IL-1 *in vivo* [17, 168]. Although prostaglandins are produced by cultured tumor cells *in vitro*, indomethacin treatment of malignancy-associated hypercalcemia is only effective on occasion [134]. Recent evidence indicates that the prostaglandin EP2 receptor mediates PGE2-mediated hypercalcemia in mice [113].

Recently RANK ligand has been directly implicated in the pathogenesis of hypercalcemia of malignancy. A novel cDNA that encodes a secreted form of an osteoclast differentiation factor/tumor necrosis factor that induces a cytokine was sequenced from 5′ RACE cDNA clones of squamous cell carcinoma cell lines, SCC-4 and T3M-1 Cl.2, parental malignant tissues of which had caused severe humoral hypercalcemia [137].

Treatment of Hypercalcemia of Malignancy

Eradication of the underlying cancer constitutes the definitive treatment of malignancy-associated hypercalcemia. However, because cure may not be possible, therapy of patients with symptomatic or life-threatening hypercalcemia must be aimed against the mediating mechanisms. Increased osteoclastic bone resorption is present in virtually all patients with hypercalcemia of malignancy. Bone resorption becomes, therefore, a key target for treatment of hypercalcemia. Two mechanisms in particular, the increase in osteoclastic bone resorption and renal tubular calcium reabsorption, are encountered in most patients with hypercalcemia of malignancy, even in cases not associated with PTHrP production [173, 203, 204]. Medical therapy should therefore be aimed at inhibiting bone resorption and promoting renal calcium excretion.

Because many hypercalcemic patients are dehydrated, this first step of therapy is to rehydrate the patient. This will enhance calciuresis by increasing the glomerular filtration rate and reduce the fractional reabsorption of calcium and sodium. The use of loop diuretics, such as furosemide, to increase calcium excretion may exacerbate fluid loss and worsen dehydration; therefore the use of loop diuretics should be limited to the volume-replete patient and only then with close monitoring of volume status [193]. Because hydration alone rarely results in full resolution of hypercalcemia [88], more aggressive therapies are usually needed.

The bisphosphonates are currently the mainstay for long-term treatment of hypercalcemia and osteolytic bone disease. They bind to bone surfaces that undergo active resorption and are released in the bone microenvironment during remodeling. Bisphosphonates decrease osteoclastic bone resorption by two mechanisms (cf. Chapter 8). The nitrogen-substituted bisphosphonates, such as alendronate, risedronate and zoledronic acid, are potent inhibitors of the enzyme farnesyldiphosphate synthase, thereby blocking protein isoprenylation. The prenylation of small GTP-binding proteins is important for maintaining structural integrity of the osteoclast: without it, the osteoclasts undergo apoptosis. The non-nitrogen-containing bisphosphonates, clodronate and etidronate, are less potent and induce osteoclastic apoptosis, but by a mechanism that differs from that of the nitrogen-substituted bisphosphates. The non-nitrogen-containing bisphosphonates are incorporated into nonhydrolyzable ATP analogs that inhibit ATP-dependent intracellular enzymes. The FDA has approved the use of bisphosphonates to treat myeloma osteolytic bone disease in 1995 and osteolytic bone disease due to breast cancer in 1996.

Several lines of evidence indicate that bisphosphonates affect osteoclastic bone resorption through their actions on osteoblasts. Bisphosphonates have multiple actions on osteoblasts such as (1) modulation of proliferation and differentiation [156]; (2) prevention of apoptosis [151]; (3) modulation of extracellular matrix protein production [69, 102]; and (4) regulation of the expression and excretion of IL-6 [70, 201]. Recently, Viereck et al. [212] presented *in vitro* evidence that bisphosphonates act directly on human osteoblasts causing them to increase the production of both osteoprotegerin (OPG) mRNA and protein. It seems reasonable to infer that by increasing OPG expression, the RANKL mediated stimulation of osteoclasts can be neutralized.

Available bisphosphonates vary in potency, but all are poorly absorbed and are most effective for treatment of hypercalcemia when used intravenously. Intravenous etidronate, the least potent of the class, normalized calcium concentration in only 30%–40% of patients when given in doses of 7.5 mg/kg on three consecutive days [76, 101, 182]. Oral etidronate, at dosages of 25 mg/kg per day for more than 6 months can cause bone mineralization defects [55]. Pamidronate combines high potency with low toxicity and has become the agent of choice for the treatment of hypercalcemia of malignancy.

When used at the recommended dose of 30–90 mg IV over 4–24 hours, pamidronate is highly effective in normalizing serum calcium concentrations and does not cause mineralization defects [87].

The clinical response to bisphosphonates is somewhat delayed. In studies that used a 90-mg infusion of pamidronate over four hours the mean time to achieve normocalcemia was approximately four days, with the resulting normocalcemia lasting 28 days [153]. By using pamidronate in combination with calcitonin, one can achieve a rapid and sustained reduction in serum calcium [197].

Zoledronic acid, the most potent bisphosphonate to date, has been approved for the treatment of hypercalcemia of malignancy. This bisphosphonate, at a dose of 4 mg and 8 mg, when compared to a single infusion of 90 mg pamidronate, was superior with respect to the time needed to normalize plasma calcium and the duration of response [121]. The FDA-approved dose is 4 mg, as 8 mg induced some renal dysfunction.

Calcitonin inhibits osteoclastic bone resorption and renal tubular calcium reabsorption within minutes of administration; this makes it an excellent agent for the acute treatment of hypercalcemia. Unfortunately, tachyphylaxis frequently develops within 48 hours as a result of down regulation of the calcitonin receptor. Concomitant use of glucocorticoids, however, can prolong treatment duration [9]. This appears to result from a glucocorticoid-mediated up-regulation of cell-surface calcitonin receptors and an increase in the de novo production of calcitonin receptors in the osteoclast [213]. Calcitonin can be administered every 6–12 hours in doses of 4–8 U/kg. Human calcitonin is available, but salmon calcitonin is more generally used. If salmon calcitonin is to be used, then a test dose of 1 unit should be administered first, to check for a possible anaphylactic reaction.

Two antineoplastic agents have been used to treat malignancy-associated hypercalcemia. Plicamycin, or mithramycin, inhibits DNA-dependent RNA synthesis and is a potent inhibitor of bone resorption. The dosage used to treat hypercalcemia (25 µg/kg) is one-tenth the usual chemotherapeutic dose and the drug should be infused over four hours. Its considerable side effects include nephrotoxicity, hepatotoxicity, thrombocytopenia, nausea, and vomiting. Gallium nitrate is another antineoplastic agent with calcium lowering effects. It is also nephrotoxic and somewhat inconvenient to use, as it must be administered continuously over a five-day period. Use of these antineoplastic agents should therefore be restricted to cases of hypercalcemia that are unresponsive to bisphosphonates.

About 30% of patients treated with glucocorticoids for malignancy-associated hypercalcemia respond with a drop in serum calcium concentration. Glucocorticoids are likely to be most effective in hypercalcemia associated with multiple myeloma or in hematologic malignancies associated with 1,25-$(OH)_2D_3$. Glucocorticoids inhibit osteoclastic bone resorption by decreasing tumor production of locally active cytokines, in addition to having direct tumorolytic effects [133]. Glucocorticoids should be given in doses equivalent to 40–60 mg of prednisone, daily. If no response is observed in 10 days, then glucocorticoid therapy should be discontinued.

Hypercalcemia in experimental animals is inhibited by antibodies to PTHrP [110]. In a search for small-molecule inhibitors of PTHrP production or effects, Gallwitz et al. [45] found that guanine-nucleotide analogs inhibit PTHrP expression by human tumor cells. In nude athymic mice these compounds reduce hypercalcemia caused by excessive PTHrP production by a lung squamous-cell carcinoma. The PTHrP gene promoter may therefore be a suitable target for treating the skeletal effects of malignancy [65].

Solid Tumor Metastasis to Bone

When cancers metastasize to bone, they often cause bone destruction, or osteolysis, which leads to bone pain, fracture, hypercalcemia, and nerve compression. Cancer patients with bone metastases often now survive several years during which they suffer bone pain and related sequelae. Breast cancer is the solid tumor that most commonly metastasizes to bone, the cells showing a marked affinity to grow in bone. The association of breast cancer with skeletal morbidity was already noted in 1889, when Stephen Paget stated "in a cancer of the breast the bones suffer in a special way, which cannot be explained by any theory of embolism alone." The mechanisms responsible for osteotropism are complex and involve both the breast cancer cells and the bone to which the tumors metastasize. Paget [148] proposed the "seed and soil" hypothesis to explain this: "When a plant goes to seed, its seeds are carried in all directions; but they can only grow if they fall on congenial soil." The bone microenvironment provides the fertile soil in which the cancer cells grow [52, 136]. The cancer cells seem to activate bone cells, thereby stimulating local bone destruction and formation.

Paget's century-old concept continues to guide the study of breast cancer metastasis and our understanding of how the vicious cycle is driven by molecules produced by bone and tumor cells [155]. The bone cell highlighted in this volume of *Topics in Bone Biology*, the osteoclast, plays an integral role in this cycle. As indicated below, osteoclast activity is stimulated by a variety of mechanisms in patients with bone metastases: (1) by tumor cell products; (2) by increased osteoblast activity which leads to increased expression of receptor activator of nuclear factor kappa B ligand (RANKL); and (3) by sex-steroid deficiency, a frequent result of cancer therapy.

Classification of Bone Metastases

Bone metastases are typically classified by their radiographic appearance as either osteolytic or osteoblastic. In reality, these classifications represent two ends of a spectrum as patients with solid tumor metastases to the skeleton often have components of both bone destruction and new bone formation. In addition to cancers of the breast, other tumors such as those of prostate, lung, kidney, and thyroid, also metastasize to the skeleton, and all but prostate cancers cause predominantly osteolytic lesions. Approximately 15% of patients with breast cancer bone metastases have osteoblastic lesions that are characterized by disorganized new bone formation [78]. A substantial fraction of skeletal metastases exhibit a mixture of osteolytic and osteoblastic responses. Although patient material containing skeletal metastases is seldom available for detailed analyses, recent autopsy studies demonstrate that cancer metastases to the skeleton display marked heterogeneity with respect to the osteolytic and osteoblastic phenotypes [165]. It is also likely that individual metastases change phenotypically with time. As tumor-bone interactions alter gene expression patterns of both, the local balance between bone formation and destruction may change. Although tumor cells can directly destroy or synthesize bone [48, 111, 115], it seems likely their stimulation of bone cells is the physiologically important factor in the etiology of bone metastases. In advanced disease direct tumor actions may contribute to existing pathological bone lesions.

Osteolytic and osteoblastic lesions are most often diagnosed by bone scans and radiographs. Biochemical markers of bone resorption and formation are often increased in both [56, 105]. In cases of pure osteolytic disease, as in myeloma, bone scans may be negative.

The major organic component of bone matrix is type I collagen. The biosynthesis of collagen by the osteoblast releases soluble pro-peptide fragments, which can serve as markers of new bone formation and osteoblastic activity. Similarly, osteoclastic bone resorption releases fragments from cross-linked collagen, which can be utilized as markers of bone destruction. Biochemical markers are used to monitor active bone remodeling in patients and their responses to treatment [67]. Markers of bone formation include bone-specific alkaline phosphatase and serum procollagen I amino-terminal propeptide (PINP). Markers of resorption are urinary collagen cross-linked N-telopeptide (NTX), collagen I carboxy-terminal telopeptide (CTX), pyridinolines (PYD), and deoxypyridinolines (DPYD). Both types of markers are increased in prostate cancer patients with osteoblastic metastases. Markers of resorption may increase when bone loss is the result of adjuvant and chemotherapy and cannot be used alone to diagnose bone metastases. NTX is not as sensitive as a bone scan for diagnosing bone metastases, but may be used as an auxiliary diagnostic index [60]. Biochemical markers are useful to monitor response to bisphosphonate treatment, with NTX the most sensitive [10]. This area of diagnostics is still under active development. Radionuclide complexes with bone-seeking bisphosphonates provide the basis for scintigraphic bone scans, an effective approach for localizing osteoblastic metastases [7]. Bone scans are not impaired in patients that have been treated with bisphosphonates [166].

Frequency of Bone Metastases

Seventy percent of patients dying of breast cancer have bone metastases [32]. Bone is the most common site of breast cancer metastases, and one of the earliest organs to be affected by metastatic disease [183]. In about 20% of cases bone metastatic lesions are isolated [16]. Skeletal metastases are virtually incurable in breast cancer patients. However, the disease, once housed in bone, is relatively indolent, with a median survival of two years and five-year survival in nearly 40% of patients 180, 183]. Since metastases to organs such as liver and brain have much poorer prognoses, it appears that bone metastases are not a major source of secondary metastases to these sites.

Skeletal Involvement in Malignant Disease

The sites within the skeleton preferentially colonized by tumor cells appear to be those which receive the most abundant vascular supply. These include regions with extensive red bone marrow within the axial skeleton, ribs, the proximal metaphyses of the long bones, and the spine. Solid tumors, such as in breast cancer, and hematological malignancies show the same distribution of sites within bone [64]. Prostate cancer displays an unusual preference for the spine. This has been attributed to anatomical access via Batson's plexus. It is more likely that specific gene expression patterns characteristic of this tumor and of the vertebral bones are the molecular basis for the preference. Breast cancer metastases are sometimes found in the posterior clinoid processes of the base of the skull. The basis for this site preference is not understood.

Metastasis of human tumors to specific sites has been modeled in immunocompromised rodents. Tumor cells are often entrapped within the capillary beds of lung or liver when injected into the venous circulation. However, many of the same tumor cell lines will form lesions limited to bone if the cells are inoculated through the left cardiac ventricle to avoid pulmonary entrapment [3]. This animal model has been used to study metastases to bone with a variety of tumor cell lines, in particular the human breast cancer cell line MD-MB-231

[228]. Similar animal models of osteoblastic metastases have recently been described, in which three human breast cancer cell lines were found to metastasize to bone [226].

Clinical Consequences of Local Metastatic Disease

Bone pain is the most common symptom of cancer metastasis to bone and may be the initial presenting symptom. Pathological fractures may occur in patients with advanced disease. Vertebral fracture as the initial presentation in an elderly patient with metastatic breast cancer may be misdiagnosed as age-related osteoporosis. Bone marrow suppression and leukopenia can occur with sufficient tumor burden within bone. Hypercalcemia caused by excessive bone destruction used to occur in up to 30% of breast cancer patients with bone involvement, but the incidence of this condition has decreased as a result of the utilization of effective bisphosphonate antiresorptive agents. Spinal cord compression can occur as a consequence of osteoblastic lesions or vertebral fractures and may be devastating for the patient. Since breast cancer patients with metastases limited to the skeleton have a median survival of 2–4 years, these patients have a high cumulative risk of skeletal-related events (SREs). Approximately 60% of these patients will suffer pathological fractures, 20% will develop hypercalcemia, and 10% will have spinal cord compression [117].

Many patients with terminal metastatic disease suffer from severe weight loss. This cachexia involves the loss of muscle and fat mass and can occur independently of anorexia or intestinal malabsorption [200]. Cancer cachexia is an area that has received insufficient attention from researchers. Rapid onset cachexia often occurs in animals with breast cancer bone metastases [228], and weight loss correlates with tumor burden in bone [226]. The results suggest that bone metastases release factors into the peripheral circulation that then stimulate wasting of skeletal muscle. Effective anti-cachectic therapies improve the quality of life and may increase the survival of patients with advanced, metastatic disease.

Bone cancer pain, whether constant or intermittent, is often intractable. In the case of osteolytic metastases, products released from bone by osteolytic resorption activate pain receptors on nerve endings in the skeleton. Inhibitors of bone resorption effectively palliate bone pain. The serious paraneoplastic syndrome of bone pain has only recently received scientific attention. A model of bone pain, based on the rodent model of Arguello et al. [3], has been used to demonstrate that antiresorptive treatment can decrease metastatic bone pain [85]. Studies with the model suggest that the mechanisms of pain in bone are specific [123]. Thus, bone pain caused by cancer is fundamentally different from inflammatory pain and shows much less response to morphine [118]. Further study of bone pain is likely to lead to approaches that would markedly improve the quality of life of patients with advanced breast cancer.

Steps in Tumor Cell Metastasis

Extravasation and Migration

Initial angiogenesis followed by tumor cell migration through extracellular matrix and extravasation into the bloodstream are general properties of all metastatic cancer cells. These steps require the expression of enzymes to degrade extracellular matrix and of autocrine factors to stimulate tumor cell motility [52, 124, 218]. Metastasis to bone is likely controlled by interactions subsequent to the exit of tumor cells from the primary site. Matrix metalloproteinases, MMPs, form a large family of proteins with roles in tumor cell invasion [120]. MMP-1, interstitial collagenase, is necessary for the initiation of bone resorption [231]. MMP inhibitors have been tested in clinical trials, with disappointing results to date [38, 146]. The lack of efficacy of these inhibitors may reflect the complexity and redundancy of the MMP family members and not their value as targets for treatment.

Chemotaxis and Homing to Bone

Bone produces factors that stimulate primary tumor cells, such as those that originate in the breast, to home to bone [126, 145]. The best-characterized example of such a factor is the chemokine stromal-derived factor, SDF-1, which is released by bone, and its tumor-expressed receptor CXCR-4 [132]. The ligand-receptor pair mediates the attraction of breast and other cancer cells to specific metastatic sites including, but not limited to, bone. CXCR-4 is a co-receptor for HIV. Small molecule inhibitors of CXCR-4 are under development and may also function to decrease breast cancer metastases. CXCR-4 expression is increased by the vascular endothelial growth factor, VEGF [4]. The mechanisms of adhesion of tumor cells to bone [124, 126] and to bone marrow endothelium [36] have been studied extensively. The surface of bone is rich in extracellular matrix components, including integrin substrates. The receptors on tumor cells for these molecules offer opportunities for inhibition of metastases to bone [27, 228]. The $\alpha v\beta 3$ integrin plays an important role in osteoclast binding and activation in bone and can regulate breast cancer metastases [50]. Antagonists of $\alpha v\beta 3$ integrin may have a therapeutic role as inhibitors of metastasis to bone [196].

Colonization of Bone

The initiation of a metastasis is believed to be a rare and inefficient process [52], although tumor cells are often detectable in patient bone marrow samples when analyzed by sensitive PCR techniques [147]. The basic mechanisms of cancer metastases to specific sites continue to evolve. Cancer cells continue to mutate *in vivo*. The ability of cancer cells to metastasize is characteristic of advanced disease and could occur only after the gradual accumulation of a necessary set of pro-metastatic mutations [52]. However, recent experiments suggest that a constellation of expressed genes necessary for metastasis to bone preexists within the primary breast tumor. [98]. The results strongly support a multi-factorial mechanism underlying organ-specific metastases. Thus, bone-specific metastases are the consequence of the selection of variants from a heterogeneous population of cells within the primary tumor, plus changes in gene expression induced by bone factors. The results of Kang et al. [98] are confirmed by gene array analyses of micro-dissected patient samples, comparing primary and metastatic breast cancer cells [176]. Cells of the osteoblastic lineage appear to be the main targets of tumor-secreted factors. In turn, bone-derived transforming growth factor-β [TGFβ] is a major factor regulating of tumor cell behavior in bone.

There are no convenient animal models where primary tumors reproducibly metastasize to bone. Many of the preclinical findings described in this chapter use an animal model in which human tumor cells are inoculated into immuno-deficient mice. Careful tumor administration directly into the left cardiac ventricle can result in 100% incidence of bone metastases with many tumor cell lines. Osteolytic lesions are detected by X-ray as early as three weeks and can be quantified by image analysis. Osteoblastic lesions may take up to six months to develop in nude mice, and the lesions cannot be quantified radiographically.

Development of Skeletal Lesions

The growth of bone metastases is usually slow [180], as is usually the progression from microscopic lesion to initial diagnosis. The initial steps in the development of bone lesions have not been investigated in depth in animal models.

Tumor cells secrete proteolytic enzymes and acid in abundance and therefore can destroy bone matrix *in vitro* [32]. During the establishment of metastases, however, bone is resorbed by osteoclasts rather than by tumor cells. Histological analysis and scanning electron microscopy of osteolytic bone metastases indicate that the bone destruction is mediated by the osteoclast [18, 195].

Cellular Mechanisms of Bone Destruction: Bone Stromal Cells Control Osteoclast Formation and Activity by Expression of RANK Ligand and Osteoprotegerin

Although the osteolytic factor, parathyroid hormone-related protein, PTHrP, is clearly a potent stimulator of bone resorption, tumor-produced PTHrP does not have direct actions on cells of the osteoclastic lineage. Thomas et al. [199] showed that a recently identified osteoclast differentiation factor indirectly mediates the effects PTHrP on bone resorption. The tumor factor acts on cells of the osteoblast lineage, which in turn regulate the formation, activity, and lifetime of osteoclasts derived from hematopoietic progenitors. The regulation of osteoclasts by osteoblasts has been recognized for over 15 years, but its molecular basis has been understood only in the last five years. Stromal cell-expressed RANK ligand, in combination with macrophage colony-stimulating factor (M-CSF) can generate osteoclasts from hematopoietic precursors in the absence of cells or other factors [192]. RANK ligand is a member of the TNF family and is a membrane-bound molecule. Opposing the actions of membrane-bound RANK ligand is soluble osteoprotegerin (Opg), a secreted TNF receptor family member whose overexpression in mice resulted in osteopetrosis [181]. Conversely, mice deficient in OPG are osteoporotic. OPG functions as a soluble inhibitory binding protein for RANK ligand [192]. Both RANK ligand and OPG are made by osteoblastic cells, which regulate osteoclast formation and activity by the ratio of the two opposing factors. Interleukin 1 and tumor necrosis factor-α have RANK-independent effects on osteoclastogenesis, but the quantitative importance of these pathways is unclear, and their contributions to bone metastasis are unknown. A variety of organic mediators (prostaglandin E2, 1,25dihydroxyvitaminD3) and protein factors (PTH, PTHrP, IL-6, IL-11) appear to exert their osteoclastogenic actions primarily via stimulation of RANK ligand expression on the surface of cells in the osteoblast lineage. Nearly all of these conclusions are based on data obtained with mice. The role of the RANK ligand pathway in bone resorption stimulated by IL-1, IL-6, and TNFα may be different in humans compared to mice [84]. The components of the central osteoclast-regulating pathway, RANK, RANK ligand, and OPG offer new opportunities for molecular therapies against metastatic bone disease.

Tumor-Produced Factors Which Stimulate Osteoclasts

Many factors that stimulate bone resorption do so not by acting directly on osteoclasts or their precursors, but by indirect actions on bone marrow stromal cells in the osteoblastic lineage, involving regulation of the ratio of RANK ligand to osteoprotegerin [166]. Pertinent to the molecular mechanisms of osteolytic metastases is experimental evidence that breast cancer-produced PTHrP mediates osteolysis via increasing RANK ligand and decreasing OPG expression by the osteoblast. Breast cancer cells express OPG and RANK, but not RANK ligand [199].

Role of Parathyroid Hormone-related Protein

The tumor-secreted factor PTHrP is often responsible for the osteoclast-stimulating activity and bone destruction caused by breast cancer [78, 227]. As noted earlier approximately 60% of human primary breast cancers express PTHrP [21, 22, 186]. Some of these retrospective studies suggested that women with PTHrP-positive tumors were more likely to develop bone metastases [21, 22, 186]. However, PTHrP expression by breast cancer at metastatic sites differs significantly from that of the primary site. PTHrP is expressed by greater than 90% of breast cancer metastases to bone compared with only 17% of non-bone metastases [152, 186, 211]. These observations suggest two possible explanations: that PTHrP, as a bone-resorbing factor, favors tumor growth in bone or that the bone microenvironment enhances the production of PTHrP. The explanations are not mutually exclusive. Interpretation of the clinical findings is limited by the data on PTHrP expression in metastatic and primary tumor tissue, which were obtained from different patients.

A prospective study of over 300 breast cancer patients indicated that those whose primary tumors were PTHrP-negative were more likely to develop bone metastases [83]. Tumor tissue from both bone metastases and primary tumor was available from three patients. In these cases, the bone metastases were PTHrP-positive and the respective primary tumors were PTHrP-negative. This is the only published study to compare PTHrP expression between primary and metastatic tumor in the same patient. Data from this small subset of patients suggest that tumor PTHrP expression is enhanced in the bone microenvironment. Studies with larger numbers of patients are needed to confirm these observations.

The clinical studies suggested a role for PTHrP as a local mediator of bone destruction by metastatic breast cancer and provided the rationale for the following experimental studies. A neutralizing monoclonal antibody to PTHrP-(1–34) inhibited the development of breast cancer metastases to bone by the human breast cancer cell line, MDA-MB-231, which produces small amounts of PTHrP [80]. This monoclonal antibody has been humanized and placed in clinical trials against humor hypercalcemia of malignancy. Examination of the long bones from tumor-bearing mice revealed significantly fewer osteoclasts at the tumor-bone interface and less tumor burden in animals treated with the PTHrP antibody compared with the controls. Similar results were obtained with PTHrP-secreting lung cancer cells [91]. Neutralizing PTHrP decreased not only osteoclastic bone resorption, but also tumor burden in bone. Experimental overexpression of PTHrP by MCF-7 breast cancer cells, which do not express PTHrP and do not cause osteolytic metastases, induced marked bone destruction and increased osteoclast formation, compared to the controls which caused no bone metastases [199].

The data together suggest that tumor production of PTHrP is important for the establishment and progression of osteolytic bone metastases. Unaddressed was the possibility that the bone microenvironment induces PTHrP expression. The regulation of PTHrP is complex, and factors such as prolactin, estrogen, epidermal growth factor (EGF), insulin, IGFs 1 and 2, TGFα, TGF-β, angiotensin II, stretch, and src have been shown to increase expression, while glucocorticoids and the active form of vitamin D3 decrease it [78]. PTHrP plays a local, paracrine role in breast cancer bone metastases, which occur in animals in the absence of detectable increases in plasma PTHrP concentrations or malignant hypercalcemia [80].

Osteoclastic resorption of bone releases high concentrations of ionized calcium and phosphate from the dissolution of the bone mineral. The calcium-sensing receptor is a G-protein coupled, seven-transmembrane domain receptor, which responds to small variations in the concentration of extracellular calcium [222]. The calcium-sensing receptor is expressed by breast cancer cells and regulates tumor secretion of PTHrP [20, 170], an effect which is enhanced by TGFβ. Thus, the high concentrations of ionized calcium in bone may contribute to the vicious cycle by increasing PTHrP production and osteolysis. Small molecule agonists and antagonists of the receptor have been developed and are in clinical trials [141]. Such agents may be effective against breast cancer bone metastasis.

Roles of Other Osteolysis-Stimulating Factors

PTHrP cannot be the only factor responsible for bone metastases, and a number of other proteins play either contributory or PTHrP-independent roles [29]. Candidate factors that may contribute to PTHrP-induced osteolytic lesions are interleukin [IL]-11, macrophage colony-stimulating factor [M-CSF], and VEGF [209]. A number of PTHrP-independent factors have also been reported, including IL-8 [6].

Kang et al. [144] compared less- and more-metastatic variants of a breast cancer cell line by gene expression profiling. They identified mRNAs whose expression strongly correlated with increased bone metastasis. Five of the mRNAs encoded IL-11, matrix metalloproteinase [MMP]-1 osteopontin, connective tissue growth factor [CTGF], and CXCR-4. MMP-1 is an interstitial collagenase made by osteoblasts. It cleaves collagen at a site resistant to osteoclastic enzyme hydrolysis and may be rate-limiting in normal bone resorption [231]. Osteopontin plays a complex role in metastasis, including modulation of anti-tumor immune responses [25, 215]. CTGF is a potent osteoblast-stimulatory factor [171] and is expressed by tumor cells. CXCR4 is the receptor for the chemokine SDF-1 and functions in the attraction of breast cancer cells to specific metastatic sites including, but not limited to bone [132]. Kang et al. [98] found that the pro-metastatic gene set was coordinately increased in cells that pre-existed in the original cell population. The authors attempted to convert low-metastatic MDA-MB-231 breast cancer cell line clones into ones highly metastatic to bone by overexpressing each of the five individual factors. They found that conversion of the cells to a phenotype of aggressive bone metastasis required co-transduction of combinations of four of the five factors. The results strongly support a multifactorial mechanism underlying organ-specific metastases. These factors may provide additional targets for therapeutic intervention to reduce breast cancer bone metastases.

Actions of Bone-Derived Factors on Tumor Cells

The effects of bone-derived factors on tumor cells remain understudied. Van der Pluim et al. [209] elegantly demonstrated that several mRNAs are increased in bone compared with non-bone sites of human breast cancer metastases in nude mice. RNA abundances were determined by species-specific RT-PCR. PTHrP, VEGFs, and M-CSF were increased specifically in bone, while several mouse markers of host angiogenesis were similarly increased. These experiments did not identify the factor(s) responsible for the bone-specific mRNA induction. Hauschka et al. [82] found that insulin-like growth factors [IGFs]-1 and -2, were most abundant in bone matrix. The second most abundant was TGFβ, whereas bone morphogenetic proteins (BMPs), fibroblast growth factors-1 and -2, and platelet-derived growth factor were at lower concentrations. Only TGFβ has been shown to play a direct role in stimulating tumor cells, although IGF signaling may regulate breast cancer cells that metastasize to bone [95]. TGFβ is growth-inhibitory in the early stages of tumorigenesis. Advanced cancers lose growth inhibition but retain TGFβ regulation of metastasis-promoting genes [214], such as CTGF and IL-11, [98], and PTHrP [227]. In the MDA-MB-231 model of breast cancer metastasis to bone, detailed experiments showed that tumor cell expression of PTHrP is the major target of TGFβ and that TGFβ is the most important regulator of PTHrP [227]. These experiments also showed that dual pathways in the tumor cells transmit TGFβ signaling to the nucleus: through p38 MAP kinase and through the Smad proteins [97]. Osteoclastic bone resorption specifically activates TGFβ from its stored form in bone matrix [40]. This step may be another point at which the efficacy of bisphosphonates against bone metastases is exerted [47]. Signaling

pathways, such as the MAP kinases, and extracellular mediators, such as TGFβ [46], offer further targets to be tested for inhibition of skeletal metastases.

Interactions Between Tumor And Bone – The Vicious Cycle

Preclinical animal models have established that bone metastases involve a vicious cycle between tumor cells and the skeleton (Figure 9.1). The cycle is fueled by four contributors: the tumor cells, bone-forming osteoblasts, bone-destroying osteoclasts, and organic bone matrix. Osteoclast formation and activity is regulated by the osteoblast, adding complexity to the vicious cycle. The mineralized matrix of bone is a vast storehouse of growth factors, such as insulin-like and transforming growth factors [82]. These are synthesized by osteoblasts and released by osteoclastic bone resorption. The factors reach high local concentrations in the bone microenvironment and can act on tumor cells to attract tumor cells [145] or to encourage metastatic growth. In turn, cancer cells secrete many factors that act on bone cells. Therapies

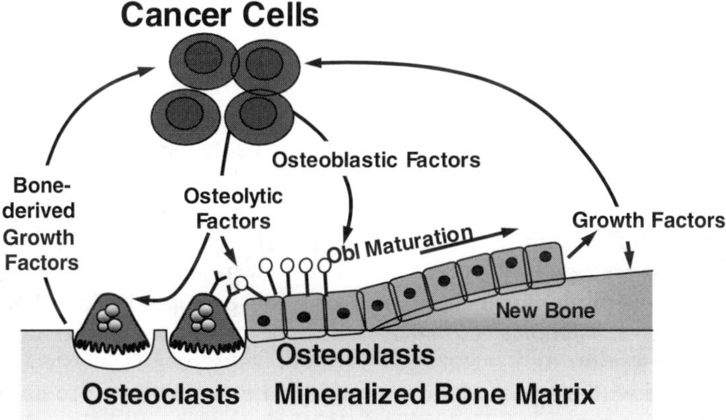

Figure 9.1 The vicious cycle between tumor cells and bone which fuels the growth of bone metastases. The major components of this vicious cycle include the cancer cells, osteoclasts, osteoblasts, and mineralized bone matrix, a major source of immobilized growth factors. Tumor products, such as ET-1, adrenomedullin, and PTHrP1–23, stimulate osteoblasts (Obl) proliferation, while full-length PTHrP, IL-11, and IL-8 stimulate osteoclastic bone resorption. Immature osteoblasts respond to osteolytic cytokines, such as PTHrP and IL-11, by expressing RANK ligand. RANK ligand stimulates osteoclastic bone resorption by binding its cognate receptor RANK (Y) on osteoclast precursors (shown here on mature osteoclasts). This bone resorption causes release of growth factors (TGFβ) and Ca++ from mineralized matrix. Mature osteoblasts synthesize growth factors, which are incorporated into bone and also enrich the local microenvironment. Growth factors stimulate tumor cells. Osteoblasts lose RANK ligand expression during maturation. The balance of osteoblast proliferation vs maturation, plus tumor production of osteolytic factors like PTHrP and IL-11, determines whether bone metastases are osteoblastic or osteolytic.

targeting the vicious cycle can decrease metastases by lowering the concentrations of growth factors in bone.

Osteoblastic and Mixed Metastases

Histomorphometric studies of prostate cancer samples indicate that osteoblastic metastases are due to tumor-produced factors that stimulate bone formation [26, 107]. The seed and soil analogy of Paget can be applied to osteoblastic metastases, which share a similar pathophysiology with osteolytic metastases. The tumor cells, the seeds, secrete factors that stimulate osteoblast activity and bone formation. The bone microenvironment is enriched with osteoblast-derived growth factors, which enhance the local growth of tumor cells.

Role of Endothelin-1

Endothelin-1, ET-1, is a 21-amino acid peptide that is a potent vasoconstrictor. It is expressed by many tissues and binds to two G-protein-coupled receptors. It is also a potent osteoblast-stimulatory factor through its activation of the ET A receptor [79]. Many receptor-selective endothelin receptor antagonists have been developed by the pharmaceutical industry for the treatment of cardiovascular conditions [158]. Endothelin plays an important role in cancer and on osteoblastic bone metastases in particular [139].

An animal model of osteoblastic metastases that uses three standard human breast cancer cell lines, ZR-75.1, T47D, and MCF7, has been established. All three lines are estrogen receptor-positive and express ET-1 but not PTHrP. The ZR75.1 cell line was studied in the greatest detail. It stimulates new bone formation in organ culture and causes osteoblastic metastases *in vivo*. Bone formation and metastases were effectively blocked with a selective antagonist of the endothelin A receptor [226]. This orally active antagonist, Atrasentan, is in clinical trials in men with advanced metastatic prostate cancer [163]. The endothelin receptor antagonist blocks the activation of osteoblasts by tumor-produced ET-1. It also decreases osteoclastic bone resorption, as indicated by a drop in bone resorption markers seen in the patient trials [140]. Bisphosphonates, on the other hand, effectively reduce skeletal-related events in prostate cancer [47]. Bisphosphonates

should therefore be effective therapy against all types of bone metastases, whereas endothelin receptor antagonists may be useful in the treatment of osteoblastic metastases.

Other factors responsible for osteoblastic metastases still need to be tested. Such factors should possess at least these two characteristics: the ability to stimulate osteoblastic new bone formation and to be expressed by cancer cells. The bone morphogenetic proteins are obvious candidates, but appear not to play a causal role in bone metastases. CTGF, identified in the experiments of Kang et al. [98], is a factor that stimulates osteoblasts [169]. Adrenomedullin, a 52-amino acid vasoactive peptide with potent bone-stimulatory actions [37], is produced by many cancers [232]. Unpublished data (Guise et al.) with lung and prostate cancer cell lines suggest that adrenomedullin increases bone metastases *in vivo*. Adrenomedullin is also an autocrine growth factor for breast cancer cells [128] and is transcriptionally regulated in endometrial cells by tamoxifen [144]. Its role in bone metastases induced by breast cancer has not been investigated.

Mixed osteolytic-osteoblastic metastases are characteristic of both breast and prostate cancers. The effects of the combined expression of osteolytic and osteoblastic factors on bone have not been studied, so the net response of bone at the metastatic site is unpredictable. As noted, osteolytic factors such as PTHrP and IL-11 act on osteoblasts to increase expression of RANK ligand. We tested the effects of introducing the osteoblastic factor ET-1 into the PTHrP-secreting MDA-MB-231 breast cancer cell line. Instead of converting the bone response from osteolytic to osteoblastic, the bone-destructive effects were enhanced by ET-1 (Yin, Chirgwin, and Guise, unpublished). Some of this effect may be caused by autocrine responses of the tumor cells to ET-1. Osteoblastic factors can stimulate osteoblast proliferation, increasing the population of early osteoblasts [31]. The enlarged pool of early osteoblasts responds to osteolytic factors by increased expression of RANK ligand [43, 68]. Recently Yi et al. [225] overexpressed platelet-derived growth factor B-chain in MDA-MB-231 cells and observed osteosclerotic rather than osteolytic metastases.

A puzzling question has been the role of PTHrP in osteoblastic metastases, especially those due to prostate cancers, which nearly always express PTHrP. A partial explanation was provided by the observation that prostate-specific antigen [PSA] is a serine proteinase, which cleaves PTHrP after residue 23 [39, 93]. The resulting fragment fails to activate the classical PTH/PTHrP receptor. It was later observed that the inactive fragment PTHrP1–16 increased cyclic AMP in cardiomyocytes by activating the endothelin A receptor. Binding was attributed to a four amino acid near-identity between the two peptides [174]. We have extended these observations to bone. PTHrP1–23, in concentrations as low as 1nM, is a potent stimulator of calvarial new bone formation. PSA is commonly expressed in breast cancer [12]. The results suggest that PSA proteolysis, rather than inactivating PTHrP, converts it from an osteolytic factor to a potent osteoblastic one. The same may occur in breast cancer bone metastases.

Tumor cells also secrete factors that oppose the development and progression of bone metastases. One such example is interleukin-18, which decreases osteoclast formation [94, 138]. Clearly these factors may hold new approaches for future anti-metastatic therapies. Similarly, the roles of angiogenesis [208] and the immune system [161] in bone metastases are not well known.

Clinical And Experimental Therapies

Bisphosphonates

Bisphosphonates are approved by the Food and Drug Administration for treatment of established bone metastases due to breast and prostate cancer, as well as other solid tumors. Bisphosphonates have many low-specificity biochemical actions that may be responsible for their effectiveness. They reduce tumor growth *in vitro* [30, 73] and invasiveness [14], as well as increase apoptosis [33]. Bisphosphonates can reduce adhesion of tumor cells to bone [210] and decrease angiogenesis [72, 217]. Angiogenesis plays an important role in bone metastases, and bisphosphonates may affect vascular endothelial cells and tumor cells in bone. Osteoblasts bind bisphosphonates, which appear to be anti-apoptotic for the cells, while they are pro-apoptotic for osteoclasts. Compound-specific effects unique to osteoblasts have been reported [59, 157], but it is unknown if these actions are important *in vivo*. The actions of bisphosphonates are limited by their

cellular concentrations *in vivo*. It is thus controversial whether they have significant effects on tumor cells, particularly at non-bone sites.

Controversy surrounds clinical data on the effects of bisphosphonates on breast cancer tumor burden at extra-skeletal sites [44, 45]. Although bisphosphonates have direct anti-tumor actions *in vitro*, it is unclear whether the compounds reach sufficiently high local concentrations in extra-skeletal sites to have such actions in the body. The bisphosphonates have the potential to enhance anti-tumor activities of known cytotoxic agents, but further and larger clinical trials are required to address the importance of the preclinical data. A major morbidity for patients with skeletal metastases is intractable bone pain, which is reduced by bisphosphonate treatment [35, 116, 226]. Interruption of the vicious cycle with bisphosphonates reduces the concentrations of pain-stimulating molecules in the microenvironment surrounding metastatic tumor cells. Although numerous bisphosphonates are in clinical use and several are approved for cancer bone metastases, they have not been shown to improve patient survival in patients with established solid tumor metastases to bone [33–35, 116].

Other Bone-targeting Agents

The affinity of the bisphosphonate chemical structure for the mineralized matrix of bone constitutes a unique mechanism by which these agents can be targeted to bone. An inhibitor of intracellular src signaling was modified by the addition of a pair of phosphonate groups and shown to inhibit osteoclastic bone resorption [179]. This may provide a new way to add specificity for bone targeting to chemotherapeutic and adjuvant compounds.

Morony et al. [130] treated mice with a modified recombinant version of osteoprotegerin (OPG), the soluble, inhibitory binding protein for RANK ligand. OPG inhibits osteoclast formation, activity, and survival. OPG, when injected into mice, decreased osteolytic destruction and tumor burden in bone, but had no effect on metastases in soft tissues [130]. OPG treatment also decreased bone pain [85]. Recombinant OPG has entered initial clinical trials [13], but it is unclear whether it will prove equal or superior to the widely used and more convenient bisphosphonate antiresorptive agents.

Therapy to neutralize PTHrP or inhibit its production is currently under investigation to treat breast cancer metastases to bone. PTHrP neutralizing antibodies, which effectively reduced breast cancer metastases to bone in a mouse model, have been changed for human application and have now entered clinical trials [80]. Similarly, small molecule inhibitors of PTHrP transcription have reduced osteolytic bone metastases in the same mouse models and offer promise as clinical treatment for osteolytic bone metastases [65]. A recent study, designed to inhibit the nuclear promoter responsible for PTHrP transcription in tumor cells, used a PTHrP promoter-luciferase reporter in a high-throughput screen of small molecules and identified two related molecules as effective inhibitors of PTHrP transcription: 6-thioguanine and 6-thioguanosine. These agents have been used for over a quarter of a century against leukemias and several inflammatory disorders. When tested in animal models of humoral hypercalcemia of malignancy and against breast cancer bone metastases, both were effective [65].

Endothelin receptor antagonists may also prove effective against osteoblastic metastases [139, 140, 163, 226]. Small molecule inhibitors of intracellular signaling in either bone or cancer cells have not been reported to be effective against bone metastases, although the range of testable targets is very wide.

Bone Loss in the Patient with Cancer and Effects of Therapy on the Skeleton

Bone metastases are not the only source of skeletal morbidity in cancer patients. Patients with prostate and breast cancer are often sex-steroid deficient due to treatment. This state results in accelerated osteoclastic bone resorption, bone loss, and increased risk of fracture [42]. Sex steroids have complex, gender-specific effects on bone through both genomic and non-genomic mechanisms [106, 122, 187] and also regulate the tumor production of bone-active factors such as PTHrP [63] and ET-1. The standard of care for patients with advanced prostate cancer, for example, is androgen ablation. However, hypogonadism causes male osteoporosis, and bisphosphonate treatment prevents bone loss or can increase bone mass [184, 185].

Women who have had breast cancer are at increased risk for osteoporosis. They are more likely to undergo early menopause due to chemotherapy-induced ovarian failure or oophorectomy. Chemotherapy may also adversely affect bone mineral density.

Tamoxifen treatment causes significant bone loss in premenopausal women, yet prevents it in postmenopausal women. In women with breast cancer the risk of vertebral fracture is markedly increased [99, 100], with incidence increased nearly five times in women from the time of first diagnosis of breast cancer and 20-fold in women with soft-tissue metastases who had no skeletal metastases. Selective estrogen-receptor modulators, SERMS, may play a particularly important role in the treatment of breast cancer without causing bone loss [34, 57, 159]. The active metabolite of vitamin D stimulates osteoblastic expression of RANK ligand and can increase osteoclastic bone resorption. At the same time, vitamin D metabolites have powerful anti-tumor effects. As with other steroid derivatives, selective receptor-modulating vitamin D analogs may be effective against breast cancer cells, while sparing bone [49].

Since bone resorption directly stimulates the vicious cycle of bone metastasis (Figure 9.1) it is possible that treatment-induced bone loss could increase skeletal metastases. This undesirable possibility has now been shown to occur in animal models (Padalecki et al, in preparation), but may be treatable with antiresorptive agents. If this is true, then it would be desirable to inhibit treatment-related bone loss, thus preserving skeletal health and decreasing bone metastases.

Acknowledgments

Work in the authors' laboratory was supported in part by funding from the Gerald D. Aurbach endowment, the Mellon Institute of the University of Virginia Cancer Center, and research grants from the NIH (R01 CA69158 and P01 CA44035) and the U.S. Army (DAMD17–99–1–9401) to T.A.G and the Veterans Administration Research Service (Merit Award) and the U.S. Army (DAMD17–98–1–8245 and DAMD17–02–1–0586) to J.M.C. The authors thank Mr. Cliff Martin for assistance in preparing the figures.

References

1. Abou-Samra AB, Juppner H, Force T, Freeman MW, Kong XF, Schipani E, et al. (1992) Expression cloning of a common receptor for parathyroid hormone and parathyroid hormone-related peptide from rat osteoblast-like cells: a single receptor stimulates intracellular accumulation of both cAMP and inositol trisphosphates and increases intracellular free calcium. Proc Natl Acad Sci USA 89(7):2732–6.
2. Adams JS, Sharma OP, Gacad MA, Singer FR (1983) Metabolism of 25-hydroxyvitamin D3 by cultured pulmonary alveolar macrophages in sarcoidosis. Journal of Clinical Investigation 72(5):1856–60.
3. Arguello F, Baggs RB, Frantz CN (1998) A murine model of experimental metastasis to bone and bone marrow. Cancer Res 48:6876–81.
4. Bachelder RE, Wendt MA, Mercurio AM (2002) Vascular endothelial growth factor promotes breast carcinoma invasion in an autocrine manner by regulating the chemokine receptor CXCR4. Cancer Res 62:7203–6.
5. Barhoum M, Hutchins L, Fonseca VA (1999) Intractable hypercalcemia due to a metastatic carcinoid secreting parathyroid hormone-related peptide and interleukin-6: response to octreotide. American Journal of the Medical Sciences 318(3):203–5.
6. Bendre MS, Gaddy-Kurten D, Mon-Foote T, Akel NS, Skinner RA, Nicholas RW, Suva LJ (2002) Expression of interleukin 8 and not parathyroid hormone-related protein by human breast cancer cells correlates with bone metastasis in vivo. Cancer Res 62:5571–9.
7. Berruti A, Dogliotti L, Tucci M, Tarabuzzi R, Guercio S, Torta M, Tampellini M, Dovio A, Poggio M, Scarpa RM, Angeli A (2002) Metabolic effects of single-dose pamidronate administration in prostate cancer patients with bone metastases. Int J Biol Markers 17:244–52.
8. Bertolini DR, Nedwin GE, Bringman TS, Smith DD, Mundy GR (1986) Stimulation of bone resorption and inhibition of bone formation in vitro by human tumour necrosis factors. Nature 319(6053):516–18.
9. Binstock ML, Mundy GR (1981) Effect of calcitonin and glutocorticoids in combination on the hypercalcemia of malignancy. Annals of Internal Medicine 93(2):269–72.
10. Bisaz S, Jung A, Fleisch H (1978) Uptake by bone of pyrophosphate, diphosphonates and their technetium derivatives. Clin Sci Mol Med 54:265–72.
11. Black K, Garrett IR, Mundy GR (1991). Chinese hamster ovarian cells transfected with the murine interleukin-6 gene cause hypercalcemia as well as cachexia, leukocytosis and thrombocytosis in tumor-bearing nude mice. Endocrinology 128(5):2657–9.
12. Black MH, Diamandis EP (2000) The diagnostic and prognostic utility of prostate-specific antigen for diseases of the breast. Breast Cancer Res Treat 59:1–14.
13. Body JJ, Greipp P, Coleman RE, Facon T, Geurs F, Fermand JP, Harousseau JL, Lipton A, Mariette X, Williams CD, Nakanishi A, Holloway D, Martin SW, Dunstan CR, Bekker PJ (2003) A phase I study of AMGN-0007, a recombinant osteoprotegerin construct, in patients with multiple myeloma or breast carcinoma related bone metastases. Cancer 97(3 Suppl):887–92.
14. Boissier S, Ferreras M, Peyruchaud O, Magnetto S, Ebetino FH, Colombel M, Delmas P, Delaisse JM, Clezardin P (2000) Bisphosphonates inhibit breast and prostate carcinoma cell invasion, an early event in the formation of bone metastases. Cancer Res 60:2949–54.
15. Botella A, Rekik M, Delvaux M, Davicco MJ, Barlet JP, Frexinos J, et al. (1994) Parathyroid hormone (PTH) and PTH-related peptide induce relaxation of smooth muscle cells from guinea pig ileum: interaction with vasoactive intestinal peptide receptors. Endocrinology 135(5):2160–7.
16. Boxer DI, Todd CE, Coleman R, Fogelman I (1989) Bone secondaries in breast cancer: the solitary metastasis. J Nucl Med 30:1318–20.
17. Boyce BF, Aufdemorte TB, Garrett IR, Yates AJ, Mundy GR (1989) Effects of interleukin-1 on bone turnover in normal mice. Endocrinology 125(3):1142–50.
18. Boyde A, Maconnachie E, Reid SA, Delling G, Mundy GR (1986) Scanning electron microscopy in bone pathology: Review of methods. Potential and applications. Scanning Electron Microscopy IV:1537–54.
19. Breslau NA, McGuire JL, Zerwekh JE, Frenkel EP, Pak CY (1984) Hypercalcemia associated with increased serum calcitriol levels in three patients with lymphoma. Annals of Internal Medicine 100(1):1–6.
20. Buchs N, Manen D, Bonjour JP, Rizzoli R (2000) Calcium stimulates parathyroid hormone related protein production in Leydig tumor cells through a putative cation-sensing mechanism. Eur J Endocrinol 142:500–5.
21. Bundred NJ, Ratcliffe WA, Walker RA, Coley S, Morrison JM, Ratcliffe JG (1991) Parathyroid hormone related protein and hypercalcaemia in breast cancer. British Medical Journal 303(6816):1506–9.
22. Bundred NJ, Walker RA, Ratcliffe WA, Warwick J, Morrison JM, Ratcliffe JG (1992) Parathyroid hormone related protein and skeletal morbidity in breast cancer. European Journal of Cancer 28(2–3):690–2.
23. Burtis WJ, Brady TG, Orloff JJ, Ersbak JB, Warrell RP, Jr., Olson BR, et al. (1990) Immunochemical characterization of circulating parathyroid hormone-related protein in patients with humoral hypercalcemia of cancer. New England Journal of Medicine 322(16):1106–12.
24. Burtis WJ, Wu T, Bunch C, Wysolmerski J, Insogna K, Weir E, Broadus AE, Stewart AF (1987) Identification of a novel 17,000-dalton parathyroid hormone-like adenylate cyclase-stimulating protein from a tumor associated with humoral hypercalcemia of malignancy. J Biol Chem 262:7151–6.
25. Chambers AF, Groom AC, MacDonald IC (2002) Dissemination and growth of cancer cells in metastatic sites. Nat Rev Cancer 2:563–72.
26. Charhon SA, Chapuy MC, Delvin EE, Valentin-Opran A, Edouard CM, Meunier PJ (1983) Histomorphometric analysis of sclerotic bone metastases from prostatic carcinoma special reference to osteomalacia. Cancer 51:918–24.
27. Chelouche Lev D, Price JE (2002) Therapeutic intervention with breast cancer metastasis. Crit Rev Eukaryot Gene Expr 12:137–50.
28. Chen HL, Demiralp B, Schneider A, Koh AJ, Silve C, Wang CY, et al. (2002) Parathyroid hormone and

parathyroid hormone-related protein exert both pro- and anti-apoptotic effects in mesenchymal cells. Journal of Biological Chemistry 277(22):19374–81.

29. Chirgwin JM, Guise TA (2000) Molecular mechanisms of tumor-bone interactions in osteolytic metastases. Crit Rev Eukaryot Gene Exp 10:159–78.

30. Clezardin P (2002) The antitumor potential of bisphosphonates. Semin Oncol 29(6 Suppl 21):33–42.

31. Coffman JA (2003) Runx transcription factors and the developmental balance between cell proliferation and differentiation. Cell Biol Int 27:315–24.

32. Coleman RE, Rubens RD (1987) The clinical course of bone metastases from breast cancer. Brit J Cancer 55:61–6.

33. Coleman RE (2002) Bisphosphonates for the prevention of bone metastases. Semin Oncol 29(6 Suppl 21):43–9.

34. Coleman RE (2003) Current and future status of adjuvant therapy for breast cancer. Cancer. 97(3 Suppl):880–6.

35. Coleman RE (2002) Efficacy of zoledronic acid and pamidronate in breast cancer patients: a comparative analysis of randomized phase III trials. Am J Clin Oncol 25(6 Suppl 1):S25–31.

36. Cooper CR, Chay CH, Gendernalik JD, Lee HL, Bhatia J, Taichman RS, McCauley LK, Keller ET, Pienta KJ (2003) Stromal factors involved in prostate carcinoma metastasis to bone. Cancer 97(3 Suppl):739–47.

37. Cornish J, Naot D, Reid IR (2003) Adrenomedullin-a regulator of bone formation. Regul Pept 112:79–86.

38. Coussens LM, Fingleton B, Matrisian LM (2002) Matrix metalloproteinase inhibitors and cancer: trials and tribulations. Science 295:2387–92.

39. Cramer SD, Chen Z, Peehl DM (1996) Prostate specific antigen cleaves parathyroid hormone-related protein in the PTH-like domain: inactivation of PTHrP-stimulated cAMP accumulation in mouse osteoblasts. J Urol 156:526–31.

40. Dallas SL, Rosser JL, Mundy GR, Bonewald LF (2002) Proteolysis of latent transforming growth factor-beta (TGF-beta)-binding protein-1 by osteoclasts. A cellular mechanism for release of TGF-beta from bone matrix. J Biol Chem 277:21352–60.

41. de la Mata J, Uy HL, Guise TA, Story B, Boyce BF, Mundy GR, et al. (1995) Interleukin-6 enhances hypercalcemia and bone resorption mediated by parathyroid hormone-related protein. Journal of Clinical Investigation 95(6):2846–52.

42. Delmas PD, Balena R, Confravreux E, Hardouin C, Hardy P, Bremond A (1997) Bisphosphonate risedronate prevents bone loss in women with artificial menopause due to chemotherapy of breast cancer: a double-blind, placebo-controlled study. J Clin Oncol 15:955–62.

43. Deyama Y, Takeyama S, Koshikawa M, Shirai Y, Yoshimura Y, Nishikata M, Suzuki K, Matsumoto A (2000) Osteoblast maturation suppressed osteoclastogenesis in coculture with bone marrow cells. Biochem Biophys Res Commun 274:249–54.

44. Diel IJ, Solomayer EF, Bastert G (2000) Bisphosphonates and the prevention of metastasis: first evidences from preclinical and clinical studies. Cancer 88(12 Suppl):3080–8.

45. Diel IJ, Solomayer EF, Bastert G (2000) Treatment of metastatic bone disease in breast cancer: bisphosphonates. Clin Breast Cancer 1:43–51.

46. Dumont N, Arteaga CL (2003) Targeting the TGFβ signaling network in human neoplasia. Cancer Cell 3:531–6.

47. Eaton CL, Coleman RE (2003) Pathophysiology of bone metastases from prostate cancer and the role of bisphosphonates in treatment. Cancer Treat Rev 29:189–98.

48. Eilon G, Mundy GR (1978) Direct resorption of bone by human breast cancer cells in vitro. Nature 276:726–8.

49. El Abdaimi K, Dion N, Papavasiliou V, Cardinal PE, Binderup L, Goltzman D, Ste-Marie LG, Kremer R (2000) The vitamin D analogue EB 1089 prevents skeletal metastasis and prolongs survival time in nude mice transplanted with human breast cancer cells. Cancer Res 60:4412–14.

50. Felding-Habermann B, O'Toole TE, Smith JW, Fransvea E, Ruggeri ZM, Ginsberg MH, Hughes PE, Pampori N, Shattil SJ, Saven A, Mueller BM (2001). Integrin activation controls metastasis in human breast cancer. Proc Natl Acad Sci USA 98:1853–8.

51. Fetchick DA, Bertolini DR, Sarin PS, Weintraub ST, Mundy GR, Dunn JF (1986) Production of 1,25-dihydroxyvitamin D3 by human T cell lymphotrophic virus-I-transformed lymphocytes. Journal of Clinical Investigation 78(2):592–6.

52. Fidler IJ (2003) The pathogenesis of cancer metastasis: the "seed and soil" hypothesis revisited. Nat Rev Cancer 3:1–6.

53. Fierabracci P, Pinchera A, Miccoli P, Conte PF, Vignali E, Zaccagnini M, et al. (2001) Increased prevalence of primary hyperparathyroidism in treated breast cancer. Journal of Endocrinological Investigation 24(5):315–20.

54. Firkin F, Seymour JF, Watson AM, Grill V, Martin TJ (1996) Parathyroid hormone-related protein in hypercalcaemia associated with haematological malignancy. British Journal of Haematology 94(3):486–92.

55. Fleisch H (1991) Bisphosphonates. Pharmacology and use in the treatment of tumour-induced hypercalcaemic and metastatic bone disease. Drugs 42(6):919–44.

56. Fontana A, Delmas PD (2000) Markers of bone turnover in bone metastases. Cancer 88(12 Suppl):2952–60.

57. Fontana A, Delmas PD (2003) Selective estrogen receptors modulators in the prevention and treatment of postmenopausal osteoporosis. Endocrinol Metab Clin North Am 32:219–32.

58. Frith JC, Rogers MJ (2003) Antagonistic effects of different classes of bisphosphonates in osteoclasts and macrophages in vitro. J Bone Miner Res 18:204–12.

59. Fromigue O, Body JJ (2002) Bisphosphonates influence the proliferation and the maturation of normal human osteoblasts. J Endocrinol Invest 25:539–46.

60. Fukumitsu N, Uchiyama M (2002) Correlation of urine type I collagen-cross-linked N telopeptide levels with bone scintigraphic results in prostate cancer patients. Metabolism 51:814–18.

61. Funk JL, Lausier J, Moser AH, Shigenaga JK, Huling S, Nissenson RA, et al. (1995) Endotoxin induces parathyroid hormone-related protein gene expression in splenic stromal and smooth muscle cells, not in splenic lymphocytes. Endocrinology 136(8):3412–21.

62. Funk JL, Shigenaga JK, Moser AH, Krul EJ, Strewler GJ, Feingold KR, et al. (1994) Cytokine regulation of

parathyroid hormone-related protein messenger ribonucleic acid levels in mouse spleen: paradoxical effects of interferon-gamma and interleukin-4. Endocrinology 135(1):351–8.

63. Funk JL, Wei H (1998) Regulation of PTHrP expression in MCF-7 breast carcinoma cells by estrogen and antiestrogens. Biochem Biophys Res Commun 251:849–54.

64. Galasko CS (1986) Skeletal metastases. Clin Orthop 210:18–30.

65. Gallwitz WE, Guise TA, Mundy GR (2002) Guanosine nucleotides inhibit different syndromes of PTHrP excess caused by human cancers in vivo. J Clin Invest 110(10):1559–72.

66. Gardella TJ, Juppner H (2001) Molecular properties of the PTH/PTHrP receptor. Trends Endocrinol Metab 12:210–17.

67. Garnero P, Buchs N, Zekri J, Rizzoli R, Coleman RE, Delmas PD (2000) Markers of bone turnover for the management of patients with bone metastases from prostate cancer. Br J Cancer 82:858–64.

68. Geoffroy V, Kneissel M, Fournier B, Boyde A, Matthias P (2002) High bone resorption in adult aging transgenic mice overexpressing cbfa1/runx2 in cells of the osteoblastic lineage. Mol Cell Biol 22:6222–33.

69. Giuliani N, Pedrazzoni M, Negri G, Passeri G, Impicciatore M, Girasole G (1998) Bisphosphonates stimulate formation of osteoblast precursors and mineralized nodules in murine and human bone marrow cultures in vitro and promote early osteoblastogenesis in young and aged mice in vivo. Bone 22(5):455–61.

70. Giuliani N, Pedrazzoni M, Passeri G, Girasole G (1998) Bisphosphonates inhibit IL-6 production by human osteoblast-like cells. Scandinavian Journal of Rheumatology 27(1):38–41.

71. Gkonos PJ, London R, Hendler ED (1984) Hypercalcemia and elevated 1,25-dihydroxyvitamin D levels in a patient with end-stage renal disease and active tuberculosis. New England Journal of Medicine 311(26):1683–5.

72. Green JR, Clezardin P (2002) Mechanisms of bisphosphonate effects on osteoclasts, tumor cell growth, and metastasis. Am J Clin Oncol 25(6 Suppl 1):S3–9.

73. Green JR (2003) Antitumor effects of bisphosphonates. Cancer 97(3 Suppl):840–7.

74. Grill V, Ho P, Body JJ, Johanson N, Lee SC, Kukreja SC, et al. (1991) Parathyroid hormone-related protein: elevated levels in both humoral hypercalcemia of malignancy and hypercalcemia complicating metastatic breast cancer. Journal of Clinical Endocrinology & Metabolism 73(6):1309–15.

75. Grill V, Martin TJ (2000) Hypercalcemia of malignancy. Reviews in Endocrine & Metabolic Disorders 1(4):253–63.

76. Gucalp R, Ritch P, Wiernik PH, Sarma PR, Keller A, Richman SP, et al. (1992) Comparative study of pamidronate disodium and etidronate disodium in the treatment of cancer-related hypercalcemia. Journal of Clinical Oncology 10(1):134–42.

77. Guise TA, Garrett IR, Bonewald LF, Mundy GR (1993) Interleukin-1 receptor antagonist inhibits the hypercalcemia mediated by interleukin-1. Journal of Bone & Mineral Research 8(5):583–7.

78. Guise TA, Mundy GR (1998) Cancer and bone. Endocr Rev 19:18–54.

79. Guise TA, Yin JJ, Mohammad KS (2003) Role of endothelin-1 in osteoblastic bone metastases. Cancer 97(3 Suppl):779–84.

80. Guise TA, Yin JJ, Taylor SD, Kumagai Y, Dallas M, Boyce BF, Yoneda T, Mundy GR (1996) Evidence for a causal role of parathyroid hormone-related protein in the pathogenesis of human breast cancer-mediated osteolysis. J Clin Invest 98:1544–9.

81. Guise TA, Yoneda T, Yates AJ, Mundy GR (1993) The combined effect of tumor-produced parathyroid hormone-related protein and transforming growth factor-alpha enhance hypercalcemia in vivo and bone resorption in vitro. J Clin Endocrinol Metab 77(1):40–5.

82. Hauschka PV, Mavrakos AE, Iafrati MD, Doleman SE, Klagsbrun M (1986) Growth factors in bone matrix. Isolation of multiple types by affinity chromatography on heparin-Sepharose. J Biol Chem 261:12665–74.

83. Henderson M, Danks J, Moseley J, Slavin J, Harris T, McKinlay M, Hopper J, Martin T (2001) Parathyroid hormone-related protein production by breast cancers, improved survival, and reduced bone metastases. J Natl Cancer Inst 93:234–7.

84. Hofbauer LC, Heufelder AE (2001) Role of receptor activator of nuclear factor-kappaB ligand and osteoprotegerin in bone cell biology. J Mol Med 79:243–53.

85. Honore P, Luger NM, Sabino MA, Schwei MJ, Rogers SD, Mach DB, O'keefe PF, Ramnaraine ML, Clohisy DR, Mantyh PW (2000) Osteoprotegerin blocks bone cancer-induced skeletal destruction, skeletal pain and pain-related neurochemical reorganization of the spinal cord. Nat Med 6:521–8.

86. Horiuchi N, Caulfield MP, Fisher JE, Goldman ME, McKee RL, Reagan JE, et al. (1987) Similarity of synthetic peptide from human tumor to parathyroid hormone in vivo and in vitro. Science 238(4833):1566–8.

87. Hortobagyi GN, Theriault RL, Porter L, Blayney D, Lipton A, Sinoff C, Wheeler H, Simeone JF, Seaman J, Knight RD, Heffernan M, Reitsma (1996) Efficacy of pamidronate in reducing skeletal complications in patients with breast cancer and lytic bone metastases. New Engl J Med 335:1785–91.

88. Hosking DJ, Cowley A, Bucknall CA (1981) Rehydration in the treatment of severe hypercalcaemia. Quarterly Journal of Medicine 50(200):473–81.

89. Ibbotson KJ, Twardzik DR, D'Souza SM, Hargreaves WR, Todaro GJ, Mundy GR (1985) Stimulation of bone resorption in vitro by synthetic transforming growth factor-alpha. Science 228(4702):1007–9.

90. Iguchi H, Miyagi C, Tomita K, Kawauchi S, Nozuka Y, Tsuneyoshi M, et al. (1998) Hypercalcemia caused by ectopic production of parathyroid hormone in a patient with papillary adenocarcinoma of the thyroid gland. Journal of Clinical Endocrinology & Metabolism 83(8):2653–7.

91. Iguchi H, Tanaka S, Ozawa Y, Kashiwakuma T, Kimura T, Hiraga T, Ozawa H, Kono A (1996) An experimental model of bone metastasis by human lung cancer cells: the role of parathyroid hormone-related protein in bone metastasis. Cancer Res 56:4040–3.

92. Ikeda K, Ohno H, Hane M, Yokoi H, Okada M, Honma T, et al. (1994) Development of a sensitive two-site immunoradiometric assay for parathyroid hormone-related peptide: evidence for elevated levels in plasma from patients with adult T-cell leukemia/lymphoma

and B-cell lymphoma. Journal of Clinical Endocrinology & Metabolism 79(5):1322–7.

93. Iwamura M, Hellman J, Cockett AT, Lilja H, Gershagen S (1996) Alteration of the hormonal bioactivity of parathyroid hormone-related protein (PTHrP) as a result of limited proteolysis by prostate-specific antigen. Urology 48:317–25.

94. Iwasaki T, Yamashita K, Tsujimura T, Kashiwamura S, Tsutsui H, Kaisho T, Sugihara A, Yamada N, Mukai M, Yoneda T, Okamura H, Akedo H, Terada N (2002) Interleukin-18 inhibits osteolytic bone metastasis by human lung cancer cells possibly through suppression of osteoclastic bone-resorption in nude mice. J Immunother 25 Suppl 1:S52–60.

95. Jackson JG, Zhang X, Yoneda T, Yee D (2001) Regulation of breast cancer cell motility by insulin receptor substrate-2 (IRS-2) in metastatic variants of human breast cancer cell lines. Oncogene 20:7318–25.

96. Johnson RA, Boyce BF, Mundy GR, Roodman GD (1989) Tumors producing human tumor necrosis factor induced hypercalcemia and osteoclastic bone resorption in nude mice. Endocrinology 124(3):1424–7.

97. Kakonen SM, Selander KS, Chirgwin JM, Yin JJ, Burns S, Rankin WA, Grubbs BG, Dallas M, Cui Y, Guise TA (2002) Transforming growth factor-beta stimulates parathyroid hormone-related protein and osteolytic metastases via Smad and mitogen-activated protein kinase signaling pathways. J Biol Chem 277:24571–8.

98. Kang Y, Siegel PM, Shu W, Drobnjak M, Kakonen SM, Cordon-Cardo C, Guise TA, Massague J (2003) A multigenic program mediating breast cancer metastasis to bone. Cancer Cell 3:537–49.

99. Kanis JA, McCloskey EV, Powles T, Paterson AH, Ashley S, Spector T (1999) A high incidence of vertebral fracture in women with breast cancer. Br J Cancer 79:1179–81.

100. Kanis JA, McCloskey EV, Powles TJ (1999) Clodronate in the treatment of neoplastic bone disease. Program and Abstracts, Second International Conference on Cancer-Induced Bone Disease 4.

101. Kanis JA, Urwin GH, Gray RE, Beneton MN, McCloskey EV, Hamdy NA, et al. (1987) Effects of intravenous etidronate disodium on skeletal and calcium metabolism. American Journal of Medicine 82(2A):55–70.

102. Klein BY, Ben-Bassat H, Breuer E, Solomon V, Golomb G (1998) Structurally different bisphosphonates exert opposing effects on alkaline phosphatase and mineralization in marrow osteoprogenitors. Journal of Cellular Biochemistry 68(2):186–94.

103. Klein DC, Raisz LG (1970) Prostaglandins: stimulation of bone resorption in tissue culture. Endocrinology 86(6):1436–40.

104. Kohno N, Kitazawa S, Fukase M, Sakoda Y, Kanbara Y, Furuya Y, et al. (1994) The expression of parathyroid hormone-related protein in human breast cancer with skeletal metastases. Surgery Today 24(3):215–20.

105. Koizumi M, Ogata E (2002) Bone metabolic markers as gauges of metastasis to bone: a review. Ann Nucl Med 16:161–8.

106. Kousteni S, Chen JR, Bellido T, Han L, Ali AA, O'Brien CA, Plotkin L, Fu Q, Mancino AT, Wen Y, Vertino AM, Powers CC, Stewart SA, Ebert R, Parfitt AM, Weinstein RS, Jilka RL, Manolagas SC (2002) Reversal of bone loss in mice by nongenotropic signaling of sex steroids. Science 298:843–6.

107. Koutsilieris M (1995) Skeletal metastases in advanced prostate cancer: cell biology and therapy. Crit Rev Oncol Hematol 18:51–64.

108. Kovacs CS, Lanske B, Hunzelman JL, Guo J, Karaplis AC, Kronenberg HM (1996) Parathyroid hormone-related peptide (PTHrP) regulates fetal-placental calcium transport through a receptor distinct from the PTH/PTHrP receptor. Proc Natl Acad Sci USA 93(26):15233–8.

109. Kremer R, Shustik C, Tabak T, Papavasiliou V, Goltzman D (1996) Parathyroid-hormone-related peptide in hematologic malignancies. American Journal of Medicine 100(4):406–11.

110. Kukreja SC, Rosol TJ, Wimbiscus SA, Shevrin DH, Grill V, Barengolts EI, Martin TJ (1990) Tumor resection and antibodies to parathyroid hormone-related protein cause similar changes on bone histomorphometry in hypercalcemia of cancer. Endocrinology Jul 127(1):305–10.

111. Lee J, Weber M, Mejia S, Bone E, Watson P, Orr W (2001) A matrix metalloproteinase inhibitor, batimastat, retards the development of osteolytic bone metastases by MDA-MB-231 human breast cancer cells in Balb C nu/nu mice. Eur J Cancer 37:106–13.

112. Li H, Seitz PK, Selvanayagam P, Rajaraman S, Cooper CW (1996) Effect of endogenously produced parathyroid hormone-related peptide on growth of a human hepatoma cell line (Hep G2). Endocrinology 137(6):2367–74.

113. Li X, Tomita M, Pilbeam CC, Breyer RM, Raisz LG (2002) Prostaglandin receptor EP2 mediates PGE2 stimulated hypercalcemia in mice in vivo. Prostaglandins Other Lipid Mediat 67(3–4):173–80.

114. Liapis H, Crouch EC, Grosso LE, Kitazawa S, Wick MR (1993) Expression of parathyroidlike protein in normal, proliferative, and neoplastic human breast tissues. American Journal of Pathology 143(4):1169–78.

115. Lin DL, Tarnowski CP, Zhang J, Dai J, Rohn E, Patel AH, Morris MD, Keller ET (2001) Bone metastatic LNCaP-derivative C4-2B prostate cancer cell line mineralizes in vitro. Prostate 47:212–21.

116. Lipton A (2003) Bisphosphonates and metastatic breast carcinoma. Cancer 97(3 Suppl):848–853.

117. Lipton A (2003) Bone metastases in breast cancer. Curr Treat Options Oncol 4:151–8.

118. Luger NM, Sabino MA, Schwei MJ, Mach DB, Pomonis JD, Keyser CP, Rathbun M, Clohisy DR, Honore P, Yaksh TL, Mantyh PW (2002) Efficacy of systemic morphine suggests a fundamental difference in the mechanisms that generate bone cancer vs inflammatory pain. Pain 99:397–406.

119. Luparello C, Burtis WJ, Raue F, Birch MA, Gallagher JA (1995) Parathyroid hormone-related peptide and 8701-BC breast cancer cell growth and invasion in vitro: evidence for growth-inhibiting and invasion-promoting effects. Molecular & Cellular Endocrinology 111(2):225–32.

120. Lynch CC, Matrisian LM (2002) Matrix metalloproteinases in tumor-host cell communication. Differentiation 70:561–73.

121. Major P, Lortholary A, Hon J, Abdi E, Mills G, Menssen HD, et al. (2001) Zoledronic acid is superior to pamidronate in the treatment of hypercalcemia of

malignancy: a pooled analysis of two randomized, controlled clinical trials. Journal of Clinical Oncology 19(2):558–67.

122. Manolagas SC, Kousteni S, Jilka RL (2002). Sex steroids and bone. Recent Prog Horm Res 57:385–409.

123. Mantyh PW, Clohisy DR, Koltzenburg M, Hunt SP (2002) Molecular mechanisms of cancer pain. Nat Rev Cancer 2:201–9.

124. Mareel M, Leroy A (2003) Clinical, cellular, and molecular aspects of cancer invasion. Physiol Rev 83:337–76.

125. Mason RS, Frankel T, Chan YL, Lissner D, Posen S (1984) Vitamin D conversion by sarcoid lymph node homogenate. Annals of Internal Medicine 100(1): 59–61.

126. Mastro AM, Gay CV, Welch DR (2003) The skeleton as a unique environment for breast cancer cells. Clin Exp Metastasis 20:275–84.

127. Mercier RJ, Thompson JM, Harman GS, Messerschmidt GL (1988) Recurrent hypercalcemia and elevated 1,25-dihydroxyvitamin D levels in Hodgkin's disease. American Journal of Medicine 84(1):165–8.

128. Miller MJ, Martinez A, Unsworth EJ, Thiele CJ, Moody TW, Elsasser T, Cuttitta F (1996) Adrenomedullin expression in human tumor cell lines. Its potential role as an autocrine growth factor. J Biol Chem 271: 23345–51.

129. Minina E, Wenzel HM, Kreschel C, Karp S, Gaffield W, McMahon AP, et al. (2001) BMP and Ihh/PTHrP signaling interact to coordinate chondrocyte proliferation and differentiation. Development 128(22): 4523–34.

130. Morony S, Capparelli C, Sarosi I, Lacey DL, Dunstan CR, Kostenuik PJ (2001) Osteoprotegerin inhibits osteolysis and decreases skeletal tumor burden in syngeneic and nude mouse models of experimental bone metastasis. Cancer Res 61:4432–6.

131. Moseley JM, Kubota M, Diefenbach-Jagger H, Wettenhall RE, Kemp BE, Suva LJ, et al. (1987) Parathyroid hormone-related protein purified from a human lung cancer cell line. Proceedings of the National Academy of Sciences of the United States of America 84(14):5048–52.

132. Muller A, Homey B, Soto H, Ge N, Catron D, Buchanan ME, McClanahan T, Murphy E, Yuan W, Wagner SN, Barrera JL, Mohar A, Verastegui E, Zlotnik A (2001) Involvement of chemokine receptors in breast cancer metastasis. Nature 410:50–6.

133. Mundy GR, Rick ME, Turcotte R, Kowalski MA (1978) Pathogenesis of hypercalcemia in lymphosarcoma cell leukemia. Role of an osteoclast activating factor-like substance and a mechanism of action for glucocorticoid therapy. American Journal of Medicine 65(4):600–6.

134. Mundy GR, Wilkinson R, Heath DA (1983) Comparative study of available medical therapy for hypercalcemia of malignancy. American Journal of Medicine 74(3):421–32.

135. Mundy GR. Hypercalcemia (1995) In: Mundy GR, editor. Bone remodeling and its disorders. London: Martin Dunitz :88–103.

136. Mundy GR (2002) Metastasis to bone: causes, consequences and therapeutic opportunities. Nat Rev Cancer 2:584–93.

137. Nagai M, Kyakumoto S, Sato N (2000) Cancer cells responsible for humoral hypercalcemia express mRNA encoding a secreted form of ODF/TRANCE that induces osteoclast formation. Biochem Biophys Res Commun 269(2):532–6.

138. Nakata A, Tsujimura T, Sugihara A, Okamura H, Iwasaki T, Shinkai K, Iwata N, Kakishita E, Akedo H, Terada N (1999) Inhibition by interleukin 18 of osteolytic bone metastasis by human breast cancer cells. Anticancer Res 19:4131–8.

139. Nelson J, Bagnato A, Battistini B, Nisen P (2003) The endothelin axis: emerging role in cancer. Nat Rev Cancer 3:110–16.

140. Nelson JB, Nabulsi AA, Vogelzang NJ, Breul J, Zonnenberg BA, Daliani DD, Schulman CC, Carducci MA (2003) Suppression of prostate cancer induced bone remodeling by the endothelin receptor A antagonist atrasentan. J Urol 169:1143–9.

141. Nemeth EF (2002) Pharmacological regulation of parathyroid hormone secretion. Curr Pharm Des 8:2077–87.

142. Nielsen PK, Rasmussen AK, Feldt-Rasmussen U, Brandt M, Christensen L, Olgaard K (1996) Ectopic production of intact parathyroid hormone by a squamous cell lung carcinoma in vivo and in vitro. Journal of Clinical Endocrinology & Metabolism 81(10):3793–6.

143. Nussbaum SR, Gaz RD, Arnold A (1990) Hypercalcemia and ectopic secretion of parathyroid hormone by an ovarian carcinoma with rearrangement of the gene for parathyroid hormone. New England Journal of Medicine 323(19).1324–8.

144. Oehler MK, Rees MC, Bicknell R (2000) Steroids and the endometrium. Curr Med Chem 7:543–60.

145. Orr W, Varani J, Gondex MK, Ward PA, Mundy GR (1978) Chemotactic responses of tumor cells to products of resorbing bone. Science 203:176–9.

146. Overall CM, Lopez-Otin C (2002) Strategies for MMP inhibition in cancer: innovations for the post-trial era. Nat Rev Cancer 2:657–72.

147. Ozbas S, Dafydd H, Purushotham AD (2003) Bone marrow micrometastasis in breast cancer. Br J Surg 90:290–301.

148. Paget S (1889) The distribution of secondary growths in cancer of the breast. Lancet 1:571–2.

149. Philbrick WM, Dreyer BE, Nakchbandi IA, Karaplis AC (1998) Parathyroid hormone-related protein is required for tooth eruption. Proc Natl Acad Sci USA 95(20):11846–51.

150. Pirola CJ, Wang HM, Strgacich MI, Kamyar A, Cercek B, Forrester JS, et al. (1994) Mechanical stimuli induce vascular parathyroid hormone-related protein gene expression in vivo and in vitro. Endocrinology 134(5):2230–6.

151. Plotkin LI, Weinstein RS, Parfitt AM, Roberson PK, Manolagas SC, Bellido T (1999) Prevention of osteocyte and osteoblast apoptosis by bisphosphonates and calcitonin. Journal of Clinical Investigation 104(10):1363–74.

152. Powell GJ, Southby J, Danks JA, Stillwell RG, Hayman JA, Henderson MA, Bennett RC, Martin TJ (1991) Localization of parathyroid hormone-related protein in breast cancer metastasis: increased incidence in bone compared with other sites. Cancer Res 51: 3059–61.

153. Purohit OP, Radstone CR, Anthony C, Kanis JA, Coleman RE (1995) A randomised double-blind comparison of intravenous pamidronate and clodronate in

the hypercalcaemia of malignancy. British Journal of Cancer 72(5):1289–93.

154. Ralston SH, Gallacher SJ, Patel U, Campbell J, Boyle IT (1990) Cancer-associated hypercalcemia: morbidity and mortality. Clinical experience in 126 treated patients. Annals of Internal Medicine 112(7):499–504.

155. Reddi AH, Roodman D, Freeman C, Mohla S (2003) Mechanisms of tumor metastasis to the bone: challenges and opportunities. J Bone Miner Res 18:190–4.

156. Reinholz GG, Getz B, Pederson L, Sanders ES, Subramaniam M, Ingle JN, et al. (2000) Bisphosphonates directly regulate cell proliferation, differentiation, and gene expression in human osteoblasts. Cancer Research 60(21):6001–7.

157. Reinholz GG, Getz B, Sanders ES, Karpeisky MY, Padyukova NSh, Mikhailov SN, Ingle JN, Spelsberg TC (2002) Distinct mechanisms of bisphosphonate action between osteoblasts and breast cancer cells: identity of a potent new bisphosphonate analogue. Breast Cancer Res Treat 71:257–68.

158. Remuzzi G, Perico N, Benigni A (2003) New therapeutics that antagonize endothelin: promises and frustrations. Nat Rev Drug Discov 1:986–1001.

159. Riggs BL, Hartmann LC (2003) Selective estrogen-receptor modulators – mechanisms of action and application to clinical practice. N Engl J Med 348: 618–29.

160. Rizzoli R, Pache JC, Didierjean L, Burger A, Bonjour JP (1994) A thymoma as a cause of true ectopic hyperparathyroidism. Journal of Clinical Endocrinology & Metabolism 79(3):912–15.

161. Roodman GD (2003) Role of stromal-derived cytokines and growth factors in bone metastasis. Cancer 97(3 Suppl):733–8.

162. Roodman GD (2001) Biology of osteoclast activation in cancer. J Clin Oncol 19:3562–71.

163. Rosenbaum E, Carducci MA (2003) Pharmacotherapy of hormone refractory prostate cancer: new developments and challenges. Expert Opin Pharmacother 4:875–87.

164. Rosenthal N, Insogna KL, Godsall JW, Smaldone L, Waldron JA, Stewart AF (1985) Elevations in circulating 1,25-dihydroxyvitamin D in three patients with lymphoma-associated hypercalcemia. Journal of Clinical Endocrinology & Metabolism 60(1):29–33.

165. Roudier MP, True LD, Higano CS, Vesselle H, Ellis W, Lange P, Vessella RL (2003). Phenotypic heterogeneity of end-stage prostate carcinoma metastatic to bone. Hum Pathol 34:646–53.

166. Roudier MP, Vessella H, True LD, et al. (2003) Bone histology at autopsy and matched bone scintigraphy findings in patients with hormone refractory prostate cancer: the effect of bisphosphonate therapy on bone scintigraphy results. Clin Exp Metastasis 20:171–80.

167. Russell RG, Rogers MJ (1999) Bisphosphonates: from the laboratory to the clinic and back again. Bone 5:97–106.

168. Sabatini M, Boyce B, Aufdemorte T, Bonewald L, Mundy GR (1988) Infusions of recombinant human interleukins 1 alpha and 1 beta cause hypercalcemia in normal mice. Proc Natl Acad Sci USA 85(14):5235–9.

169. Safadi FF, Xu J, Smock SL, Kanaan RA, Selim AH, Odgren PR, Marks SC Jr, Owen TA, Popoff SN (2003) Expression of connective tissue growth factor in bone: Its role in osteoblast proliferation and differentiation in vitro and bone formation in vivo. J Cell Physiol1 96:51–62.

170. Sanders JL, Chattopadhyay N, Kifor O, Yamaguchi T, Brown EM (2000) Extracellular calcium-sensing receptor (CaR) expression and its potential role in parathyroid hormone-related peptide (PTHrP) secretion in the H-500 rat Leydig cell model of humoral hypercalcemia of malignancy. Biochem Biophys Res Commun 269:427–32.

171. Sasaki A, Boyce BF, Story B, Wright KR, Chapman M, Boyce R, Mundy GR, Yoneda T (1995) The bisphosphonate residronate reduces metastatic human breast cancer burden in bone in nude mice. Cancer Res 55:3551–7.

172. Sato K, Fujii Y, Kasono K, Ozawa M, Imamura H, Kanaji Y, Kurosawa H, Tsushima T, Shizume K (1989) Parathyroid hormone-related protein and interleukin-1 alpha synergistically stimulate bone resorption in vitro and increase the serum calcium concentration in mice in vivo. Endocrinology 124(5):2172–8.

173. Sato K, Onuma E, Yocum RC, Ogata E (2003) Treatment of malignancy-associated hypercalcemia and cachexia with humanized anti-parathyroid hormone-related protein antibody. Semin Oncol. 30(5 Suppl 16):167–73.

174. Schluter KD, Katzer C, Piper HM (2001) A N-terminal PTHrP peptide fragment void of a PTH/PTHrP-receptor binding domain activates cardiac ET(A) receptors. Br J Pharmacol1 32:427–32.

175. Schluter KD, Piper HM (1998) Cardiovascular actions of parathyroid hormone and parathyroid hormone-related peptide. Cardiovascular Research 37(1):34–41.

176. Schmidt-Kittler O, Ragg T, Daskalakis A, Granzow M, Ahr A, Blankenstein TJ, Kaufmann M, Diebold J, Arnholdt H, Muller P, Bischoff J, Harich D, Schlimok G, Riethmuller G, Eils R, Klein CA (2003) From latent disseminated cells to overt metastasis: Genetic analysis of systemic breast cancer progression. Proc Natl Acad Sci USA 100:7737–42.

177. Seymour JF, Gagel RF, Hagemeister FB, Dimopoulos MA, Cabanillas F (1994) Calcitriol production in hypercalcemic and normocalcemic patients with non-Hodgkin lymphoma. Annals of Internal Medicine 121(9):633–40.

178. Seymour JF, Grill V, Martin TJ, Lee N, Firkin F (1993) Hypercalcemia in the blastic phase of chronic myeloid leukemia associated with elevated parathyroid hormone-related protein. Leukemia 7(10):1672–5.

179. Shakespeare W, Yang M, Bohacek R, Cerasoli F, Stebbins K, Sundaramoorthi R, Azimioara M, Vu C, Pradeepan S, Metcalf C 3rd, Haraldson C, Merry T, Dalgarno D, Narula S, Hatada M, Lu X, van Schravendijk MR, Adams S, Violette S, Smith J, Guan W, Bartlett C, Herson J, Iuliucci J, Weigele M, Sawyer T (2000) Structure-based design of an osteoclast-selective, nonpeptide src homology 2 inhibitor with in vivo antiresorptive activity. Proc Natl Acad Sci USA 97:9373–8.

180. Sherry MM, Greco FA, Johnson DH, Hainsworth JD (1986) Metastatic breast cancer confined to the skeletal system. An indolent disease. Am J Med. 81:381–6.

181. Simonet WS, Lacey DL, Dunstan CR, Kelley M, Chang MS, Luthy R, Nguyen HQ, Wooden S, Bennett L, Boone T, Shimamoto G, DeRose M, Elliott R, Colombero A, Tan HL, Trail G, Sullivan J, Davy E, Bucay N, Renshaw-Gegg L, Hughes TM, Hill D, Pattison W, Campbell P, Boyle WJ (1997) Osteoprotegerin: a novel secreted

protein involved in the regulation of bone density. Cell 89:309–19.

182. Singer FR, Ritch PS, Lad TE, Ringenberg QS, Schiller JH, Recker RR, et al. (1991) Treatment of hypercalcemia of malignancy with intravenous etidronate. A controlled, multicenter study. The Hypercalcemia Study Group. [erratum appears in Arch Intern Med (1991) Oct 151(10):2008]. Archives of Internal Medicine 151(3):471–6.

183. Singletary SE, Walsh G, Vauthey JN, Curley S, Sawaya R, Weber KL, Meric F, Hortobagyi GN (2003) A role for curative surgery in the treatment of selected patients with metastatic breast cancer. Oncologist 8:241–51.

184. Smith MR, Eastham J, Gleason DM, Shasha D, Tchekmedyian S, Zinner N (2003) Randomized Controlled Trial of Zoledronic Acid to Prevent Bone Loss in Men Receiving Androgen Deprivation Therapy for Nonmetastatic Prostate Cancer. J Urol 169:2008–12.

185. Smith MR (2003) Management of treatment-related osteoporosis in men with prostate cancer. Cancer Treat Rev 29:211–18.

186. Southby J, Kissin MW, Danks JA, Hayman JA, Moseley JM, Henderson MA, et al. (1990) Immunohistochemical localization of parathyroid hormone-related protein in human breast cancer. Cancer Research 50(23):7710–16.

187. Spelsberg TC, Subramaniam M, Riggs BL, Khosla S (1999) The actions and interactions of sex steroids and growth factors/cytokines on the skeleton. Mol Endocrinol 13.819–28.

188. Stewart AF, Horst R, Deftos LJ, Cadman EC, Lang R, Broadus AE (1981) Biochemical evaluation of patients with cancer-associated hypercalcemia: evidence for humoral and nonhumoral groups. New England Journal of Medicine 303(24):1377–83.

189. Strewler GJ, Budayr AA, Clark OH, Nissenson RA (1993) Production of parathyroid hormone by a malignant nonparathyroid tumor in a hypercalcemic patient. Journal of Clinical Endocrinology & Metabolism 76(5):1373–5.

190. Strewler GJ, Stern PH, Jacobs JW, Eveloff J, Klein RF, Leung SC, et al. (1987) Parathyroid hormonelike protein from human renal carcinoma cells. Structural and functional homology with parathyroid hormone. Journal of Clinical Investigation 80(6):1803–7.

191. Strewler GJ (2000) The physiology of parathyroid hormone-related protein. New England Journal of Medicine 342(3):177–85.

192. Suda T, Takahashi N, Udagawa N, Jimi E, Gillespie MT, Martin TJ (1999) Modulation of osteoclast differentiation and function by the new members of the tumor necrosis factor receptor and ligand families. Endocr Rev 20:345–57.

193. Suki WN, Yium JJ, Von Minden M, Saller-Hebert C, Eknoyan G, Martinez-Maldonado M (1970) Actue treatment of hypercalcemia with furosemide. New England Journal of Medicine 283(16):836–40.

194. Suva LJ, Winslow GA, Wettenhall RE, Hammonds RG, Moseley JM, Diefenbach-Jagger H, et al. (1987) A parathyroid hormone-related protein implicated in malignant hypercalcemia: cloning and expression. Science 237(4817):893–6.

195. Taube T, Elomaa I, Blomqvist C, Beneton MNC, Kanis JA (1994) Histomorphometric evidence for osteoclast-mediated bone resorption in metastatic breast cancer. Bone 15:161–6.

196. Teti A, Migliaccio S, Baron R (2002) The role of the alphaVbeta3 integrin in the development of osteolytic bone metastases: a pharmacological target for alternative therapy? Calcif Tissue Int 71:293–9.

197. Thiebaud D, Jacquet AF, Burckhardt P (1990) Fast and effective treatment of malignant hypercalcemia. Combination of suppositories of calcitonin and a single infusion of 3-amino 1-hydroxypropylidene-1-bisphosphonate. Archives of Internal Medicine 150(10):2125–8.

198. Thiede MA, Daifotis AG, Weir EC, Brines ML, Burtis WJ, Ikeda K, et al. (1990) Intrauterine occupancy controls expression of the parathyroid hormone-related peptide gene in preterm rat myometrium. Proc Natl Acad Sci USA 87(18):6969–73.

199. Thomas RJ, Guise TA, Yin JJ, Elliott J, Horwood NJ, Martin TJ, Gillespie MT (1999) Breast cancer cells interact with osteoblasts to support osteoclast formation. Endocrinol 140:4451–8.

200. Tisdale MJ. Cancer (2002) Cachexia in cancer patients. Nat Rev 2:862–71.

201. Tokuda H, Kozawa O, Harada A, Uematsu T (1998) Tiludronate inhibits interleukin-6 synthesis in osteoblasts: inhibition of phospholipase D activation in MC3T3-E1 cells. Journal of Cellular Biochemistry 69(3):252–9.

202. Torring O, Turner RT, Carter WB, Firek AF, Jacobs CA, Health H 3rd (1992) Inhibition by human interleukin-1 alpha of parathyroid hormone-related peptide effects on renal calcium and phosphorus metabolism in the rat. Endocrinology 131(1):5–13.

203. Truong NU, deB Edwardes MD, Papavasiliou V, Goltzman D, Kremer R (2003) Parathyroid hormone-related peptide and survival of patients with cancer and hypercalcemia. Am J Med. 115(2):115–21.

204. Tuttle KR, Kunau RT, Loveridge N, Mundy GR (1991) Altered renal calcium handling in hypercalcemia of malignancy Journal of the American Society of Nephrology 2(2):191–9.

205. Ueno M, Ban S, Nakanoma T, Tsukamoto T, Nonaka S, Hirata R, et al. (2000) Hypercalcemia in a patient with renal cell carcinoma producing parathyroid hormone-related protein and interleukin-6 International Journal of Urology 7(6):239–42.

206. Uy HL, Guise TA, De La Mata J, Taylor SD, Story BM, Dallas MR, et al. (1995) Effects of parathyroid hormone (PTH)-related protein and PTH on osteoclasts and osteoclast precursors in vivo Endocrinology 136(8): 3207–12.

207. Uy HL, Mundy GR, Boyce BF, Story BM, Dunstan CR, Yin JJ, et al. (1997) Tumor necrosis factor enhances parathyroid hormone-related protein-induced hypercalcemia and bone resorption without inhibiting bone formation in vivo Cancer Research 57(15): 3194–9.

208. van der Pluijm G, Lowik C, Papapoulos S (2000) Tumour progression and angiogenesis in bone metastasis from breast cancer: new approaches to an old problem Cancer Treat Rev 26:11–27.

209. van der Pluijm G, Sijmons B, Vloedgraven H, Deckers M, Papapoulos S, Lowik C (2001) Monitoring metastatic behavior of human tumor cells in mice with species-specific polymerase chain reaction: elevated expression of angiogenesis and bone resorption stimulators by breast cancer in bone metastases. J Bone Miner Res 16:1077–91.

210. van der Pluijm G, Vloedgraven HJM, Ivanov B, Robey FA, Grzesik WJ, Robey PG, Papapoulos SE, Löwik CWGM (1996) Bone sialoprotein peptides are potent inhibitors of breast cancer cell adhesion to bone. Cancer Res. 56:1948–55.

211. Vargas SJ, Gillespie MT, Powell GJ, Southby J, Danks JA, Moseley JM, Martin TJ (1992) Localization of parathyroid hormone-related protein mRNA expression and metastatic lesions by in situ hybridization. J Bone Miner Res 7:971–80.

212. Viereck V, Emons G, Lauck V, Frosch KH, Blaschke S, Grundker C, et al. (2002) Bisphosphonates pamidronate and zoledronic acid stimulate osteoprotegerin production by primary human osteoblasts. Biochemical & Biophysical Research Communications 291(3):680–6.

213. Wada S, Yasuda S, Nagai T, Maeda T, Kitahama S, Suda S, et al. (2001) Regulation of calcitonin receptor by glucocorticoid in human osteoclast-like cells prepared in vitro using receptor activator of nuclear factor-kappaB ligand and macrophage colony-stimulating factor. Endocrinology 142(4):1471–8.

214. Wakefield LM, Roberts AB (2002) TGF-beta signaling: positive and negative effects on tumorigenesis. Curr Opin Genet Dev 12:22–9.

215. Weber GF (2001) The metastasis gene osteopontin: a candidate target for cancer therapy. Biochim Biophys Acta 1552:61–85.

216. Weissglas M, Schamhart D, Lowik C, Papapoulos S, Vos P, Kurth KH (1995) Hypercalcemia and cosecretion of interleukin-6 and parathyroid hormone related peptide by a human renal cell carcinoma implanted into nude mice. Journal of Urology 153(3 Pt 1):854–7.

217. Wood J, Bonjean K, Ruetz S, Bellahcene A, Devy L, Foidart JM, Castronovo V, Green JR (2002) Novel antiangiogenic effects of the bisphosphonate compound zoledronic acid. J Pharmacol Exp Ther 302:1055–61.

218. Woodhouse EC, Chuaqui RF, Liotta LA (1997) General mechanisms of metastasis. Cancer 80(8 Suppl):1529–37.

219. Wysolmerski JJ, Broadus AE, Zhou J, Fuchs E, Milstone LM, Philbrick WM (1994) Overexpression of parathyroid hormone-related protein in the skin of transgenic mice interferes with hair follicle development. Proc Natl Acad Sci USA 91(3):1133–7.

220. Wysolmerski JJ, Carucci JM, Broadus AE, Philbrick WM (1994) PTH and PTHrP antagonize mammary gland growth and development in transgenic mice. Journal of Bone & Mineral Research 9(Suppl 1):S121.

221. Wysolmerski JJ, Philbrick WM, Dunbar ME, Lanske B, Kronenberg H, Broadus AE (1998) Rescue of the parathyroid hormone-related protein knockout mouse demonstrates that parathyroid hormone-related protein is essential for mammary gland development. Development 125(7):1285–94.

222. Yamaguchi T, Chattopadhyay N, Brown EM (2000) G protein-coupled extracellular Ca2+ (Ca2+o)-sensing receptor (CaR): roles in cell signaling and control of diverse cellular functions. Adv Pharmacol 47:209–53.

223. Yamamoto M, Harm SC, Grasser WA, Thiede MA (1992) Parathyroid hormone-related protein in the rat urinary bladder: a smooth muscle relaxant produced locally in response to mechanical stretch. Proc Natl Acad Sci USA 89(12):5326–30.

224. Yates AJ, Boyce BF, Favarato G, Aufdemorte TB, Marcelli C, Kester MB, et al. (1992) Expression of human transforming growth factor alpha by Chinese hamster ovarian tumors in nude mice causes hypercalcemia and increased osteoclastic bone resorption. Journal of Bone & Mineral Research 7(7):847–53.

225. Yi B, Williams PJ, Niewolna M, Wang Y, Yoneda T (2002) Tumor-derived platelet-derived growth factor-BB plays a critical role in osteosclerotic bone metastasis in an animal model of human breast cancer. Cancer Res 62:917–23.

226. Yin JJ, Mohammad KS, Käkönen S-M, Harris S, Wu-Wong RJ, Wessale J, Padley RJ, Garrett IR, Chirgwin JM, Guise TA (2003) A causal role for endothelin-1 in the pathogenesis of osteoblastic bone metastases. Proc Natl Acad Sci USA 100(19):10588–9.

227. Yin JJ, Selander KS, Chirgwin JM, Dallas M, Grubbs BG, Wieser R, Massague J, Mundy GR, Guise TA (1999) TGFb signaling blockade inhibits parathyroid hormone-related protein secretion by breast cancer cells and bone metastases development. J Clin Invest 103:197–206.

228. Yoneda T (2000) Cellular and molecular basis of preferential metastasis of breast cancer to bone. J Orthop Sci 5:75–81.

229. Yoshimoto K, Yamasaki R, Sakai H, Tezuka U, Takahashi M, Iizuka M, et al. (1989) Ectopic production of parathyroid hormone by small cell lung cancer in a patient with hypercalcemia. Journal of Clinical Endocrinology & Metabolism 68(5):976–81.

230. Zehnder D, Bland R, Williams MC, McNinch RW, Howie AJ, Stewart PM, et al. (2001) Extrarenal expression of 25-hydroxyvitamin d(3)-1 alpha-hydroxylase. Journal of Clinical Endocrinology & Metabolism 86(2):888–94.

231. Zhao W, Byrne MH, Boyce BF, Krane SM (1999) Bone resorption induced by parathyroid hormone is strikingly diminished in collagenase-resistant mutant mice. J Clin Invest 103:517–24.

232. Zudaire E, Martinez A, Cuttitta F (2003) Adrenomedullin and cancer. Regul Pept 112:175–83.

Index